Advances in Diagnostic Dermatopathology, from Histopathologic to Molecular Studies

Advances in Diagnostic Dermatopathology, from Histopathologic to Molecular Studies

Editor

Yasuhiro Sakai

MDPI • Basel • Beijing • Wuhan • Barcelona • Belgrade • Manchester • Tokyo • Cluj • Tianjin

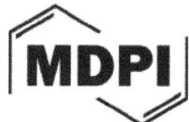

Editor
Yasuhiro Sakai
Fujita Health University
School of Medicine
Japan

Editorial Office
MDPI
St. Alban-Anlage 66
4052 Basel, Switzerland

This is a reprint of articles from the Special Issue published online in the open access journal *Diagnostics* (ISSN 2075-4418) (available at: https://www.mdpi.com/journal/diagnostics/special_issues/Diagnostic_Dermatopathology).

For citation purposes, cite each article independently as indicated on the article page online and as indicated below:

LastName, A.A.; LastName, B.B.; LastName, C.C. Article Title. *Journal Name* **Year**, *Volume Number*, Page Range.

ISBN 978-3-0365-6620-7 (Hbk)
ISBN 978-3-0365-6621-4 (PDF)

© 2023 by the authors. Articles in this book are Open Access and distributed under the Creative Commons Attribution (CC BY) license, which allows users to download, copy and build upon published articles, as long as the author and publisher are properly credited, which ensures maximum dissemination and a wider impact of our publications.

The book as a whole is distributed by MDPI under the terms and conditions of the Creative Commons license CC BY-NC-ND.

Contents

About the Editor vii

Preface to "Advances in Diagnostic Dermatopathology, from Histopathologic to Molecular Studies" ix

Yasuhiro Sakai
The Philosophy of Dermatopathology
Reprinted from: *Diagnostics* 2022, *12*, 3091, doi:10.3390/diagnostics12123091 1

Azusa Ogita and Shin-ichi Ansai
What Is a Solitary Keratoacanthoma? A Benign Follicular Neoplasm, Frequently Associated with Squamous Cell Carcinoma
Reprinted from: *Diagnostics* 2021, *11*, 1848, doi:10.3390/diagnostics11101848 3

Noritaka Oyama and Minoru Hasegawa
Lichen Sclerosus: A Current Landscape of Autoimmune and Genetic Interplay
Reprinted from: *Diagnostics* 2022, *12*, 3070, doi:10.3390/diagnostics12123070 17

Tomomitsu Miyagaki
Diagnosis of Early Mycosis Fungoides
Reprinted from: *Diagnostics* 2021, *11*, 1721, doi:10.3390/diagnostics11091721 31

Catharina Sagita Moniaga, Mitsutoshi Tominaga and Kenji Takamori
The Pathology of Type 2 Inflammation-Associated Itch in Atopic Dermatitis
Reprinted from: *Diagnostics* 2021, *11*, 2090, doi:10.3390/diagnostics11112090 41

Monica-Cristina Pânzaru, Lavinia Caba, Laura Florea, Elena Emanuela Braha and Eusebiu Vlad Gorduza
Epidermolysis Bullosa—A Different Genetic Approach in Correlation with Genetic Heterogeneity
Reprinted from: *Diagnostics* 2022, *12*, 1325, doi:10.3390/diagnostics12061325 57

Shun Ohmori, Yu Sawada, Natsuko Saito-Sasaki, Sayaka Sato, Yoko Minokawa, Hitomi Sugino, et al.
A Positive Dermcidin Expression Is an Unfavorable Prognostic Marker for Extramammary Paget's Disease
Reprinted from: *Diagnostics* 2021, *11*, 1086, doi:10.3390/diagnostics11061086 79

Takashi Morikura and Shogo Miyata
Mechanical Intermittent Compression Affects the Progression Rate of Malignant Melanoma Cells in a Cycle Period-Dependent Manner
Reprinted from: *Diagnostics* 2021, *11*, 1112, doi:10.3390/diagnostics11061112 89

Megumi Kishimoto, Mayumi Komine, Miho Sashikawa-Kimura, Tuba Musarrat Ansary, Koji Kamiya, Junichi Sugai, et al.
STAT3 Activation in Psoriasis and Cancers
Reprinted from: *Diagnostics* 2021, *11*, 1903, doi:10.3390/diagnostics11101903 103

Noha Z. Tawfik, Hoda Y. Abdallah, Ranya Hassan, Alaa Hosny, Dina E. Ghanem, Aya Adel and Mona A. Atwa
PSORS1 Locus Genotyping Profile in Psoriasis: A Pilot Case-Control Study
Reprinted from: *Diagnostics* 2022, *12*, 1035, doi:10.3390/diagnostics12051035 113

Sohshi Morimura, Yasuhiko Tomita, Shinichi Ansai and Makoto Sugaya
Secondary Malignant Tumors Arising in Nevus Sebaceus: Two Case Reports
Reprinted from: *Diagnostics* **2022**, *12*, 1448, doi:10.3390/diagnostics12061448 . . . . **129**

About the Editor

Yasuhiro Sakai

Yasuhiro Sakai, M.D., Ph.D., F.I.A.C. is a Japanese dermatopathologist and a qualified expert surgical pathologist, molecular pathologist, and clinical laboratory physician in Japan. He has been recognized by the International Board of Cytopathology, certified by International Academy of Cytology (IAC). He graduated Shinshu University School of Medicine in 2009 and obtained a medical license. He received a Doctor of Philosophy from Shinshu University Graduate School of Medicine in 2014. He was honoured to receive the Japanese Society of Pathology's Centennial Anniversary Award for Young Scientists in 2013. He is active in the area of immunopathology, with topics of interest ranging from immune response dynamics to tumorigenesis associated with immunological DNA repair factors. He is also interested in researching the application of immunologic signal molecules to useful markers in pathologic diagnosis.

Preface to "Advances in Diagnostic Dermatopathology, from Histopathologic to Molecular Studies"

Dermatopathology is the most sophisticated area in anatomic pathology; we can easily observe superficial skin lesions using our eyes without the need for an invasive approach and can easily compare gross configurations to microscopic findings. Meanwhile, dermatopathology has recently focused on the study of various cutaneous diseases at the molecular biology level. Here, we introduce original research articles as well as review articles that reveal novel findings of diagnostic dermatopathology, such as diagnosable new morphological (histopathologic) findings, immunohistochemical and immunofluorescent markers, and molecular techniques for dermatologists and pathologists, in the Special Issue.

Yasuhiro Sakai
Editor

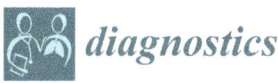

Editorial

The Philosophy of Dermatopathology

Yasuhiro Sakai

Department of Joint Research Laboratory of Clinical Medicine, Fujita Health University School of Medicine, Aichi 470-1192, Japan; ya-sakai@fujita-hu.ac.jp; Tel.: +81-562-93-9934

Diagnostic pathology involves studying sample cells and tissues obtained from the specific lesions of interest. It is designed not only to observe changes occurring in actual cells and tissues using morphologic, immunologic, microbiologic, and molecular biologic techniques but also to explain the reasons underlying these changes and ultimately to confirm the diagnosis.

Dermatopathology is one of the most sophisticated areas of diagnostic pathology; we can easily observe superficial skin lesions using only our eyes without invasive techniques such as an endoscopic or operational approach. For example, more than one hundred kinds of "dermatitis" are now being subclassified and studied because dermatologists have been making detailed gross observations of cardinal inflammatory signs, including heat, pain, redness, and swelling, for two thousand years—ever since Aulus Cornelius Celsus first provided descriptions. Henry Seguin Jackson originally coined the term *dermato-pathologia* in 1792, and since then, these visual signs have been compared to microscopic findings.

Thereafter, pathologists such as Rudolph Ludwig Karl Virchow, one of the greatest pathologists in history, paid very little attention to dermatopathology. While dermatopathology was originally developed based on dermatologists' significant efforts, as a result of this lack of attention, even now many general pathologists barely understand the specialty of dermatopathology, such as the many classifications of cutaneous disorders, pathoetiologic wavelength, clinicopathological relationship, and glossaries unique to dermatopathology.

In order to further promote "dermatopathology", we should bridge the divide between dermatology and pathology using morphologic, immunologic, microbiologic, and molecular techniques, even if only in small steps. For example, keratoacanthoma is one of the most "divided" cutaneous disorders. It is pathologically difficult to distinguish from well-differentiated invasive squamous cell carcinoma; however, it exhibits a distinct clinical behavior and may regress spontaneously. Ogita and Ansai deepen the morphological consideration and focus on the "large pale pink cells", which are the key criteria for keratoacanthoma [1]. They sharpen the classification of crateriform tumors, including keratoacanthoma, in the view of both dermatologists and pathologists, which may result in changes to the WHO's criteria. Another difficult example is mycosis fungoides. Mycosis fungoides, particularly in its erythematous phase, is sometimes pathologically indistinguishable from eczematous dermatitis, a benign inflammatory disorder. Miyagaki summarizes the novel diagnostic tools for early mycosis fungoides: novel immunohistochemical markers, such as thymocyte selection-associated high mobility group box factor; cell adhesion molecule 1; the next-generation sequencing of T-cell receptor genes; and microRNA profiles [2].

Recently, dermatology and pathology have been brought together through molecular biology, and dermatopathology has focused on the study of various cutaneous diseases at the molecular level. Dozens and dozens of these are now being well-researched, including melanocytic nevus, malignant melanoma, extramammary Paget disease, atopic dermatitis, psoriasis, epidermolysis bullosa, and lichen sclerosus (et atrophicus). For example, Morikura and Miyata note that mechanical intermittent compression promotes malignant melanoma progression by melanoma cell proliferation and collagen degradation [3]. Acral

---

Citation: Sakai, Y. The Philosophy of Dermatopathology. *Diagnostics* **2022**, *12*, 3091. https://doi.org/10.3390/diagnostics12123091

Received: 2 December 2022
Accepted: 6 December 2022
Published: 8 December 2022

Publisher's Note: MDPI stays neutral with regard to jurisdictional claims in published maps and institutional affiliations.

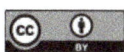

Copyright: © 2022 by the author. Licensee MDPI, Basel, Switzerland. This article is an open access article distributed under the terms and conditions of the Creative Commons Attribution (CC BY) license (https://creativecommons.org/licenses/by/4.0/).

melanomas in non-sun-exposed skin, such as planta may be associated with mechanical stress. Ohmori et al. show that dermcidin, which is expressed in normal eccrine glands and provides antimicrobial action in sweat, is expressed in Paget cells and is closely associated with a poor prognosis in extramammary Paget diseases [4]. Moniaga et al. review the molecular mechanism of atopic dermatitis. Neuroimmune crosstalk by cytokines associated with type 2 inflammation, such as interleukin (IL)-4, IL-5, IL-13, and IL-31, which stimulates cutaneous sensory neurons and causes itching [5]. Kishimoto et al. note that STAT3 is not closely related to extracutaneous cancers in patients with psoriasis, although STAT3 is activated in psoriatic cutaneous lesions as well as multiple cancerous tissues [6]. Tawfik et al. demonstrate that various single-nucleotide polymorphisms in the PSORS1 locus are significantly associated with psoriasis in an Egyptian cohort [7]. Pânzaru et al. review the clinical and genetic heterogeneity of epidermolysis bullosa and summarize the genotype–phenotype correlation [8]. Oyama and Hasegawa review the dermatophysiology and functional importance of extracellular matrix protein 1 (ECM1) and explain the etiopathological relationship between ECM1 and lichen sclerosus [9].

Dermatopathology is an academic discipline which systematizes human skin diseases by unifying dermatology and pathology, and we should continuously add new and ever-evolving knowledge into the system of dermatopathology. We should also seriously consider reorganizing the system of dermatopathology because molecular biology is so rapidly developing. This Special Issue aims to focus on advances in diagnostic dermatopathology from histopathologic to molecular studies, and we hope that it serves as a trigger to promote the study of dermatopathology.

Institutional Review Board Statement: Not applicable.

Acknowledgments: The author thanks all those scholars who wrote an original and review article for the Special Issue "Advances in Diagnostic Dermatopathology, from Histopathologic to Molecular Studies" in *Diagnostics*.

Conflicts of Interest: The author declares no conflict of interest.

References

1. Ogita, A.; Ansai, S. What is solitary keratoacanthoma? A benign follicular neoplasm, frequently associated with squamous cell carcinoma. *Diagnostics* **2021**, *11*, 1848. [CrossRef] [PubMed]
2. Miyagaki, T. Diagnosis of early mycosis fungoides. *Diagnostics* **2021**, *11*, 1721. [CrossRef] [PubMed]
3. Morikura, T.; Miyata, S. Mechanical intermittent compression affects the progression rate of malignant melanoma cells in a cycle period-dependent manner. *Diagnostics* **2021**, *11*, 1112. [CrossRef] [PubMed]
4. Ohmori, S.; Saito-Sasaki, N.; Sato, S.; Minokawa, Y.; Sugino, H.; Nanamori, H.; Yamamoto, K.; Okada, E.; Nakamura, M. A positive dermcidin expression is an unfavorable prognostic marker for extramammary Paget's disease. *Diagnostics* **2021**, *11*, 1086. [CrossRef] [PubMed]
5. Moniaga, C.S.; Tominaga, M.; Takamori, K. The pathology of type 2 inflammation-associted itch in atopic dermatitis. *Diagnostics* **2021**, *11*, 2090. [CrossRef] [PubMed]
6. Kishimoto, M.; Komine, M.; Sashikawa-Kimura, M.; Ansary, T.M.; Kamiya, K.; Sugai, J.; Mieno, M.; Kawata, H.; Sekimoto, R.; Fukushima, N.; et al. STAT3 activation in psoriasis and cancers. *Diagnostics* **2021**, *11*, 1903. [CrossRef] [PubMed]
7. Tawfik, N.Z.; Abdallah, H.Y.; Hassan, R.; Hosny, A.; Ghanem, D.E.; Adel, A.; Atwa, M.A. PSORS1 locus genotyping profile in psoriasis: A pilot case-control study. *Diagnostics* **2022**, *12*, 1035. [CrossRef] [PubMed]
8. Pânzaru, M.; Caba, L.; Florea, L.; Braha, E.E.; Gorduza, E.V. Epidermolysis bullosa——a different genetic approach in correlation with genetic heterogeneity. *Diagnostics* **2022**, *12*, 1325. [CrossRef] [PubMed]
9. Oyama, N.; Hasegawa, M. Lichen sclerosus: A current landscape of autoimmune and genetic interplay. *Diagnostics* **2022**, *12*, 3070. [CrossRef]

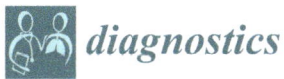

Review

What Is a Solitary Keratoacanthoma? A Benign Follicular Neoplasm, Frequently Associated with Squamous Cell Carcinoma

Azusa Ogita and Shin-ichi Ansai *

Division of Dermatology and Dermatopathology, Nippon Medical School Musashi Kosugi Hospital, Kawasaki 211-8533, Japan; azu@nms.ac.jp
* Correspondence: shin8113@nms.ac.jp; Tel.: +81-44-733-5181

Citation: Ogita, A.; Ansai, S.-i. What Is a Solitary Keratoacanthoma? A Benign Follicular Neoplasm, Frequently Associated with Squamous Cell Carcinoma. *Diagnostics* **2021**, *11*, 1848. https://doi.org/10.3390/diagnostics11101848

Academic Editor: Yasuhiro Sakai

Received: 27 August 2021
Accepted: 5 October 2021
Published: 7 October 2021

Publisher's Note: MDPI stays neutral with regard to jurisdictional claims in published maps and institutional affiliations.

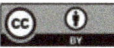

Copyright: © 2021 by the authors. Licensee MDPI, Basel, Switzerland. This article is an open access article distributed under the terms and conditions of the Creative Commons Attribution (CC BY) license (https://creativecommons.org/licenses/by/4.0/).

Abstract: We present histopathological criteria for diagnosing keratoacanthoma (KA). In KA, four histological stages are recognized, which are the early/proliferative stage, well-developed stage, regressing stage and regressed stage. In diagnosing KA, we emphasize that KA consists of the proliferation of enlarged pale pink cells with ground glass-like cytoplasm without nuclear atypia, other than crateriform architecture. KA sometimes exhibits malignant transformation within the lesions. We describe the characteristics of benign and malignant epithelial crateriform tumors that should be differentiated from KA. We also present the data of histopathological diagnosis of lesions clinically diagnosed as KA, its natural course and related lesions after partial biopsy, and incidence of crateriform epithelial neoplasms. Based on these data, we recommend complete excision of the lesion when KA is clinically suspected, especially when the lesion is located on a sun-exposed area of an elderly patient. If complete excision is impossible, partial excision of a sufficient specimen with intact architecture is required. In such a case, however, careful investigation after biopsy will be needed, even if the histopathological diagnosis is KA, because there is some possibility that a conventional SCC lesion remains in the residual tissue.

Keywords: keratoacanthoma; squamous cell carcinoma (SCC); keratoacanthoma-like SCC; keratoacanthoma with malignant transformation; crateriform neoplasms; crateriform verruca; crateriform seborrheic keratosis; crateriform Bowen disease; crateriform SCC arising from actinic keratosis; crater form of infundibular SCC

1. Introduction

Keratoacanthoma (KA) often occurs in a solitary form and exhibits a distinct clinical and histopathological presentation [1]. Whether KA is benign or malignant, i.e., squamous cell carcinoma (SCC) that is one of the most common malignant tumors affecting the akin and of which characteristic is the abnormal and quick growth of keratinocytes in the epidermis, often secondary to ultraviolet or sunlight exposure [2], or not, has been a controversial issue for many years, although there have been many studies concerning the differentiation of KA and SCC [3]. Such confusion is mainly based on similarity of histopathological findings between KA and SCC and lack of accepted reliable histopathological criteria in diagnosing KA [4]. Furthermore, few cases of KA exhibit distant metastasis and tumor-related death [5,6]. Therefore, KA was classified into low-grade SCC in the recent WHO classification of cutaneous tumors [1]. On the other hand, Misago and colleagues suggested that KA is either a benign lesion or a distinct borderline malignant entity that is fundamentally different from conventional SCC and features follicular (infundibular/isthmic) differentiation characterized by the involvement of continuous multi-follicular infundibula [7–12]. They also emphasized that KA consists of the proliferation of enlarged pale pink cells with ground glass-like cytoplasm without nuclear atypia, at least in a part of the lesion, and it relatively frequently exhibits malignant transformation. We think that this opinion explains most phenomena about the relationship between KA and SCC. From such points of view, we consider the discussion concerning whether KA is SCC to be meaningless. We are convinced that KA is a benign epithelial neoplasm with follicular differentiation that sometimes grows conventional SCC within the lesion.

In this article, we want to present the true characteristics of solitary KA based on its distinctive histopathological criteria, in addition to histopathological findings of other epithelial crateriform tumors that should be differentiated from KA. Our classification of epithelial crateriform tumors is stated in Table 1.

Table 1. Our classification of epithelial crateriform tumors.

Benign Neoplasms	Malignant Neoplasms
Crateriform verruca (CFV)	Crateriform (Papillated) Bowen disease
Crateriform seborrheic keratosis (CSK)	
Keratoacanthoma (KA)	KA with conventional SCC component (KASCC)
	Crateriform SCC arising from actinic keratosis (cSCC)
	Crater form of infundibular SCC

SCC: squamous cell carcinoma.

2. Clinical and Histopathological Characteristics of Solitary KA

2.1. Clinical Findings

Solitary KA usually develops on sun-exposed areas of elderly patients. Its clinical findings are characterized by a flesh to pink colored crater-like nodule with a central keratotic plug. An essential clinical characteristic of solitary KA is its self-limiting course, with rapid enlargement within several weeks and spontaneous regression within several months. Such a clinical course is highly important in diagnosing KA.

2.2. Histopathological Findings

2.2.1. Histopathological Stages

Solitary KA has different histopathological features depending on the stage of the lesion at the time of biopsy or resection [7,12,13]. Four histological stages of KA are recognized, which are the early/proliferative stage, well-developed stage, regressing stage and regressed stage. It is highly important that excisional biopsy or partial biopsy including the center and both sides of KA be performed for correct histopathological diagnosis.

2.2.2. Mutual Findings among Stages

KA histopathologically exhibits characteristic findings through all stages except in the regressed stage. These include an exo-endophytic architecture, a relatively well-defined, almost symmetrical outline and a multilobular lesion with a central keratinous plug. It also presents overhanging epithelial lips covered with normal epidermis. Furthermore, other findings should be emphasized: (i) presence of invaginated infundibular structures (laminated keratinization) and lobules with enlarged pale pink cells with ground glass-like cytoplasm, which generally lack nuclear atypia; (ii) lobules of large pale eosinophilic cells with a few layers of basophilic cells at their periphery; (iii) possible nuclear atypia or mitotic figures, limited to the peripheral areas of the basophilic cells; and (iv) minimally infiltrating borders. In particular, proliferation of enlarged pale pink cells with ground glass-like cytoplasm without nuclear atypia is the most important finding in diagnosing KA and differentiating KA from SCC. In KA, the crateriform architecture is characteristic and can be recognized in most cases, but that is not essential. We previously reported cases having the same components as conventional KA without the crateriform architecture as keratoacanthoma en plaque/nodule [14] (Figure 1).

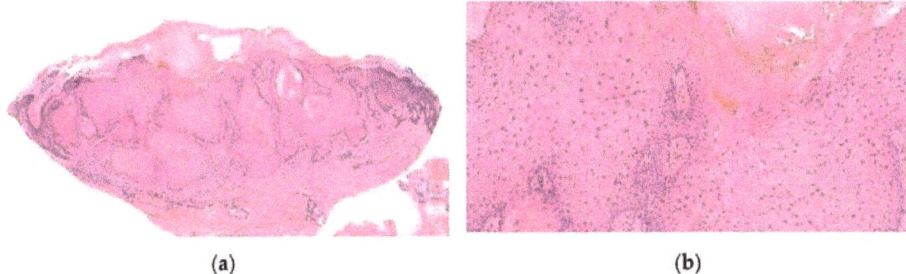

Figure 1. Histopathological findings of KA en plaque/nodule. Gross findings of the lesion reveal an exo-endophytic and non-crateriform architecture (**a**). The lesion consisted of proliferation of large pale eosinophilic cells with a few layers of basophilic cells at their periphery (**b**). Large pale eosinophilic cells show no nuclear atypia (**b**).

2.2.3. Early/Proliferative Stage

The early/proliferative stage of KA is histopathologically characterized by several keratin-filled invaginations of the epidermis or infundibulum, demonstrating a laminated pattern of keratinization, often with prominent keratohyalin granules. In the deeper areas, pale pink keratinocytes with a glassy appearance are observed. The deeper areas of the lesion are sometimes poorly demarcated from the surrounding stroma and exhibit slightly invasive growth (Figure 2).

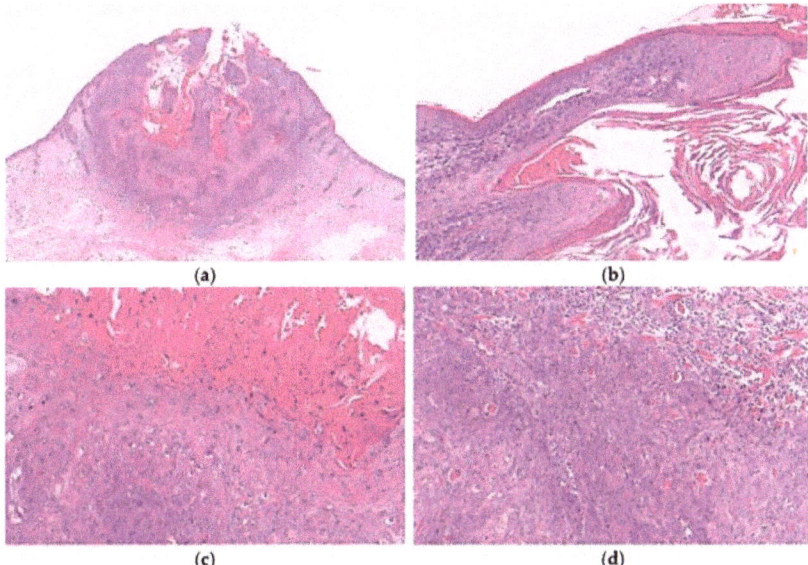

Figure 2. Histopathological findings of KA at the early/proliferative stage. Gross findings of the lesion include crateriform architecture with a central keratinous plug (**a**). A lip-like structure is observed (**b**). Pale pink keratinocytes with a glassy appearance are observed. In the deeper areas, pale pink keratinocytes with a glassy appearance are noted (**c**). The deeper areas of the lesion are poorly demarcated from the surrounding stroma and exhibit slightly invasive growth (**d**).

2.2.4. Well-Developed Stage

The well-developed stage of KA exhibits the following histopathological findings: (i) characteristic symmetric, crateriform, exo-endophytic architecture; (ii) contiguous, dilated infundibular structures (multilocular and multilobular) with a central large keratotic horn situated above isthmic differentiation; (iii) overhanging epithelial lips with a normal overlying epidermis; and (iv) characteristic neoplastic lobules with isthmic differentiation (proliferation of large pale pink cells with a glassy appearance demonstrating compact keratinization) in most parts (Figure 3). There are also sometimes fine keratohyalin granules or focal parakeratosis.

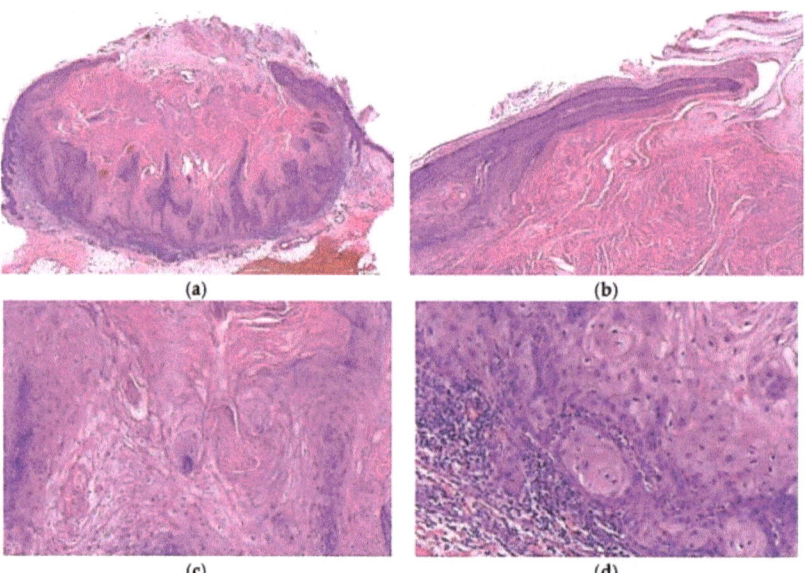

Figure 3. Histopathological findings of KA at the well-developed stage. Gross findings of the lesion include crateriform and exo-endophytic architecture with a central keratinous plug (**a**). Overhanging epithelial lips with a normal overlying epidermis are observed (**b**). Characteristic proliferation of large pale pink cells with a glassy appearance showing compact keratinization is observed in most parts of the lesion (**c**). The deeper areas of the lesion are slightly poorly demarcated from the surrounding stroma and exhibit slightly invasive growth (**d**).

2.2.5. Regressing Stage

The regressing stage of KA maintains a crateriform architecture, but it becomes one or two keratin-filled and shallow crateriform structures (Figure 4). The regressing stage KA again exhibits infundibular characteristics of laminated keratinization and the pale pink keratinocytes with a glassy appearance are often lost. Fibrosis in the dermal papillae and mixed cell inflammation are also noted (Figure 4).

2.2.6. Regressed Stage

The regressed stage of KA is a depressed epidermal lesion with overhanging or rising edges, and the epidermis is flattened and atrophic with loss of rete ridges (Figure 5).

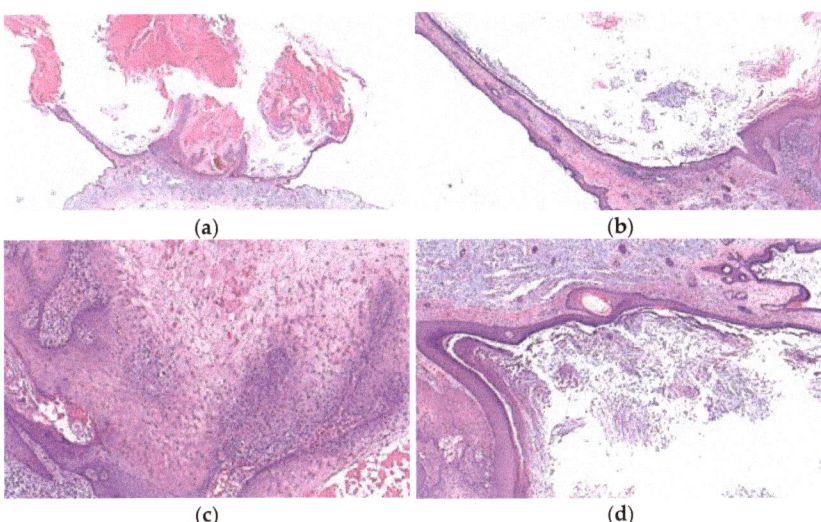

Figure 4. Histopathological findings of KA at the regressing stage. Gross findings of the lesion include crateriform architecture (**a**) and a lip-like structure (**b**). The lesion shows infundibular characteristics of laminated keratinization (**b**,**d**) and often loses the pale pink keratinocytes with a glassy appearance (**c**). Fibrosis in the dermal papillae and mixed cell inflammation are also observed (**b**).

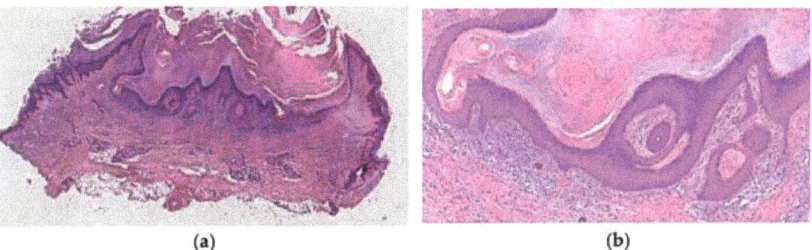

Figure 5. Histopathological findings of KA at the regressed stage. A depressed epidermal lesion with overhanging and rising edges is observed (**a**), and the epidermis is flattened and atrophic with loss of rete ridges (**b**).

3. Diagnostically Problematic Lesions, KA with a Conventional SCC Component (KASCC)

KA-like SCC [9] and KA with malignant transformation (mKA) [15,16] are types of KASCC [10,12,13]. Both types have a component with the histopathological features of KA, e.g., an exo-endophytic lesion formed by invaginated infundibulum and lobules with large pale pink cells having a glassy appearance, generally without nuclear atypia. In KA-like SCC, conventional KA components and SCC components are relatively ill-demarcated and often admixed (Figures 6 and 7). On the other hand, mKA exhibits a well-demarcated contrast between typical KA and SCC sections (nests of anaplastic cells of different shapes and sizes). However, differentiation between these two conditions is often difficult and we found no difference between them in clinical course; therefore, we recommend these tumors be unified as KA with a conventional SCC component (KASCC). KA has a somewhat asymmetrical outline and focally prominent infiltrating border. KA-like SCC is also diagnosed when nuclear atypia is observed in most of the cells constituting the KA-like component (invaginated infundibular structures and lobules of large, pale pink cells). The KA components may be in any stage: early/proliferative, well-developed or regressing. Ratios of the KA and SCC components can vary in each lesion or even in different sections of a single lesion [9,12].

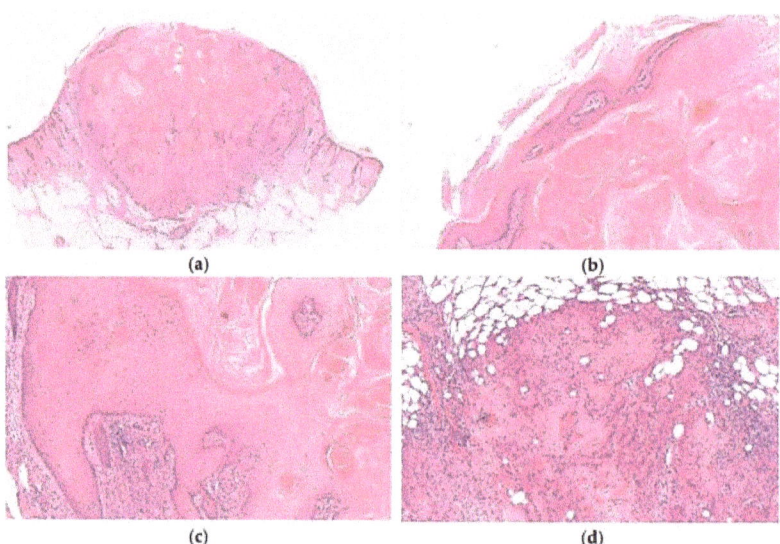

Figure 6. Histopathological findings of KA-like SCC. Gross findings of the lesion include crateriform architecture with a central keratinous plug (**a**). In part of the lesion, the histopathological features of KA are observed (**b**,**c**), whereas the SCC component is composed of tumor cells with keratinocytic differentiation and apparent nuclear atypia and shows invasive growth pattern (**d**).

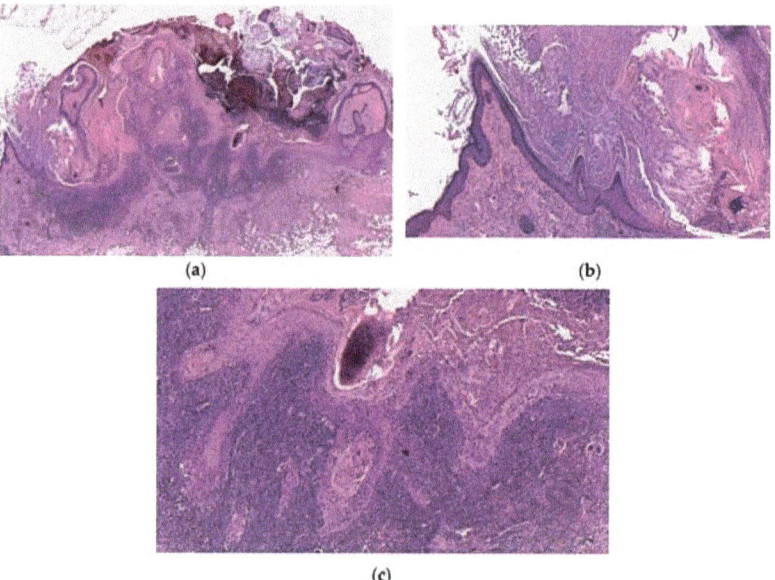

Figure 7. Histopathological findings of mKA. Crateriform architecture is observed, and there is a clear distinction between KA and SCC (**a**). Both sides of the lesion show regressing KA (**b**), whereas the SCC component is in the center (**c**). The boundary between the two components is clear-cut (**a**).

4. Other Crateriform Tumors

4.1. Benign Neoplasms

4.1.1. Crateriform Verruca (CFV)

We previously reported crateriform epithelial tumors exhibiting some histopathological overlap with KA that failed to meet all of the histological criteria for a diagnosis of KA and had some verrucous features, and we proposed the term crateriform verruca (CFV) to differentiate these verrucous neoplasms from KA [17]. CFV often is diagnosed as KA or verruca. Compared clinically with KA, CFV is smaller despite its longer duration. The common sites of CFV are sun-exposed areas, especially the face and neck [17].

Histopathologically, CFV is characterized by finger-like exophytic projections associated with hyperkeratosis (parakeratosis or orthokeratosis), focal hypergranulosis (koilocytes are not always prominent) and acanthosis, together with epithelial lip-like structures at the periphery (Figure 8). Characteristic inturning of elongated rete ridges (arborization) is usually observed (Figure 8). CFV can be differentiated from KA because it consists of several lobular structures composed of the proliferation of keratinocytes of a similar size and regular arrangement and because the base of CFV is well demarcated without endophytic growth. Cells with a large eosinophilic cytoplasm may be found in some parts of CFV, but these cells exhibit no downward proliferation unlike in KA (Figure 8). There is generally no nuclear atypia in the basal cell layer, or it is very mild if present, in contrast to the obvious nuclear atypia and mitosis of proliferating keratinocytes at the periphery of early-stage KA. There is either no inflammatory cell infiltration or slight infiltration (mainly lymphocytes and plasma cells), whereas KA in the regressing stage demonstrates fibrosis of dermal papillae and mixed inflammatory cell infiltration. CFV with large pink cytoplasm and trichilemmal keratinization is also histopathologically similar to so-called trichilemmal keratosis (horn) [18,19], the main histological features of which are trichilemmal keratinization and verrucous epidermal hyperplasia composed of large pale staining keratinocytes.

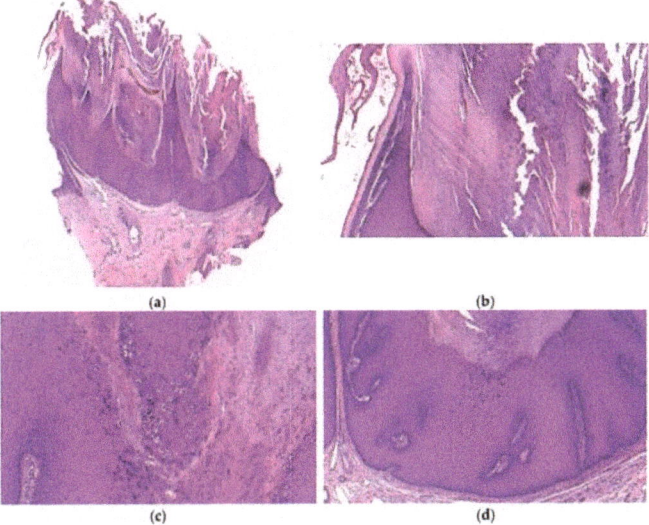

Figure 8. Histopathological findings of CFV. A crateriform configuration with finger-like exophytic projections accompanied (**a**) by epithelial lip-like structures at the periphery (**b**) is exhibited. Arborization is observed and the base is well demarcated without endophytic growth (**a**). Focal hypergranulosis and koilocytes are visible between the papillary projections (**c**). The lesion consists of several lobular structures composed of the proliferation of keratinocytes of a similar size and regular arrangement (**d**).

4.1.2. Crateriform Seborrheic Keratosis (CSK)

CSK is an exo-endophytic lesion, often having finger-like exophytic projections, which features hyperkeratosis and acanthosis with the proliferation of basaloid cells. Pseudohorn cysts are often evident (Figure 9).

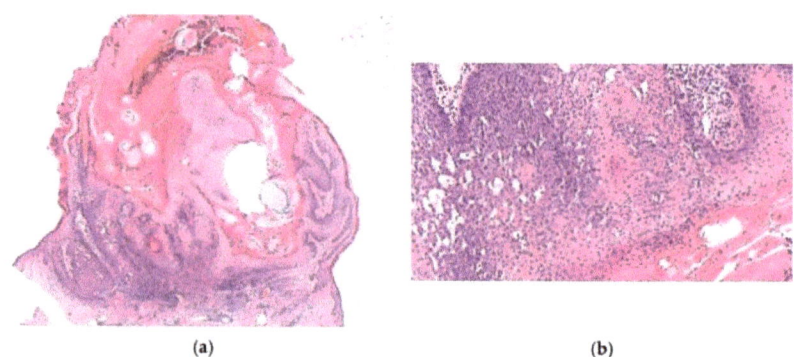

Figure 9. Histopathological findings of CSK. The lesion is crateriform with finger-like exophytic projections (**a**), showing hyperkeratosis and acanthosis with proliferation of basaloid cells (**b**). Pseudohorn cysts (**a**) and squamous eddies (**b**) are evident.

4.2. Other Malignant Neoplasms

4.2.1. Crateriform (Papillated) Bowen Disease

Crateriform Bowen's disease is an exo-endophytic lesion with a central keratotic horn [9,20]. It is formed from contiguous, keratinizing lobules and has overhanging epithelial lip-like structures (Figure 10). The typical features of Bowen's disease (full-thickness dysplasia of the epidermis with markedly atypical keratinocytes, including multinucleated cells and dyskeratotic cells, with sparing of the basal cell layer) are observed at the sides of the epithelial lip-like structures and in the neoplastic lobules (Figure 10).

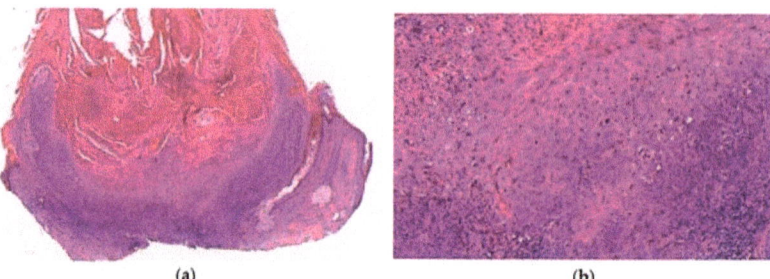

Figure 10. Histopathological findings of crateriform Bowen disease. The lesion shows crateriform and exo-endophytic proliferation with a central keratotic plug and overhanging epithelial lip-like structures (**a**). Typical features of Bowen's disease, which are full-thickness dysplasia with markedly atypical keratinocytes, are seen in the epidermis (**b**).

4.2.2. Crateriform SCC Arising from Actinic Keratosis (cSCC)

This type of SCC is an exo-endophytic lesion exhibiting the full thickness of atypical keratinocytes with bowenoid features in the epidermis and into the dermis [9,15] (Figure 11). Epithelial lip-like structures may also be observed (Figure 11). There is no follicular (isthmic) differentiation, namely, no large pale pink keratinizing cells with a glassy appearance, in the lobules. A solar keratosis (bowenoid type) maybe be noted in the lesion or at its periphery (Figure 11).

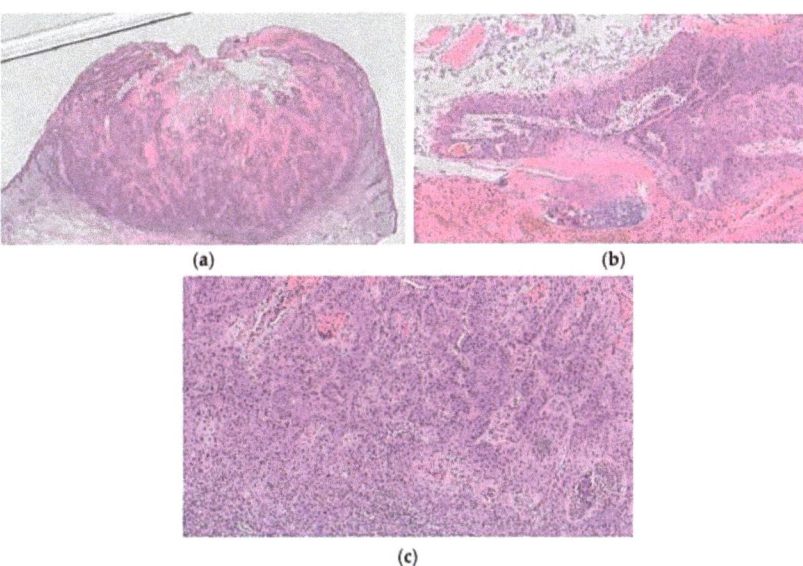

Figure 11. Histopathological findings of cSCC. A multilobular crateriform lesion (**a**) with epithelial lip-like structures (**b**) is observed. The full epidermal thickness of atypical keratinocytes with bowenoid features is evident at the base of the crater (**c**). There are no large, pale pink keratinizing cells with a glassy appearance featuring isthmic differentiation in the lobules (**c**). The histopathological features of solar keratosis are also observed in the periphery of the lesion (**b**).

4.2.3. Crater Form of Infundibular SCC

The term follicular SCC was first proposed for folliculocentric SCC [21], and Kossard et al. [22] were the first to advocate the concept of SCC with infundibular differentiation as a subset of follicular carcinoma and introduced the descriptive term infundibulocystic SCC. Then, Misago et al. [20] focused on crater/ulcerated infundibular SCC, which was originally described as poorly differentiated infundibulocystic SCC by Kossard and colleagues [19]. The crater form of infundibular SCC has an exo-endophytic configuration with central ulceration or crusting and exhibits neoplastic aggregates of SCC expanding from a follicular infundibulum and neoplastic cells invade deeply into the dermis (Figure 12) [11]. On one or both sides of the lesion, epithelial lip-like structures may sometimes be noted in the periphery. Two or three contiguous follicular infundibula are involved along with proliferation of atypical keratinocytes. The neoplastic infundibular canal-like structures are composed of atypical bowenoid keratinocytes with parakeratosis, in contrast with the laminated keratinization of infundibular canals without nuclear atypia in KA. It is essential to confirm the absence of features of KA or features of bowenoid dysplasia (solar keratosis or Bowen's disease) in the interfollicular epidermis (Figure 12) [11,23].

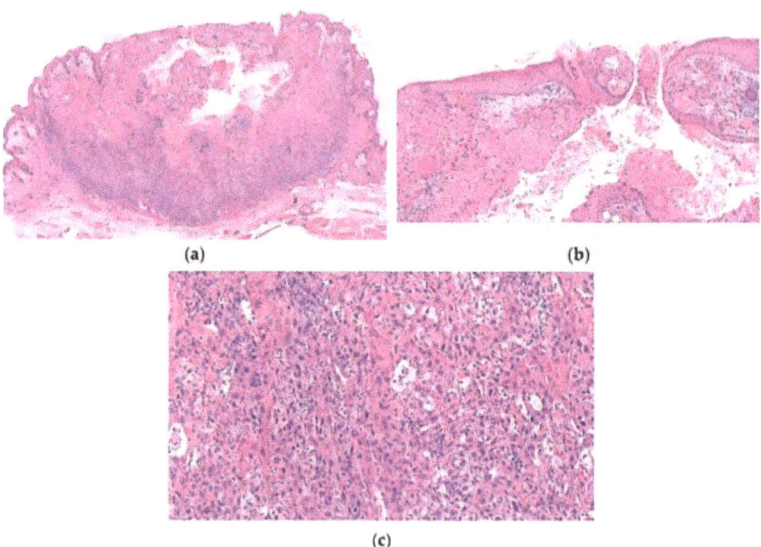

Figure 12. Histopathological findings of crater form of infundibular SCC. The lesion has a crateriform KA-like configuration with a central low keratin-filled ulcer (**a**). The tumor shows neoplastic aggregates of SCC expanding from a follicular infundibulum (**b**) and neoplastic cells invade deeply into the dermis (**a**,**c**). The features of KA or features of bowenoid dysplasia (solar keratosis or Bowen's disease) are absent in the interfollicular epidermis (**a**).

5. Data of Histopathological Diagnosis of Lesions Clinically Diagnosed as KA

Ansai, the co-author, reported the histopathological diagnosis of 1527 patients who were clinically diagnosed with KA at a Japanese institution [24]. Those lesions were most frequently located on the face (in approximately two-thirds). In 999 patients (65.4%), the histopathological architecture of KA was observed (KA lesion). The mean age at resection of the KA lesion (68.3 ± 15.1 years old) was significantly higher for these patients than for those without KA histopathological architecture (non-KA lesion) (61.0 ± 20.5 years old). In sun-exposed areas, the rate of KA lesions was high; 28.5% of the patients had malignant neoplasms, including SCC, especially patients over 60 years old, and 39.0% of cases were malignant. The rate of malignant lesions was higher in sun-exposed areas in elderly patients. The mean age at resection of malignant lesions (77.5 ± 11.5 years old) was significantly higher than that for benign lesions (61.1 ± 17.3 years old). The 1527 cases included 1397 (85.9%) epithelial tumors (including KA, verruca vulgaris, inverted follicular keratosis, trichofolliculoma and molluscum contagiosa) 99 (8.5%) non-epithelial tumors (including dermatofibroma, pyogenic granuloma, neurofibroma, xanthogranuloma, etc.), and 31 (2.0%) inflammatory lesions (including prurigo nodularis, etc.). Based on our impression, clinical differential diagnosis of crateriform epithelial tumors is very difficult. We consider that there is no certain clinical feature that differentiate benign crateriform tumors, especially solitary KA, from malignant ones, other than clinical course of the lesion, although CFV that is frequently observed benign crateriform tumor, shows long-standing course. Based on these findings, lesions clinically suspected as KA should be totally resected as soon as possible, especially on the faces of elderly patients.

6. Natural Course of KA and Related Lesions after Partial Biopsy

Takai and colleagues reported the clinical courses in 66 cases of KA and related lesions after partial biopsy [10]. They histopathologically classified these lesions into five types: (1) solitary KA at various stages (53 lesions); (2) KA-like SCC (3 lesions); (3) KA with malignant transformation (3 lesions); (4) infundibular SCC (5 lesions); and (5) crateriform

SCC arising from solar keratosis (2 lesions). They analyzed the clinical course in each group. The regression rate of KA was 98.1% and that of KA-like SCC/KA with malignant transformation was 33.3%. No regression was observed in either infundibular SCC or crateriform SCC arising from solar keratosis. Thus, KA is a distinct entity that should be distinguished from other types of SCC with crateriform architecture based on the high frequency of regression. The regression rate of 33.3% in KA-like SCC/KA with malignant transformation indicated that KA lesions with a SCC component retain the potential for regression. However, this also suggested that KA is biologically unstable and some KA evolves into conventional SCC with a gradual loss of the capacity for the spontaneous regression. Infundibular SCC and crateriform SCC arising from solar keratosis are fundamentally different from KA, not only according to the histopathological findings, but also based on the biological properties. Thus, the classification we present in this article is reasonable in terms of the biological behavior of each neoplasm.

7. Incidence of Crateriform Epithelial Neoplasms

We previously reported the incidence of 380 epidermal crateriform tumors using our classification [12]. There were 214 cases of KA (56.3%), 76 cases of CFV (20%), 45 cases of KA with a conventional SCC component (11.8%), 12 cases of CSK and crateriform Bowen's disease (3.2%), 11 cases of cSCC (2.9%) and 10 cases of infundibular SCC (2.6%). Benign crateriform neoplasms (CFV and CSK) and malignant crateriform neoplasms (KA with a conventional SCC component, Crateriform Bowen's disease, cSCC and infundibular SCC) accounted for 88 lesions (23.3%) and 78 lesions (20.5%), respectively (Table 2). A total of 259 lesions at least partly had histopathological features of KA (KA and KA with a conventional SCC component), among which 45 (17.4%) had a SCC component. The incidence of SCC developing in KA was influenced by the patient's age, being 8.3% in patients younger than 70 years old and increasing to 24.3% in those over 70. In this case, cSCC developed much more frequently in women than in men, CSK exhibited no sex difference, and the other lesions displayed a male predominance. The average age of the patients with malignant crateriform neoplasms was 70 years or older, whereas the average age of patients with benign crateriform neoplasms or KA was under 70 years. The average size of all types of lesions was approximately 1 cm. The mean duration of CFV was 14 months, which was the longest among the 7 types of neoplasms. Data for KA suggested that it progresses to the next stage every 2–3 months. The mean duration of infundibular SCC was 3.4 months, suggesting that it grows faster than the other malignant crateriform neoplasms. The sites of 366/380 lesions are summarized in Table 2. Most of the lesions developed on sun-exposed areas (head, face, neck, dorsum of hand and forearm). In particular, malignant crateriform neoplasms developed on sun-exposed areas (94.7%, 71/75). Of the 366 lesions, 232 (63.4%) were on the face, among which 138 (59.5%), 65 (28%) and 29 (12.5%) were KA, malignant crateriform neoplasms and benign crateriform neoplasms, respectively. All 10 infundibular SCCs developed on the face in elderly patients (mean age: 73 years, range: 59 to 87 years).

Table 2. Incidence of crateriform epithelial neoplasms.

Tumor			Case
	CFV		76 (20.0%)
	CSK		12 (3.2%)
KA		early/proliferative	85 (22.4%)
		well-developed	82 (21.6%)
		regressing/regressed	47 (12.4%)
		total	214 (56.3%)
	Crateriform Bowen disease		12 (3.2%)
	KAs with a conventional SCC		45 (11.8%)
	cSCC		11 (2.9%)
	Crateriform infundibular SCC		10 (2.6%)

8. Conclusions

Complete surgical excision of the lesion is the most effective therapy for solitary KA. Therefore, we recommend complete excision of the lesion when KA is clinically suspected, especially when the lesion is located on a sun-exposed area in an elderly patient. If complete excision is impossible, partial excision of a sufficient specimen with intact architecture is required. In such a case, however, careful investigation after biopsy will be needed, even if the histopathological diagnosis is KA, because there is some possibility that a conventional SCC lesion remains in the residual tissue [25].

As mentioned above, solitary KA is a benign epithelial neoplasm with follicular differentiation that sometimes grows conventional SCC within it and is different from conventional SCC. We consider these to be the true characteristics of solitary KA.

Funding: This research received no external funding.

Data Availability Statement: The data presented in this study are available in reference [10,12,24].

Acknowledgments: The authors wish to thank Misago who gave us motive, encouragement and valuable advice in this work.

Conflicts of Interest: The authors declare no conflict of interest.

References

1. Murphy, G.F.; Beer, T.W.; Cerio, R.; Kao, G.F.; Nagore, E.; Pulitzer, M.P. Squamous cell carcinoma. In *World Health Organization Classification of Tumours*, 4th ed.; Elder, D.E., Massi, D., Scolyer, R.A., Willemze, R., Eds.; IARC Press: Lyon, France, 2018; pp. 35–45.
2. Bennardo, L.; Bennardo, F.; Giudice, A.; Passante, M.; Dastoli, S.; Morrone, P.; Provensano, E.; Patruno, C.; Nisticò, S.P. Local chemotherapy as an adjuvant treatment in unresectable squamous cell carcinoma: What do we know so far? *Curr. Oncol.* **2021**, *28*, 2317–2325. [CrossRef]
3. Tisak, A.; Fotouhi, A.; Fidai, C.; Fridman, B.J.; Ozog, D.; Veenstra, J. A clinical and biological review of keratoacanthoma. *Br. J. Dermatol.* **2021**, *185*, 487–498. [CrossRef]
4. Cribier, B.; Asch, P.-H.; Grosshans, E. Differentiating squamous cell carcinoma from keratoacanthoma using histopathological criteria. Is it possible? A study of 296 cases. *Dermatology* **1999**, *199*, 208–212. [CrossRef]
5. Hodak, E.; Jones, R.E.; Ackerman, A.B. Solitary keratoacanthoma is a squamous-cell carcinoma: Three examples with metastasis. *Am. J. Dermatopathol.* **1993**, *15*, 332–342. [CrossRef]
6. Ansai, S.; Manabe, M. Possible spontaneous regression of a metastatic lesion of keratoacanthoma-like squamous cell carcinoma in a regional lymph node. *J. Dermatol.* **2005**, *32*, 899–903. [CrossRef]
7. Misago, N.; Takai, T.; Toda, S.; Narisawa, Y. The histopathologic changes in keratoacanthoma depend on its stage. *J. Cutan. Pathol.* **2014**, *41*, 617–619. [CrossRef] [PubMed]
8. Misago, N.; Takai, T.; Toda, S.; Narisawa, Y. The changes in the expression levels of follicular markers in keratoacanthoma depend on the stage: Keratoacanthoma is a follicular neoplasm exhibiting infundibular/isthmic differentiation without expression of CK15. *J. Cutan. Pathol.* **2014**, *41*, 437–446. [CrossRef] [PubMed]
9. Misago, N.; Inoue, T.; Koba, S.; Narisawa, Y. Keratoacanthoma and other types of squamous cell carcinoma with crateriform architecture: Classification and identification. *J. Dermatol.* **2013**, *40*, 443–452. [CrossRef] [PubMed]
10. Takai, T.; Misago, N.; Murata, Y. Natural course of keratoacanthoma and related lesions after partial biopsy: The clinical analysis of the 66 lesions. *J. Dermatol.* **2015**, *42*, 353–362. [CrossRef]
11. Misago, N.; Inoue, T.; Nagase, K.; Tsuruta, N.; Tara-Hashimoto, A.; Kimura, H.; Takahara, K.; Narita, T.; Narisawa, Y. Crater/ulcerated form of infundibular squamous cell carcinoma: A possible distinct entity as a malignant (or high-grade) counterpart to keratoacanthoma. *J. Dermatol.* **2015**, *42*, 667–673. [CrossRef]
12. Ogita, A.; Ansai, S.; Misago, N.; Anan, T.; Fukumoto, T.; Saeki, H. Histopathological diagnosis of epithelial crateriform tumors: Keratoacanthoma and other epithelial crateriform tumors. *J. Dermatol.* **2016**, *43*, 1321–1331. [CrossRef]
13. Takai, T. Advances in histopathological diagnosis of keratoacanthoma. *J. Dermatol.* **2017**, *44*, 304–314. [CrossRef]
14. Misago, N.; Ansai, S.; Fukumoto, T.; Anan, T.; Nakao, T. Keratoacanthoma en plaque/nodule: A brief report of the clinicopathological features of five cases. *J. Dermatol.* **2017**, *44*, 803–807. [CrossRef]
15. Sáchez Yus, E.; Simón, P.; Requena, L.; Ambrojo, P.; de Eusebio, E. Solitary keratoacanthoma: A self-healing proliferation that frequently becomes malignant. *Am. J. Dermatopathol.* **2000**, *22*, 305–310.
16. Weedon, D.D.; Malo, J.; Brooks, D.; Williamson, R. Squamous cell carcinoma arising in keratoacanthoma: A neglected phenomenon in the elderly. *Am. J. Dermatopathol.* **2010**, *32*, 423–426. [CrossRef]
17. Ogita, A.; Ansai, S.; Misago, N.; Anan, T.; Fukumoto, T.; Saeki, H. Clinicopathological study of crateriform verruca: Crateriform epithelial lesions histopathologically distinct from keratoacanthoma. *J. Dermatol.* **2016**, *43*, 1154–1159. [CrossRef]

18. Poblet, E.; Jimenez-Reyes, J.; Gonzalez-Herrada, C.; Granados, R. Trichilemmal keratosis. A clinicopathologic and immunohistochemical study of two cases. *Am. J. Dermatopathol.* **1996**, *18*, 543–547. [CrossRef]
19. Kimura, S. Trichilemmal keratosis (horn): A light and electron microscopic study. *J. Cutan. Pathol.* **1983**, *10*, 59–67. [CrossRef] [PubMed]
20. Sun, J.D.; Barr, R.J. Papillated Bowen disease, a distinct variant. *Am. J. Dermatopathol.* **2006**, *28*, 395–398. [CrossRef] [PubMed]
21. Diaz-Cascajo, C.; Borghi, S.; Weyers, W.; Bastida-Inarrea, J. Follicular squamous cell carcinoma of the skin: A poorly recognized neoplasm arising from the wall of hair follicles. *J. Cutan. Pathol.* **2004**, *31*, 19–25. [CrossRef] [PubMed]
22. Kossard, S.; Tan, K.B.; Choy, C. Keratoacanthoma and infundibulocystic squamous cell carcinoma. *Am. J. Dermatopathol.* **2008**, *30*, 127–134. [CrossRef] [PubMed]
23. Misago, N.; Inoue, T.; Toda, S.; Narisawa, Y. Infundibular (follicular) and infundibulocystic squamous cell carcinoma: A clinicopathological and immunohistochemical study. *Am. J. Dermatopahtol.* **2011**, *33*, 687–694. [CrossRef]
24. Ansai, S.; Fukumoto, T.; Anan, T.; Kimura, T.; Kawana, S. Histopathological diagnosis of lesions clinically diagnosed as keratoacanthoma. *Jpn. J. Dermmtol.* **2013**, *123*, 1775–1784.
25. Ansai, S.; Umebayashi, Y.; Katsumata, N.; Kato, H.; Kadono, T.; Takai, T.; Namiki, T.; Nakagawa, M.; Soejima, T.; Koga, H.; et al. Japanese dermatological association guidelines: Outlines of guidelines for cutaneous squamous cell carcinoma 2020. *J. Dermatol.* **2021**, *48*, e288–e311. [CrossRef] [PubMed]

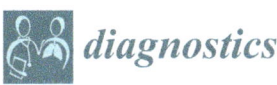

Review

Lichen Sclerosus: A Current Landscape of Autoimmune and Genetic Interplay

Noritaka Oyama * and Minoru Hasegawa

Department of Dermatology, Faculty of Medical Sciences, University of Fukui, 23-3 Matsuoka-Shimoaizuki, Eiheiji, Fukui 910-1193, Japan
* Correspondence: norider@u-fukui.ac.jp; Tel.: +81-(0)776-61-3111

Abstract: Lichen sclerosus (LS) is an acquired chronic inflammatory dermatosis predominantly affecting the anogenital area with recalcitrant itching and soreness. Progressive or persistent LS may cause urinary and sexual disturbances and an increased risk of local skin malignancy with a prevalence of up to 11%. Investigations on lipoid proteinosis, an autosomal recessive genodermatosis caused by loss-of-function mutations in the extracellular matrix protein 1 (*ECM1*) gene, led to the discovery of a humoral autoimmune response to the identical molecule in LS, providing evidence for an autoimmune and genetic counterpart targeting ECM1. This paper provides an overview of the fundamental importance and current issue of better understanding the immunopathology attributed to ECM1 in LS. Furthermore, we highlight the pleiotropic action of ECM1 in homeostatic and structural maintenance of skin biology as well as in a variety of human disorders possibly associated with impaired or gained ECM1 function, including the inflammatory bowel disease ulcerative colitis, Th2 cell-dependent airway allergies, T-cell and B-cell activation, and the demyelinating central nervous system disease multiple sclerosis, to facilitate sharing the concept as a plausible therapeutic target of this attractive molecule.

Keywords: lichen sclerosus; extracellular matrix protein 1; lipoid proteinosis; basement membrane zone; laminin-332; collagen IV; collagen VII; glycosaminoglycan

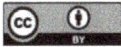

1. Introduction

Lichen sclerosus (LS), also known as 'lichen sclerosus et atrophicus', 'balanitis xerotica obliterans', 'kraurosis vulvae', or 'hypoplastic dystrophy', is an acquired chronic inflammatory disease that primarily affects the skin and mucous membranes, with a high occurrence in the anogenital area [1–3]. LS represents one of the most common referrals for pruritis and structural alteration in the vulva [1,4]. The predilection sites of the disease often cause serious urinary and sexual dysfunction, including dyspareunia and psychological impairments. In addition, LS has been associated with an increased risk of malignancy, mostly squamous cell carcinoma, in long-standing lesions in both sexes [5–8]. For therapeutic remedies, the topical application of potent corticosteroids is a primary mainstay [4,9,10]. Treatment options for refractories to the standard treatment regimens include systemic or local immunosuppressants (e.g., oral or topical calcineurin inhibitors), retinoids, phototherapy, and photodynamic therapy [11–15]. The mechanisms of action of these agents imply the possible involvement of an immunological disturbance in LS.

Although the pathogenesis of LS has yet to be elucidated, a series of etiological and epidemiological studies have suggested a possible genetic susceptibility and an autoimmune basis for the disease. For example, LS has a higher familial predisposition [16,17]; of 1052 individual cases with LS, 126 (~12%) had family histories. In addition, there have been increasing reports of monozygotic and dizygotic twins with LS. Genetic assessment of reliable numbers of LS cohorts identified a high association with the presence of particular human leukocyte antigens (HLAs) and haplotypes [18–20], such as DQ7, DR12, DRB1*12, and DRB1*13. Clinically, LS tends to coincide with various promiscuous autoimmune diseases with serum autoantibodies, such as morphea, Hashimoto's thyroiditis, rheumatoid arthritis, pernicious anemia, type I diabetes mellitus, alopecia areata, vitiligo, morphea, and immuno-bullous mucocutaneous diseases [21–27]. Of these, serum anti-thyroid antibodies were highly detectable in female LS (11–12%), compared to normal females. A series of clinical evidence has gradually suggested a scenario for the possible involvement of autoimmune imbalance, particularly autoimmune response to skin antigen(s), in LS.

More critically, loss-of-function mutations in the extracellular matrix protein 1 (*ECM1*) gene were demonstrated in an autosomal recessive genodermatosis referred to as lipoid proteinosis (LiP), a counterpart disease that is a similar skin pathology to LS [28]. This clinical rationale has led to the identification of humoral autoimmunity to ECM1 protein in patients with female anogenital LS [29], which was also applicable in the immunopathogenesis of male penile LS [2]. Furthermore, the similar clinicopathology between LS and LiP has allowed for considerable progress in addressing the in vivo biological function of this attractive molecule in animal model studies using a passive transfer of anti-ECM1 antibodies, and gene knockout and transgenic systems targeted for ECM1 in mice and zebrafish [30–33]. In addition, recent studies have demonstrated the role of ECM1 in the genetic predisposition to the inflammatory bowel disease (IBD) ulcerative colitis [34,35], the acquisition of immune tolerance and allergic responses via particular T-cell subsets such as CD4+CD25+ regulatory T cells and Th2 cells [31,36], and activation of abundant B-cell biology [33]. Thus, the biology of ECM1 positions it as an attractive core candidate to interconnect disease-specific pathophysiology.

2. Clinical Characteristics of LS

2.1. Clinical Features

LS mostly affects the anogenital skin and mucous membranes in the vast majority of cases (85–98%), typically female [1–3]. In male patients, the site-specific predisposition has been associated with a high occurrence rate of LS on normal penile skin grafts whose original diseases were unrelated to LS [37], but this is not a fate of the original skin sites. Without regard to gender, the typical clinical picture includes erosions as well as whitish-pale, indurative polygonal (porcelain-like) papules and plaques, which later change to atrophic scarring (Figure 1). An itching sensation, among various symptoms, is primary and inevitable [38]. The lesion may account for the bullous and hemorrhagic appearance, but it causes a potential difficulty in arriving at an accurate diagnosis [39,40]. Several reports for extragenital LS cases have suggested a variety of affected skin sites including the head, neck, scalp, palms and soles, periorbital area, tongue, lip, and peristoma skin [41] (Figure 2). Interestingly, extragenital LS, unlike genital disease, seldom develops local skin malignancies, giving way to the assumption that genital circumstances can be a primary extrinsic factor in the development of LS. The proposed candidate may include occasional herpes virus infection, urine and/or fecal irritation, constitutive colonization of gram-negative bacteria, or any combination of these.

2.2. Epidemiology and Etiology

Results from epidemiological studies indicated that LS was probably underreported and may have had a prevalence of approximately 0.1–0.3%, with a male-to-female ratio of 1:10 [42,43]. LS can develop at any age; however, a bimodal peak has been found in prepubertal girls and postmenopausal women as well as in middle-aged men [2,42,44–46]. A retrospective analysis using a large number (n = 411) of uncharacterized penile dermatoses revealed that ~10% of the foreskin biopsy samples showed the typical LS pathology [47]. Therefore, LS may occur far more frequently than previously expected, although the gender bias remains unchanged (~3% in females and >0.07% in males) [46,48]. The significant sex ratio and age bimodality indicates a possible association with hormonal imbalance, particularly estrogen deficiency, but hormone replacement therapy neither improves existing disease nor provides any protective effects against the disease. Persistent LS may result in severe scarring, which can lead to impairments in micturition and sexual activity, urethral stricture, and associated physical morbidities [49,50], and more importantly an increased risk of malignancy, particularly non-differentiated squamous cell carcinoma (4.7–10.7%) [51,52] (Figure 1).

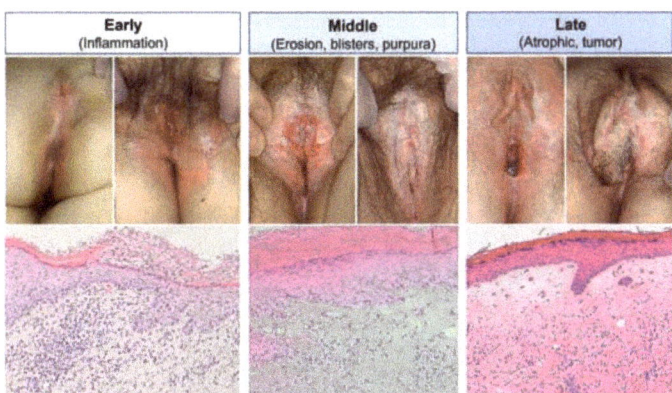

Figure 1. Stage-specific clinical and pathological features of female genital LS. In the early clinical stage of LS (**left columns**), it initiates as erythema and mild erosion, mostly covering the entire perivaginal and perianal area. Pathologically, early LS shows parakeratotic scales, irregular epidermal thickening, and intense inflammatory infiltrates in the upper dermis with faint homogenization of dermal collagen bundles. The condition fluctuates and gradually exacerbates into persistent erosions with focal blistering and induration, leading to a whitish-pale appearance in the middle clinical stage (**middle columns**). Note that dermal hyalinosis is more apparent with dilated blood vessels. The chain of these inflammatory events finally results in scarring and irreversible adhesion of external genital parts, and abruptly develops squamous cell carcinoma in the late clinical stage (**right columns**). The preexisting dermal hyalinosis in the skin pathology further extends diffusely, becoming more prone to eosinophilic staining and a thinner color. Dilated blood vessels in the upper dermis look atrophic, narrowing in size with thickening vessel walls.

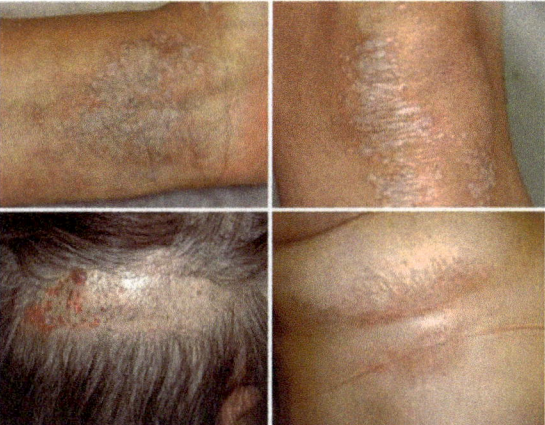

Figure 2. Clinical features of LS developed on the extragenital skin. The extragenital LS occurs at any skin sites, including extremities (**upper left and right**), scalp (**lower left**), and trunk (**lower right**).

2.3. Histopathological Features

Typical LS pathology displays a thickening epidermis with hyperkeratosis and follicular plugging, particularly in the early clinical stage, consequently followed by atrophic flattening of the epidermal rete ridges (Figure 3). The dermis underneath undergoes zonal hyalinization, intermingled with amorphous eosinophilic materials, homogeneous collagen bundles, and telangiectasia. A band-like infiltration of inflammatory cells may be present along with and/or separate from the hyalinizing dermis, which becomes sparser and more focal during the clinical course. However, each of these pathological findings often coexists at differing frequencies and degrees. Skin biopsies may therefore provide inconsistent pictures and result in difficulty differentiating other mimicking dermatoses affected in the anogenital area, resulting in the dilemma of diagnostic inaccuracy and delay [53,54].

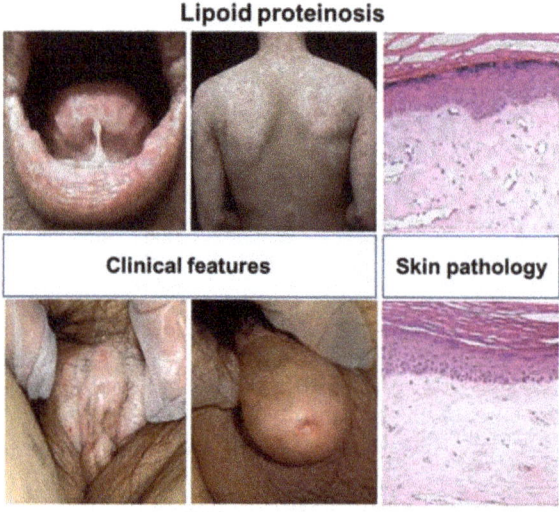

Figure 3. Clinicopathology of lipoid proteinosis (an ECM1-lacking genodermatosis: **upper panels**) and lichen sclerosus (an anti-ECM1 autoantibody-carrying condition in females and males; **left and right in the lower panels, respectively**). Irrespective of a predilection to different skin sites between the two diseases, their skin pathologies display similar features (**right columns**), including packed and parakeratotic hyperkeratosis, epidermal atrophy, and diffuse hyaline changes and dilated blood vessels in the upper dermis. Of these, dermal hyalinosis is a hallmark of both diseases.

3. Molecular Characteristics of ECM1: A Secretory Glycoprotein

3.1. Historical Background for the Discovery of the ECM1 Gene: What It Means

The human *ECM1* gene was first isolated in 1997 and was mapped to chromosome 1q21.2, located centromerically to the gene cluster termed epidermal differentiation complex (EDC) [55,56]. Comparing the plane structure to the previously discovered mouse *Ecm1* gene in 1994 [57], the human counterpart represents one exon fewer than the mouse gene; the sequence is homologous to the sixth shortest mouse exon [55]. The upstream regulatory sequences of the human gene contain putative binding sites for various major transcription factors, such as GATA, Sp1, AP-1, and ETS family members, all of which, except for the potential GATA-binding motifs, are highly conserved with the equivalent portion of the mouse *Ecm1* gene [58]. The *ECM* gene is highly conserved and expressed in most eukaryotes and their various cell types [59], supporting the concept of potential significance in the evolutionary process, as was the discovery of a genetic disease caused by mutations in this gene, lipoid proteinosis [28].

3.2. Gene Structure and Variants

The human *ECM1* gene is located on chromosome 1q21.2 and encodes four splice variants, ECM1a–d [55,56]. ECM1a (1.8-kb, 540 amino acids) comprises 10 exons, whereas

ECM1b (1.4-kb, 415 amino acids) only lacks exon 7. ECM1c (1.85-kb, 559 amino acids) contains an additional exon (5a) within intron 5 of ECM1a. These three major variants show widespread and differential expression patterns in human tissues [58,60]. For example, ECM1a is ubiquitously expressed in major organs including the skin, liver, intestine, lung, ovary, prostate, testis, skeletal muscle, pancreas, and kidney, with the greatest expression levels observed in the placenta and heart. ECM1b expression seems to be restricted to the tonsils and epidermal keratinocytes, whereas the tissue/cell type-specific expression of ECM1c remains to be identified [61]. ECM1d comprises a minimum splicing variant, with an out-of-frame insertion of 71 nucleotides at the 5′ end of exon 2, resulting in a truncated protein of 57 amino acids [62] and an enigmatic biological significance. In skin, ECM1a was expressed in the epidermal basal layer, dermal blood vessels, outer root sheath of hair follicles, sebaceous lobules, and sweat gland epithelia, whereas ECM1b was localized to the suprabasal layers of the epidermis [60,61,63]. Thus, in vivo associations between each of the ECM1 splicing variants and skin biology are gradually forming.

3.3. Protein Structure and Function

ECM1 is an 85-kDa-secreted glycoprotein known to play pivotal roles in the structural and homeostatic organization of various skin components through direct binding with various extracellular molecules, such as perlecan, matrix metalloproteinase family members, fibulins, fibrillins, fibronectin, laminin-332, type IV and type VII collagens, cartilage-derived oligomeric matrix protein (COMP), proteoglycans, glycosaminoglycans, phospholipids (particularly phospholipid scramblase 1), and progranulin chondrogenic growth factor (PGRN) [61,64–69]. Of note, these molecules co-localize immunohistologically with in vivo ECM1 in human skin. The multifocal interaction between skin structural molecules contributes to the biological significance of ECM1 in epidermal growth and differentiation, basement membrane integrity, angiogenesis, endochondral development, and certain malignancies, as well as in the structural maintenance of the dermis (Figure 4). Most of these biological activities are associated with positive regulation of cell proliferation, migration, and differentiation, resulting in tissue formation and organization; however, negative effects on chondrocyte hypertrophy, matrix mineralization, and endochondral bone formation have been described as well [70–72]. ECM1 thus penetrates into the fundamental skin biology via complex organization with surrounding microstructural molecules, and mutations of their corresponding genes are responsible for a hereditary genodermatosis LiP [28].

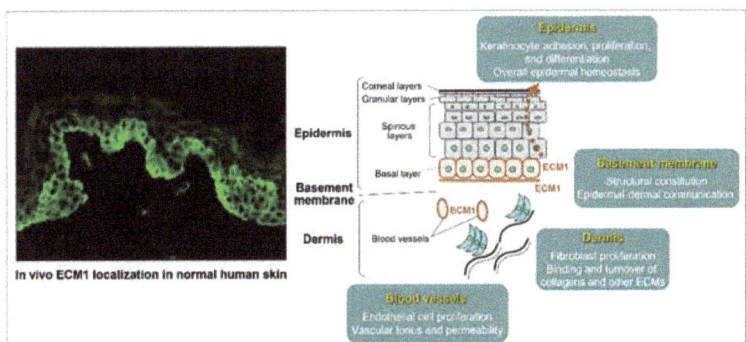

Figure 4. Multifocal interaction of in vivo ECM1 with surrounding extracellular matrix and structural molecules in the skin. ECM1 is expressed in the major skin components (particularly the epidermal basal layer and basement membranes) and adjunct appendages (blood vessel walls and follicular epithelium), as immunostained in normal human skin (**left panel**), and regulates the different in vivo turnover and feedback productivity of binding partners as a 'biological glue', contributing to the integrity and maintenance of skin homeostasis (**right panel**).

4. Autoimmune Response in LS

4.1. Etiological Scenario for Autoimmunity to ECM1 in LS

Although no plausible evidence regarding the local and systemic autoimmune reactions characteristic of LS has been put forth, recent progress on the screening of disease-specific serum autoantibodies in LS is extrapolated from bipolar evidence for possible genetic susceptibility and a humoral autoimmune basis for the disease. Specifically, study findings have identified variable intra-familial cases with LS [16,73], an association with particular HLA class II antigens (DQ7-9, DR11, DR12, and DQ17) [18,20], and a high coexistence of various autoimmune diseases, such as morphea, Hashimoto's thyroiditis, rheumatoid arthritis, pernicious anemia, type I diabetes mellitus, alopecia areata, vitiligo, bullous pemphigoid, and mucous membrane pemphigoid [21–25,27]. Of these autoantibody- and/or T-cell-driven diseases, anti-thyroid antibodies were highly detectable in female LS patients (11.1–40%) compared with other organ- and tissue-specific autoantibodies. However, the autoantibodies mostly do not correlate with either severity or duration of the corresponding diseases, proving irrelevant as a consequence of LS [74].

A century ago, evidence implicating a humoral autoimmune response in LS was demonstrated in a case where probable LS was induced through the injection of an autologous serum from an affected individual into non-lesional skin [75]. More critically, the skin pathology of LS shares considerable overlap with that of LiP (OMIM 247100), an ECM1-deficient genetic skin disease [28], for example, trauma-induced inflammation (also known as Koebner's phenomenon) and lesional skin microscopy showing the atrophic epidermis with hyperkeratosis, disruption and duplication of the basement membrane, and hyaline (glassy-like) collagen changes and telangiectasia in the upper dermis (Figure 3). Altogether, this clinicopathological evidence straightforwardly implicates a counterpart disease concept targeting ECM1 in both LS and LiP [76].

4.2. Identification of IgG Autoantibodies Reactive with ECM1 in LS

Primary screening using immunoblotting with cultured normal human keratinocyte substrates identified detectable levels of serum IgG-class antibodies to three of the four ECM1 isoforms, namely ECM1a–c in ~70% of female patients with genital LS [29]. The fidelity of the seroreactivity was confirmed using a bacterially generated full-length recombinant ECM1a protein. Thereafter, antigen-specific enzyme-linked immunosorbent assays (ELISAs) utilizing a highly antigenic portion of the recombinant ECM1 protein (359–559 amino acids) optimized the immunoreactivity of serum anti-ECM1 antibodies in 74–80% of female patients with genital LS, with 94% specificity in discriminating LS from other autoimmune diseases and healthy controls [30]. In another cohort study, ECM1 seroreactivity was also detectable in male patients with male penile LS [2]. The update series has further accelerated the serological diagnostic accuracy in individual cases suspicious of LS [39,75]. Irrespective of gender, humoral autoimmunity to ECM1 needs to be considered on the basis of its pathogenic significance in LS.

5. Issues that Need to be Addressed to Better Understand ECM1 Autoimmunity in LS

5.1. Lack of In Vivo-Bound Anti-ECM1 IgG in the LS Skin

Debate continues regarding the difficulties in detecting the anti-ECM1 autoantibody in LS lesional skin. For example, direct immunofluorescence studies of LS skin have shown no signals [44,77]. In addition, indirect immunofluorescence studies using LS patients' sera on normal human skin sections also showed negative (with standard dilutions of the sera) or only faintly positive signals along with the lower epidermis and basement membrane. These controversial observations may be attributable to differences in affinity and/or avidity of antigen-specific serum IgG to the in vivo-native ECM1 antigen, because the IgG fraction of affinity purified from LS sera exhibits intense immuno-reactivity in the lower epidermis, and similar observations were made from immuno-labeling with rabbit anti-ECM1 polyclonal antibodies on normal human skin [29] (Figure 4). Based on our recognition, ECM1 is considered a secretory glycoprotein that acts as a biological 'glue' to stabilize robust structural proteins [78], such as BPAG I/II, laminin-332, and collagens. One may consider that the flowability and turnover of in vivo ECM1, in part, affect the accessibility and reactivity of the antibody. Considering these technical limitations, the standard immunohistochemical approach using patients' skin or sera remains less valuable in a routine laboratory workup, and the ELISA system specific for ECM1—or at least immunoblotting using recombinant ECM1 protein—may currently be a preferable tool for a noninvasive and objective serodiagnosis in LS [30].

5.2. Difficulty in the Establishment of Mouse Models for LS and LiP

The pathogenic relevance of autoimmunity to ECM1 in LS has been reevaluated by mouse passive-transfer experiments using intra-cutaneous injections of either a rabbit anti-ECM1 polyclonal antibody or an affinity-purified IgG from ECM1 ELISA-positive LS patients' sera [30]. Both antibodies recognize the regions of the ECM1 protein that are highly homologous between humans and mice, and when injected into the skin, both IgGs were indeed accessible to native mouse ECM1 in vivo, as was identical immunoreactivity to human skin. The mouse skin sites injected either with a rabbit anti-ECM1 polyclonal antibody or an affinity-purified IgG from LS sera exhibited a clinicopathology compatible with the early clinical stage of LS, including erythematous swelling (dermal inflammation) and dilated blood vessels (telangiectasia) for up to two weeks after the initial injection. However, this approach failed to reproduce dermal hyalinosis or scarring, both of which are histological hallmarks of the well-established (late) stage of LS. This incomplete observation raises possible interpretations for how hyalinosis and/or sclerotic events in LS skin are indeed consequences of complex and sensitive events. For example, the sensitivity may depend on the particular genetic background(s) of the mouse strain(s) or the HLA class II haplotypes of the patients [18,20]. In addition, it may be affected by the constitutive impairment of in vivo ECM1 function, e.g., more prolonged exposure to anti-ECM1 antibodies. Considering the clinical aspect that (i) the vast majority of LS affects anogenital skin and (ii) extragenital LS sometimes develops around utero-abdominal fistula [41,79], urinary irritation and/or local infection with gram-negative bacteria may be (a) confounding factor(s).

Additional experiments have explored the fact that conventional/targeted disruptions of the *Ecm1* gene in mice (ECM1$^{-/-}$) render it lethal (surviving for no more than 6–8 weeks) [31,80], strongly suggesting that ECM1 is indispensable for at least early embryonic development. In contrast, LiP patients represent an ECM1-knockout condition in humans who can survive and show no evidence of short life spans or disease-related mortality. In addition to this discrepancy, a systematic disease translational study comparing gene transcriptional responses to inflammatory insults in mice and humans detected disparities in the gene expression profiles between the mouse models and their human counterparts [80]. Species-specific gene regulation may thus represent a challenge to reproducing typical LS pathology in mice.

5.3. Establishment of ECM1-Knockdown Human Dermal Fibroblasts

A series of our failures for recapitulating LS and LiP phenotypes in mouse models led us to re-recognize what happens to the impaired ECM1 function in vitro. ECM1 siRNA knockdown in human dermal fibroblasts showed a significant delay of growth and migratory activities, as well as collagen gel contraction, compared to control fibroblasts [69]. Also, the ECM1 knockdown upregulated genes related to structural, fibrogenic, and carcinogenic properties, some of which shared the skin structural molecules that are major binding partners for ECM1, such as laminin-332, and type IV and VII collagens [64,67,69]. All of the binders displayed altered immunolabeling at the basement membrane zone and dermal vessels in the LS lesional skin (Figure 4), where ECM1 is highly expressed. Combining these in vitro data with the ECM1 autoantibody scenario, one may speculate that the antibody-dependent impairment of ECM1 function disrupts a biological interconnection with the in vivo binding partners, resulting in their functional behavior to maintain the structural integrity responsible for the LS pathology (Figure 5).

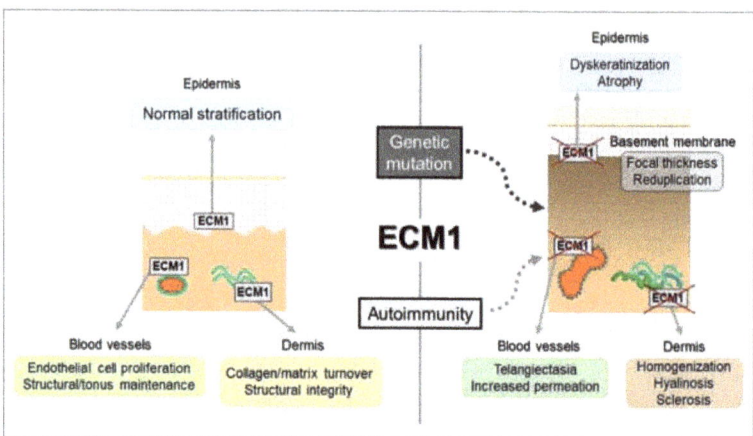

Figure 5. Schematic image for autoimmune and genetic impairment of ECM1 function in the skin. Genetic ablation and autoantibody targeting of the skin ECM1 cause dysregulation of its binding partners, as listed in Figure 3, contributing to the homeostatic imbalance or collapse in the epidermis (dyskeratosis and atrophy), dermis (collagen homogenization and sclerosis), and blood vessels (telangiectasia and impermeability). The chain of these statements finally establishes the pathological features seen in LiP and LS.

6. Lessens from Novel ECM1 Function in Other Animal Models

6.1. Th2 Cell-Dependent Allergic Response in the Airway

DNA microarray assays have disclosed the expression of the *Ecm1* gene in mouse hematopoietic cells, particularly in T cells [81,82], although the transcription levels considerably differ in the T-cell differentiation- and lineage-dependent manner; it was much higher in CD4+ helper T cells and CD4+CD25+ T cells (Tregs) but relatively lower in CD8+ cytotoxic T cells and CD3-negative naïve T cells. Of the CD4+ helper T-cell lineage, the ECM1 expression was almost prone to Th2 cells [31], indicating the possible association between ECM1 and allergic reactions. This scenario was also compounded through the finding that chimeric BALB/c mice transplanted with ECM1-deficient bone marrow cells showed a decrease in inflammatory response in experimentally induced airway allergy. Functional analysis for several T-cell lineages from ECM1-knockout mice exhibited no substantial differences in the proliferation activity, cytokine/chemokine profiles, and polarization of their differentiation, suggesting the direct action of ECM1 in Th2 cell trafficking from lymph nodes into circulation.

In Th2 cells, ECM1 mRNA and protein expression were detectable three days after antigen-dependent engagement of the T-cell receptor. Subsequently, ECM1 can bind with an IL-2 receptor subunit (CD122), but with neither CD25 nor CD132, to inhibit the phosphorylation and activation of the downstream-signaling molecules, such as STAT5, KLF2, and S1P1 [31], resulting in the downregulation of Th2 cell trafficking to the local inflammatory sites.

On the other hand, freshly isolated and activated CD4+ CD25+ Tregs highly express ECM1 transcription [83]. CD4+ CD25+Tregs are well-known to regulate innate and adaptive immune responses, tumor immunity, and a potent anti-inflammatory capacity in autoimmune and chronic inflammatory diseases, such as autoimmune encephalitis, diabetes, thyroiditis, IBDs, and contact skin hypersensitivity [84–88]. Naturally occurring Tregs, the other Treg phenotype that comprises up to 5% of the peripheral CD4+ T-cell pool, have also been shown to express ECM1 [87]. More critically, the ECM1 transcription was significantly increased in naïve T cells by transient transduction of forkhead box P3 (FOXP3), a transcription factor that acts as a master control molecule for the development and function of CD4+CD25+ Tregs in the thymus and periphery [88].

6.2. Macrophage Polarization in Inflammatory Bowel Diseases (IBDs)

Genotyping using a reliable number of ulcerative colitis cohorts (n = 905) determined a strong disease susceptibility locus at the ECM1 gene [34]. The foothold identification further accelerated the research activity concerning ECM1-targeted culprit cells in the disease. Mice transplanted with ECM1 knocked-down macrophages, a phenotype unable to polarize towards M1 macrophage, decreased pathological inflammation of colitis in experimental IBD mice [34], raising a direct interpretation of ECM1 function to regulate the IBD-dependent macrophage lineage. However, data from several trials determining ECM1 gene mutation and/or polymorphism in IBD cohorts remains unstable as the genetic signature [88,89], which may be impacted by racial difference. Also, there has been no available evidence of a relationship between ECM1 and the intestinal epithelial barrier, as well as permeability balance and luminal antigen absorption in the intestine interface.

6.3. Miscellaneous

6.3.1. Multiple Sclerosis

Multiple sclerosis is a chronic inflammatory condition in the central nervous system characterized by demyelination and axonal damage through Th17-dependent innate immunity. Administration of recombinant ECM1 ameliorated the severity of encephalomyelitis with cerebral demyelination and inflammation, accompanied by a decrease in the Th17 response, in an experimental model for multiple sclerosis [90]. Inversely, in vivo overexpression of ECM1 successfully inhibited encephalomyelitis with Th17 cell activation. The protective action of ECM1 is mediated in part by its direct interaction with av-integrin on dendritic cells, blocking the integrin-mediated activation of TGF-β. Data support a possible engagement in a replacement therapy targeting ECM1.

6.3.2. B Cell Function

Follicular helper T cells (T_{FH}) are a subset of the $CD4^+$ helper T-cell lineage that enables a variety of B-cell responses, i.e., the formation of germinal centers (GCs), affinity maturation of GC B cells, differentiation of high-affinity antibody-producing plasma cells, and production of memory B cells. All the B cell-specific reactions were impaired by an ECM1 knockout in antigen-immunized mice [33]. Exogenously injected ECM1 into mice infected with influenza virus exhibited a protective immune response via enhancing differentiation towards T_{FH} cells and production of virus-neutralizing antibodies. ECM1 can therefore promote T_{FH} cell differentiation and antibody production, both of which are indispensable for humoral autoimmunity.

7. Conclusions

Considerable progress has recently been made in both clinical and animal studies designed to elucidate the in vivo function of ECM1. Novel insights regarding this molecule in the restricted T-cell repertoire, B-cell activation, organ-specific allergic reaction, and genetic susceptibility to ulcerative colitis have been condensed during the last decade. In addition, much attention has been paid to the role of ECM1 in tumor biology, particularly its microenvironment as an alternative to tumor-directed therapy [72,91,92]. Notwithstanding these updates, genetic ablation of ECM1 and passive transfer of ECM1-specific antibodies in mice has yet to fully explain the characteristic pathophysiology in human diseases LiP and LS, respectively. Future studies concerning the establishment of animal models for LS now await sophistication of the overall technical processes.

Clinical observation shows that LiP patients are viable without an inherent susceptibility to any type of cancer, unlike LS patients. ECM1 can therefore be dispensable or at least compensable spatially and temporally for the development of certain organs, including the skin. Future studies will encourage research on the tissue and organ developmental stage-specific significance of ECM1 action.

Author Contributions: Conceptualization, structure, and writing, N.O.; conceptualization and correction, M.H. All authors have read and agreed to the published version of the manuscript.

Funding: This research received no external funding.

Institutional Review Board Statement: Not available.

Informed Consent Statement: Not applicable.

Data Availability Statement: Not applicable.

Acknowledgments: This work was supported by JSPS KAKENHI Grant Numbers JP21K08321 (N.O.) and JP22K08426 (M.H.).

Conflicts of Interest: The authors declare no conflict of interest.

References

1. Goldstein, A.T.; Marinoff, S.C.; Christopher, K.; Srodon, M. Prevalence of Vulvar Lichen Sclerosus in a General Gynecology Practice. *J. Reprod. Med.* **2005**, *50*, 477–480. [PubMed]
2. Edmonds, E.V.J.; Hunt, S.; Hawkins, D.; Dinneen, M.; Francis, N.; Bunker, C.B. Clinical Parameters in Male Genital Lichen Sclerosus: A Case Series of 329 Patients. *J. Eur. Acad. Dermatology Venereol.* **2012**, *26*, 730–737. [CrossRef] [PubMed]
3. Hagedorn, M.; Buxmeyer, B.; Schmitt, Y.; Bauknecht, T. Survey of Genital Lichen Sclerosus in Women and Men. *Arch. Gynecol. Obstet.* **2002**, *266*, 86–91. [CrossRef] [PubMed]
4. Kirtschig, G.; Becker, K.; Günthert, A.; Jasaitiene, D.; Cooper, S.; Chi, C.C.; Kreuter, A.; Rall, K.K.; Aberer, W.; Riechardt, S.; et al. Evidence-Based (S3) Guideline on (Anogenital) Lichen Sclerosus. *J. Eur. Acad. Dermatol. Venereol.* **2015**, *29*, e1–e43. [PubMed]
5. Bleeker, M.C.G.; Visser, P.J.; Overbeek, L.I.H.; Van Beurden, M.; Berkhof, J. Lichen Sclerosus: Incidence and Risk of Vulvar Squamous Cell Carcinoma. *Cancer Epidemiol. Biomark. Prev.* **2016**, *25*, 1224–1230. [CrossRef]
6. Davick, J.; Samuelson, M.; Krone, J.; Stockdale, C. The Prevalence of Lichen Sclerosus in Patients with Vulvar Squamous Cell Carcinoma. *Int. J. Gynecol. Pathol.* **2017**, *36*, 305–309. [CrossRef]
7. Micheletti, L.; Preti, M.; Radici, G.; Boveri, S.; Di Pumpo, O.; Privitera, S.S.; Ghiringhello, B.; Benedetto, C. Vulvar Lichen Sclerosus and Neoplastic Transformation: A Retrospective Study of 976 Cases. *J. Low. Genit. Tract. Dis.* **2016**, *20*, 180–183. [CrossRef]
8. Leis, M.; Singh, A.; Li, C.; Ahluwalia, R.; Fleming, P.; Lynde, C.W. Risk of Vulvar Squamous Cell Carcinoma in Lichen Sclerosus and Lichen Planus: A Systematic Review. *J. Obstet. Gynaecol. Canada* **2022**, *44*, 182–192. [CrossRef]
9. Hasegawa, M.; Ishikawa, O.; Asano, Y.; Sato, S.; Jinnin, M.; Takehara, K.; Fujimoto, M.; Yamamoto, T.; Ihn, H. Diagnostic Criteria, Severity Classification and Guidelines of Lichen Sclerosus et Atrophicus. *J. Dermatol.* **2018**, *45*, 891–897. [CrossRef]
10. Neill, S.M.; Lewis, F.M.; Tatnall, F.M.; Cox, N.H. British Association of Dermatologists' Guidelines for the Management of Lichen Sclerosus 2010. *Br. J. Dermatol.* **2010**, *163*, 672–682. [CrossRef]
11. Funaro, D.; Lovett, A.; Leroux, N.; Powell, J. A Double-Blind, Randomized Prospective Study Evaluating Topical Clobetasol Propionate 0.05% versus Topical Tacrolimus 0.1% in Patients with Vulvar Lichen Sclerosus. *J. Am. Acad. Dermatol.* **2014**, *71*, 84–91. [CrossRef] [PubMed]
12. Bulbul Baskan, E.; Turan, H.; Tunali, S.; Toker, S.C.; Saricaoglu, H. Open-Label Trial of Cyclosporine for Vulvar Lichen Sclerosus. *J. Am. Acad. Dermatol.* **2007**, *57*, 276–278. [CrossRef] [PubMed]
13. Virgili, A.; Corazza, M.; Bianchi, A.; Mollica, G.; Califano, A. Open Study of Topical 0.025% Tretinoin in the Treatment of Vulvar Lichen Sclerosus: One Year of Therapy. *J. Reprod. Med. Obstet. Gynecol.* **1995**, *40*, 614–618.
14. Terras, S.; Gambichler, T.; Moritz, R.K.C.; Stücker, M.; Kreuter, A. UV-A1 Phototherapy vs Clobetasol Propionate, 0.05%, in the Treatment of Vulvar Lichen Sclerosus: A Randomized Clinical Trial. *JAMA Dermatol.* **2014**, *150*, 621–627. [CrossRef] [PubMed]
15. Sotiriou, E.; Panagiotidou, D.; Ioannidis, D. An Open Trial of 5-Aminolevulinic Acid Photodynamic Therapy for Vulvar Lichen Sclerosus. *Eur. J. Obstet. Gynecol. Reprod. Biol.* **2008**, *141*, 187–188. [CrossRef]
16. Thomas, R.H.M.; Kennedy, C.T.C. The Development of Lichen Sclerosus et Atrophicus in Monozygotic Twin Girls. *Br. J. Dermatol.* **1986**, *114*, 377–379. [CrossRef]
17. Sahn, E.E.; Bluestein, E.L.; Oliva, S. Familial Lichen Sclerosus et Atrophicus in Childhood. *Pediatr. Dermatol.* **1994**, *11*, 160–163. [CrossRef]
18. Azurdia, R.M.; Luzzi, G.A.; Byren, I.; Welsh, K.; Wojnarowska, F.; Marren, P.; Edwards, A. Lichen Sclerosus in Adult Men: A Study of HLA Associations and Susceptibility to Autoimmune Disease. *Br. J. Dermatol.* **1999**, *140*, 79–83. [CrossRef]
19. Marren, P.; Jell, J.; Charnock, F.M.; Bunce, M.; Welsh, K.; Wojnarowska, F. The Association between Lichen Sclerosus and Antigens of the HLA System. *Br. J. Dermatol.* **1995**, *132*, 197–203. [CrossRef]
20. Gao, X.H.; Barnardo, M.C.M.N.; Winsey, S.; Ahmad, T.; Cook, J.; Agudelo, J.D.; Zhai, N.; Powell, J.J.; Fuggle, S.V.; Wojnarowska, F. The Association between HLA DR, DQ Antigens, and Vulval Lichen Sclerosus in the UK: HLA DRB112 and Its Associated DRB112/DQB10301/04/09/010 Haplotype Confers Susceptibility to Vulval Lichen Sclerosus, and HLA DRB10301/04 and Its Associated DRB10301/04/DQB10201/02/03 Haplotype Protects from Vulval Lichen Sclerosus. *J. Investig. Dermatol.* **2005**, *125*, 895–899.

21. Khan Mohammad Beigi, P. The Immunogenetics of Morphea and Lichen Sclerosus. *Adv. Exp. Med. Biol.* **2022**, *1367*, 155–172. [PubMed]
22. Guarneri, F.; Giuffrida, R.; Di Bari, F.; Cannavò, S.P.; Benvenga, S. Thyroid Autoimmunity and Lichen. *Front. Endocrinol.* **2017**, *8*, 146. [CrossRef] [PubMed]
23. García-Bravo, B.; Sánchez-Pedreño, P.; Rodríguez-Pichardo, A.; Camacho, F. Lichen Sclerosus et Atrophicus. A Study of 76 Cases and Their Relation to Diabetes. *J. Am. Acad. Dermatol.* **1988**, *19*, 482–485. [CrossRef] [PubMed]
24. Harrington, C.I.; Dunsmore, I.R. An Investigation into the Incidence of Auto-immune Disorders in Patients with Lichen Sclerosus and Atrophicus. *Br. J. Dermatol.* **1981**, *104*, 563–566. [CrossRef] [PubMed]
25. Thomas, R.H.M.; Ridley, C.M.; McGibbon, D.H.; Black, M.M. Lichen Sclerosus et Atrophicus and Autoimmunity—a Study of 350 Women. *Br. J. Dermatol.* **1988**, *118*, 41–46. [CrossRef]
26. Baldo, M.; Bailey, A.; Bhogal, B.; Groves, R.W.; Ogg, G.; Wojnarowska, F. T Cells Reactive with the NC16A Domain of BP180 Are Present in Vulval Lichen Sclerosus and Lichen Planus. *J. Eur. Acad. Dermatol. Venereol.* **2010**, *24*, 186–190. [CrossRef]
27. Walsh, M.L.; Leonard, N.; Shawki, H.; Bell, H.K. Lichen Sclerosus and Immunobullous Disease. *J. Low. Genit. Tract Dis.* **2012**, *16*, 468–470. [CrossRef]
28. Hamada, T.; McLean, W.H.I.; Ramsay, M.; Ashton, G.H.S.; Nanda, A.; Jenkins, T.; Edelstein, I.; South, A.P.; Bleck, O.; Wessagowit, V.; et al. Lipoid Proteinosis Maps to 1q21 and Is Caused by Mutations in the Extracellular Matrix Protein 1 Gene (ECM1). *Hum. Mol. Genet.* **2002**, *11*, 833–840. [CrossRef]
29. Oyama, N.; Chan, I.; Neill, S.M.; Hamada, T.; South, A.P.; Wessagowit, V.; Wojnarowska, F.; D'Cruz, D.; Hughes, G.J.; Black, M.M.; et al. Autoantibodies to Extracellular Matrix Protein 1 in Lichen Sclerosus. *Lancet* **2003**, *362*, 118–123. [CrossRef]
30. Oyama, N.; Chan, I.; Neill, S.M.; South, A.P.; Wojnarowska, F.; Kawakami, Y.; D'Cruz, D.; Mepani, K.; Hughes, G.J.; Bhogal, B.S.; et al. Development of Antigen-Specific ELISA for Circulating Autoantibodies to Extracellular Matrix Protein 1 in Lichen Sclerosus. *J. Clin. Investig.* **2004**, *113*, 1550–1559. [CrossRef]
31. Li, Z.; Zhang, Y.; Liu, Z.; Wu, X.; Zheng, Y.; Tao, Z.; Mao, K.; Wang, J.; Lin, G.; Tian, L.; et al. ECM1 Controls T(H)2 Cell Egress from Lymph Nodes through Re-Expression of S1P(1). *Nat. Immunol.* **2011**, *12*, 178–185. [CrossRef] [PubMed]
32. Li, Q.; Donahue, A.; Smith, S.; McGrath, J.A.; Oyama, N.; Uitto, J. Zebrafish Model of Lipoid Proteinosis. *J. Investig. Dermatol.* **2011**, *131*, S70.
33. He, L.; Gu, W.; Wang, M.; Chang, X.; Sun, X.; Zhang, Y.; Lin, X.; Yan, C.; Fan, W.; Su, P.; et al. Extracellular Matrix Protein 1 Promotes Follicular Helper T Cell Differentiation and Antibody Production. *Proc. Natl. Acad. Sci. USA* **2018**, *115*, 8621–8626. [CrossRef] [PubMed]
34. Fisher, S.A.; Tremelling, M.; Anderson, C.A.; Gwilliam, R.; Bumpstead, S.; Prescott, N.J.; Nimmo, E.R.; Massey, D.; Berzuini, C.; Johnson, C.; et al. Genetic Determinants of Ulcerative Colitis Include the ECM1 Locus and Five Loci Implicated in Crohn's Disease. *Nat. Genet.* **2008**, *40*, 710–712. [CrossRef] [PubMed]
35. Zhang, Y.; Li, X.; Luo, Z.; Ma, L.; Zhu, S.; Wang, Z.; Wen, J.; Cheng, S.; Gu, W.; Lian, Q.; et al. ECM1 Is an Essential Factor for the Determination of M1 Macrophage Polarization in IBD in Response to LPS Stimulation. *Proc. Natl. Acad. Sci. USA* **2020**, *117*, 3083–3092. [CrossRef]
36. Sugimoto, N.; Oida, T.; Hirota, K.; Nakamura, K.; Nomura, T.; Uchiyama, T.; Sakaguchi, S. Foxp3-Dependent and -Independent Molecules Specific for CD25+CD4+ Natural Regulatory T Cells Revealed by DNA Microarray Analysis. *Int. Immunol.* **2006**, *18*, 1197–1209. [CrossRef]
37. Abdelbaky, A.M.; Aluru, P.; Keegan, P.; Greene, D.R. Development of Male Genital Lichen Sclerosus in Penile Reconstruction Skin Grafts after Cancer Surgery: An Unreported Complication. *BJU Int.* **2012**, *109*, 776–779. [CrossRef]
38. Virgili, A.; Borghi, A.; Toni, G.; Minghetti, S.; Corazza, M. Prospective Clinical and Epidemiologic Study of Vulvar Lichen Sclerosus: Analysis of Prevalence and Severity of Clinical Features, Together with Historical and Demographic Associations. *Dermatology* **2014**, *228*, 145–151. [CrossRef]
39. Kawakami, Y.; Oyama, N.; Hanami, Y.; Kimura, T.; Kishimoto, K.; Yamamoto, T. A Case of Lichen Sclerosus of the Scalp Associated with Autoantibodies to Extracellular Matrix Protein 1. *Arch. Dermatol.* **2009**, *145*, 1458–1460. [CrossRef]
40. Khatib, J.; Wargo, J.J.; Krishnamurthy, S.; Travers, J.B. Hemorrhagic Bullous Lichen Sclerosus: A Case Report. *Am. J. Case Rep.* **2020**, *21*, e919353-1. [CrossRef]
41. Al-Niaimi, F.; Lyon, C. Peristomal Lichen Sclerosus: The Role of Occlusion and Urine Exposure? *Br. J. Dermatol.* **2013**, *168*, 643–646. [CrossRef] [PubMed]
42. Lansdorp, C.A.; Van Den Hondel, K.E.; Korfage, I.J.; Van Gestel, M.J.; Van Der Meijden, W.I. Quality of Life in Dutch Women with Lichen Sclerosus. *Br. J. Dermatol.* **2013**, *168*, 787–793. [CrossRef] [PubMed]
43. Wallace, H.J. Lichen Sclerosus et Atrophicus. *Trans. St. Johns. Hosp. Dermatol. Soc.* **1971**, *57*, 9–30. [PubMed]
44. Powell, J.; Wojnarowska, F. Childhood Vulvar Lichen Sclerosus: An Increasingly Common Problem. *J. Am. Acad. Dermatol.* **2001**, *44*, 803–806. [CrossRef] [PubMed]
45. Nelson, D.M.; Peterson, A.C. Lichen Sclerosus: Epidemiological Distribution in an Equal Access Health Care System. *J. Urol.* **2011**, *185*, 522–525. [CrossRef]
46. Kizer, W.S.; Prarie, T.; Morey, A.F. Balanitis Xerotica Obliterans: Epidemiologic Distribution in an Equal Access Health Care System. *South. Med. J.* **2003**, *96*, 9–11. [CrossRef]

47. West, D.S.; Papalas, J.A.; Selim, M.A.; Vollmer, R.T. Dermatopathology of the Foreskin: An Institutional Experience of over 400 Cases. *J. Cutan. Pathol.* **2013**, *40*, 11–18. [CrossRef]
48. Leibovitz, A.; Kaplun, V.; Saposhnicov, N.; Habot, B. Vulvovaginal Examinations in Elderly Nursing Home Women Residents. *Arch. Gerontol. Geriatr.* **2000**, *31*, 1–4. [CrossRef]
49. Vittrup, G.; Westmark, S.; Riis, J.; Mørup, L.; Heilesen, T.; Jensen, D.; Melgaard, D. The Impact of Psychosexual Counseling in Women With Lichen Sclerosus: A Randomized Controlled Trial. *J. Low. Genit. Tract Dis.* **2022**, *26*, 258–264. [CrossRef]
50. Haefner, H.K.; Aldrich, N.Z.; Dalton, V.K.; Gagné, H.M.; Marcus, S.B.; Patel, D.A.; Berger, M.B. The Impact of Vulvar Lichen Sclerosus on Sexual Dysfunction. *J. Women's Health* **2014**, *23*, 765–770. [CrossRef] [PubMed]
51. Halonen, P.; Jakobsson, M.; Heikinheimo, O.; Riska, A.; Gissler, M.; Pukkala, E. Lichen Sclerosus and Risk of Cancer. *Int. J. Cancer* **2017**, *140*, 1998–2002. [CrossRef] [PubMed]
52. Lee, A.; Bradford, J.; Fischer, G. Long-Term Management of Adult Vulvar Lichen Sclerosus: A Prospective Cohort Study of 507 Women. *JAMA Dermatol.* **2015**, *151*, 1061–1067. [CrossRef] [PubMed]
53. Regauer, S.; Liegl, B.; Reich, O. Early Vulvar Lichen Sclerosus: A Histopathological Challenge. *Histopathology* **2005**, *47*, 340–347. [CrossRef] [PubMed]
54. Niamh, L.; Naveen, S.; Hazel, B. Diagnosis of Vulval Inflammatory Dermatoses: A Pathological Study with Clinical Correlation. *Int. J. Gynecol. Pathol.* **2009**, *28*, 554–558. [CrossRef]
55. Smits, P.; Ni, J.; Feng, P.; Wauters, J.; Van Hul, W.; El Boutaibi, M.; Dillon, P.J.; Merregaert, J. The Human Extracellular Matrix Gene 1 (ECM1): Genomic Structure, CDNA Cloning, Expression Pattern, and Chromosomal Localization. *Genomics* **1997**, *45*, 487–495. [CrossRef] [PubMed]
56. Johnson, M.R.; Wilkin, D.J.; Vos, H.L.; Ortiz De Luna, R.I.; Dehejia, A.M.; Polymeropoulos, M.H.; Francomano, C.A. Characterization of the Human Extracellular Matrix Protein 1 Gene on Chromosome 1q21. *Matrix Biol.* **1997**, *16*, 289–292. [CrossRef]
57. Mathieu, E.; Meheus, L.; Raymackers, J.; Merregaert, J. Characterization of the Osteogenic Stromal Cell Line MN7: Identification of Secreted MN7 Proteins Using Two-Dimensional Polyacrylamide Gel Electrophoresis, Western Blotting, and Microsequencing. *J. Bone Miner. Res.* **1994**, *9*, 903–913. [CrossRef]
58. Smits, P.; Bhalerao, J.; Merregaert, J. Molecular Cloning and Characterization of the Mouse Ecm1 Gene and Its 5′ Regulatory Sequences. *Gene* **1999**, *226*, 253–261. [CrossRef]
59. Sercu, S.; Oyama, N.; Merregaert, J. Importance of Extracellular Matrix Protein 1 (ECM1) in Maintaining the Functional Integrity of the Human Skin. *Undefined* **2009**, *3*, 44–51. [CrossRef]
60. Sander, C.S.; Sercu, S.; Ziemer, M.; Hipler, U.C.; Elsner, P.; Thiele, J.; Merregaert, J. Expression of Extracellular Matrix Protein 1 (ECM1) in Human Skin Is Decreased by Age and Increased upon Ultraviolet Exposure. *Br. J. Dermatol.* **2006**, *154*, 218–224. [CrossRef]
61. Mongiat, M.; Fu, J.; Oldershaw, R.; Greenhalgh, R.; Gown, A.M.; Iozzo, R.V. Perlecan Protein Core Interacts with Extracellular Matrix Protein 1 (ECM1), a Glycoprotein Involved in Bone Formation and Angiogenesis. *J. Biol. Chem.* **2003**, *278*, 17491–17499. [CrossRef]
62. Horev, L.; Potikha, T.; Ayalon, S.; Molho-Pessach, V.; Ingber, A.; Gany, M.A.; Edin, B.S.; Glaser, B.; Zlotogorski, A. A Novel Splice-Site Mutation in ECM-1 Gene in a Consanguineous Family with Lipoid Proteinosis. *Exp. Dermatol.* **2005**, *14*, 891–897. [CrossRef] [PubMed]
63. Smits, P.; Poumay, Y.; Karperien, M.; Tylzanowski, P.; Wauters, J.; Huylebroeck, D.; Ponec, M.; Merregaert, J. Differentiation-Dependent Alternative Splicing and Expression of the Extracellular Matrix Protein 1 Gene in Human Keratinocytes. *J. Investig. Dermatol.* **2000**, *114*, 718–724. [CrossRef] [PubMed]
64. Sercu, S.; Zhang, M.; Oyama, N.; Hansen, U.; Ghalbzouri, A.E.L.; Jun, G.; Geentjens, K.; Zhang, L.; Merregaert, J.H. Interaction of Extracellular Matrix Protein 1 with Extracellular Matrix Components: ECM1 Is a Basement Membrane Protein of the Skin. *J. Investig. Dermatol.* **2008**, *128*, 1397–1408. [CrossRef] [PubMed]
65. Kong, L.; Tian, Q.; Guo, F.; Mucignat, M.T.; Perris, R.; Sercu, S.; Merregaert, J.; Di Cesare, P.E.; Liu, C.-J. Interaction between Cartilage Oligomeric Matrix Protein and Extracellular Matrix Protein 1 Mediates Endochondral Bone Growth. *Matrix Biol.* **2010**, *29*, 276–286. [CrossRef]
66. Merregaert, J.; Van Langen, J.; Hansen, U.; Ponsaerts, P.; El Ghalbzouri, A.; Steenackers, E.; Van Ostade, X.; Sercu, S. Phospholipid Scramblase 1 Is Secreted by a Lipid Raft-Dependent Pathway and Interacts with the Extracellular Matrix Protein 1 in the Dermal Epidermal Junction Zone of Human Skin. *J. Biol. Chem.* **2010**, *285*, 37823–37837. [CrossRef]
67. Sercu, S.; Lambeir, A.M.; Steenackers, E.; El Ghalbzouri, A.; Geentjens, K.; Sasaki, T.; Oyama, N.; Merregaert, J. ECM1 Interacts with Fibulin-3 and the Beta 3 Chain of Laminin 332 through Its Serum Albumin Subdomain-like 2 Domain. *Matrix Biol.* **2009**, *28*, 160–169. [CrossRef]
68. Fujimoto, N.; Terlizzi, J.; Brittingham, R.; Fertala, A.; McGrath, J.A.; Uitto, J. Extracellular Matrix Protein 1 Interacts with the Domain III of Fibulin-1C and 1D Variants through Its Central Tandem Repeat 2. *Biochem. Biophys. Res. Commun.* **2005**, *333*, 1327–1333. [CrossRef]
69. Utsunomiya, N.; Utsunomiya, A.; Chino, T.; Hasegawa, M.; Oyama, N. Gene Silencing of Extracellular Matrix Protein 1 (ECM1) Results in Phenotypic Alterations of Dermal Fibroblasts Reminiscent of Clinical Features of Lichen Sclerosus. *J. Dermatol. Sci.* **2020**, *100*, 99–109. [CrossRef]

70. Han, Z.; Ni, J.; Smits, P.; Underhill, C.B.; Xie, B.; Chen, Y.; Liu, N.; Tylzanowski, P.; Parmelee, D.; Feng, P.; et al. Extracellular Matrix Protein 1 (ECM1) Has Angiogenic Properties and Is Expressed by Breast Tumor Cells. *FASEB J.* **2001**, *15*, 988–994. [CrossRef]
71. Deckers, M.M.L.; Smits, P.; Karperien, M.; Ni, J.; Tylzanowski, P.; Feng, P.; Parmelee, D.; Zhang, J.; Bouffard, E.; Gentz, R.; et al. Recombinant Human Extracellular Matrix Protein 1 Inhibits Alkaline Phosphatase Activity and Mineralization of Mouse Embryonic Metatarsals in Vitro. *Bone* **2001**, *28*, 14–20. [CrossRef] [PubMed]
72. Sercu, S.; Zhang, L.; Merregaert, J. The Extracellular Matrix Protein 1: Its Molecular Interaction and Implication in Tumor Progression. *Cancer Investig.* **2008**, *26*, 375–384. [CrossRef] [PubMed]
73. Sherman, V.; McPherson, T.; Baldo, M.; Salim, A.; Gao, X.; Wojnarowska, F. The High Rate of Familial Lichen Sclerosus Suggests a Genetic Contribution: An Observational Cohort Study. *J. Eur. Acad. Dermatol. Venereol.* **2010**, *24*, 1031–1034. [CrossRef] [PubMed]
74. Goolamali, S.K.; Shuster, S.; Barnes, E.W.; Irvine, W.J. Organ-Specific Antibodies in Patients with Lichen Sclerosus. *Br. Med. J.* **1974**, *4*, 78–79. [CrossRef] [PubMed]
75. Irvine, H. Idiopathic Atrophy of the Skin. *JAMA* **1913**, *61*, 396–400. [CrossRef]
76. Chan, I. The Role of Extracellular Matrix Protein 1 in Human Skin. *Clin. Exp. Dermatol.* **2004**, *29*, 52–56. [CrossRef]
77. Bushkell, L.L.; Friedrich, E.G.; Jordon, R.E. An Appraisal of Routine Direct Immunofluorescence in Vulvar Disorders. *Acta Derm. Venereol.* **1981**, *61*, 157–161.
78. Chan, I.; Liu, L.; Hamada, T.; Sethuraman, G.; Mcgrath, J.A. The Molecular Basis of Lipoid Proteinosis: Mutations in Extracellular Matrix Protein 1. *Exp. Dermatol.* **2007**, *16*, 881–890. [CrossRef]
79. Kirby, L.; Gran, S.; Kreuser-Genis, I.; Owen, C.; Simpson, R. Is Urinary Incontinence Associated with Lichen Sclerosus in Females? A Systematic Review and Meta-Analysis. *Ski. Health Dis.* **2021**, *1*, e13. [CrossRef]
80. Sercu, S.; Liekens, J.; Umans, L.; Van De Putte, T.; Beek, L.; Huyleboreck, D.; Zwijsen, A.; Merregaert, J. The Extracellular Matrix 1 Gene Is Essential for Early Mouse Development. *FEBS J.* **2005**, *272*, 571.
81. Liu, Z.; Kim, J.H.; Falo, L.D.; You, Z. Tumor Regulatory T Cells Potently Abrogate Antitumor Immunity. *J. Immunol.* **2009**, *182*, 6160–6167. [CrossRef]
82. Maul, J.; Loddenkemper, C.; Mundt, P.; Berg, E.; Giese, T.; Stallmach, A.; Zeitz, M.; Duchmann, R. Peripheral and Intestinal Regulatory CD4+CD25high T Cells in Inflammatory Bowel Disease. *Gastroenterology* **2005**, *128*, 1868–1878. [CrossRef] [PubMed]
83. Marazuela, M.; García-López, M.A.; Figueroa-Vega, N.; De La Fuente, H.; Alvarado-Sánchez, B.; Monsiváis-Urenda, A.; Sánchez-Madrid, F.; Gonzalez-Amaro, R. Regulatory T Cells in Human Autoimmune Thyroid Disease. *J. Clin. Endocrinol. Metab.* **2006**, *91*, 3639–3646. [CrossRef] [PubMed]
84. Vocanson, M.; Hennino, A.; Cluzel-Tailhardat, M.; Saint-Mezard, P.; Benetiere, J.; Chavagnac, C.; Berard, F.; Kaiserlian, D.; Nicolas, J.F. CD8+ T Cells Are Effector Cells of Contact Dermatitis to Common Skin Allergens in Mice. *J. Investig. Dermatol.* **2006**, *126*, 815–820. [CrossRef] [PubMed]
85. Shapira, E.; Brodsky, B.; Proscura, E.; Nyska, A.; Erlanger-Rosengarten, A.; Wormser, U. Amelioration of Experimental Autoimmune Encephalitis by Novel Peptides: Involvement of T Regulatory Cells. *J. Autoimmun.* **2010**, *35*, 98–106. [CrossRef] [PubMed]
86. Zhang, Y.; Bandala-Sanchez, E.; Harrison, L.C. Revisiting Regulatory T Cells in Type 1 Diabetes. *Curr. Opin. Endocrinol. Diabetes. Obes.* **2012**, *19*, 271–278. [CrossRef] [PubMed]
87. Fontenot, J.D.; Gavin, M.A.; Rudensky, A.Y. Foxp3 Programs the Development and Function of CD4+CD25+ Regulatory T Cells. *Nat. Immunol.* **2003**, *4*, 986–992. [CrossRef]
88. Prager, M.; Buettner, J.; Buening, C. Genes Involved in the Regulation of Intestinal Permeability and Their Role in Ulcerative Colitis. *J. Dig. Dis.* **2015**, *16*, 713–722. [CrossRef]
89. Adali, G.; Tunali, N.E.; Yorulmaz, E.; Tiryakioğlu, N.O.; Mungan, S.G.; Ulaşoğlu, C.; Enç, F.Y.; Tuncer, I. Extracellular Matrix Protein 1 Gene Rs3737240 Single Nucleotide Polymorphism Is Associated with Ulcerative Colitis in Turkish Patients. *Turk. J. Gastroenterol.* **2017**, *28*, 254–259. [CrossRef]
90. Su, P.; Chen, S.; Zheng, Y.H.; Zhou, H.Y.; Yan, C.H.; Yu, F.; Zhang, Y.G.; He, L.; Zhang, Y.; Wang, Y.; et al. Novel Function of Extracellular Matrix Protein 1 in Suppressing Th17 Cell Development in Experimental Autoimmune Encephalomyelitis. *J. Immunol.* **2016**, *197*, 1054–1064. [CrossRef]
91. Lee, K.M.; Nam, K.; Oh, S.; Lim, J.; Kim, R.K.; Shim, D.; Choi, J.H.; Lee, S.J.; Yu, J.H.; Lee, J.W.; et al. ECM1 Regulates Tumor Metastasis and CSC-like Property through Stabilization of β-Catenin. *Oncogene* **2015**, *34*, 6055–6065. [CrossRef] [PubMed]
92. Wang, L.; Yu, J.; Ni, J.; Xu, X.-M.; Wang, J.; Ning, H.; Pei, X.-F.; Chen, J.; Yang, S.; Underhill, C.B.; et al. Extracellular Matrix Protein 1 (ECM1) Is over-Expressed in Malignant Epithelial Tumors. *Cancer Lett.* **2003**, *200*, 57–67. [CrossRef] [PubMed]

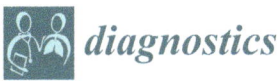

Review

Diagnosis of Early Mycosis Fungoides

Tomomitsu Miyagaki

Department of Dermatology, St. Marianna University School of Medicine, 2-16-1 Sugao, Miyamae-ku, Kawasaki 216-8511, Kanagawa, Japan; asahikari1979@gmail.com; Tel.: +81-44-977-8111; Fax: +81-44-977-3540

Abstract: Mycosis fungoides (MF), the most common type of cutaneous T-cell lymphomas, generally has a favorable clinical course. Early MF typically presents erythematous patches and/or plaques and lasts for many years without affecting the life expectancy. Only limited cases progress to develop skin tumors, with subsequent lymph nodes and rarely visceral organ involvement. One of the clinical problems in early MF is the difficulty in differentiating the disease from benign inflammatory disorders (BIDs), such as atopic dermatitis, chronic eczema, and psoriasis. In some MF cases, clinical and pathological findings are similar to those of BIDs. However, the accurate diagnosis of early MF is quite important, as inappropriate treatment including immunosuppressants can cause unfavorable or even fatal outcomes. This article focuses on general methods and novel tools for diagnosis of early MF.

Keywords: mycosis fungoides; early stage; diagnostic algorithm; T-cell receptor rearrangement; tumor-specific marker; microRNA

1. Introduction

Mycosis fungoides (MF) is the most common type of cutaneous T-cell lymphomas (CTCLs), a heterogenous group of non-Hodgkin lymphoma of T-cell origin that is defined to primarily present in the skin, representing almost 50% of all CTCL cases [1,2]. MF is characterized by malignant proliferation of $CD4^+$ T cells with epidermotropism in the skin and generally has a prolonged clinical course. In early stages, the disease typically presents in the form of erythematous patches and/or plaques and this stage can last for many years without clinical progression and affecting the life expectancy of patients [1,3–6]. A part, but not all, of such patients progress to develop skin tumors, with subsequent lymph node and rarely visceral organ involvement and they are regarded as having advanced-stage disease [1,3–6]. Guidelines describing the diagnosis of MF are created by various professional societies [2,7–9], and the methods for diagnosis are mostly consistent in those guidelines. Generally, the diagnosis of MF is made comprehensively based on clinical presentation, clinical course, pathological and immunohistochemical analysis, and occasionally molecular biological analysis. Nevertheless, the diagnosis of MF, especially early MF, is still challenging. It is sometimes hard to differentiate early MF from benign inflammatory disorders (BIDs), such as atopic dermatitis (AD), chronic eczema, and psoriasis [10–12], because in some MF cases, clinical and pathological findings are similar to those of BIDs. In addition, the difficulty in differential diagnosis can also be caused by the lack of tumor cell-specific markers and not enough sensitivity and specificity of genetic tests detecting clonality of tumor cells. The accurate diagnosis of early MF is quite important in selecting therapeutic strategy. There have been many MF cases that follow an unfavorable or even fatal outcome due to inappropriate treatment including immunosuppressants and dupilumab based on the misdiagnosis as BIDs [10,11,13]. Here, I summarize the general features, algorithm for diagnosis, and novel suggested diagnostic tools of early MF.

Citation: Miyagaki, T. Diagnosis of Early Mycosis Fungoides. *Diagnostics* 2021, 11, 1721. https://doi.org/10.3390/diagnostics11091721

Academic Editor: Yasuhiro Sakai

Received: 27 July 2021
Accepted: 18 September 2021
Published: 19 September 2021

Publisher's Note: MDPI stays neutral with regard to jurisdictional claims in published maps and institutional affiliations.

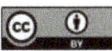

Copyright: © 2021 by the author. Licensee MDPI, Basel, Switzerland. This article is an open access article distributed under the terms and conditions of the Creative Commons Attribution (CC BY) license (https://creativecommons.org/licenses/by/4.0/).

2. General Features of Early MF for Diagnosis

Clinical presentation is one of significant factors in the diagnosis of early MF, although similar findings can be seen in some BID cases. The presence of a rare MF variant with a single lesion, unilesional MF, is well-known [14], whereas most MF cases show multiple lesions. Early MF typically presents well-demarcated erythematous patches and/or plaques with occasionally poikiloderma and the lesions are characterized by variability in the size, shape, and color (Figure 1A). Initially, MF lesions have predilection to non-sun-exposed areas, such as buttock, flanks, inner thighs, and inner arms. However, in folliculotropic MF, the most common variant of MF, lesions may appear on the face or scalp early in the clinical course [15]. Clinical course can also help the diagnosis of MF and the most important feature is the persistent nature of the disease. MF lesions tend to increase in size and number over time without treatment or even under the treatment with topical corticosteroids. Complete response rates by class I topical steroid were reported to be 63% and 25% in early MF patients with T1 stage (less than 10% of skin involved) and T2 stage (10% or more of skin involved), respectively [16]. Therefore, in many MF patients, topical steroids fail to clear the lesions completely. Moreover, in cases with complete remission, the lesions usually recur when the treatment is stopped or newly develop in the untreated areas.

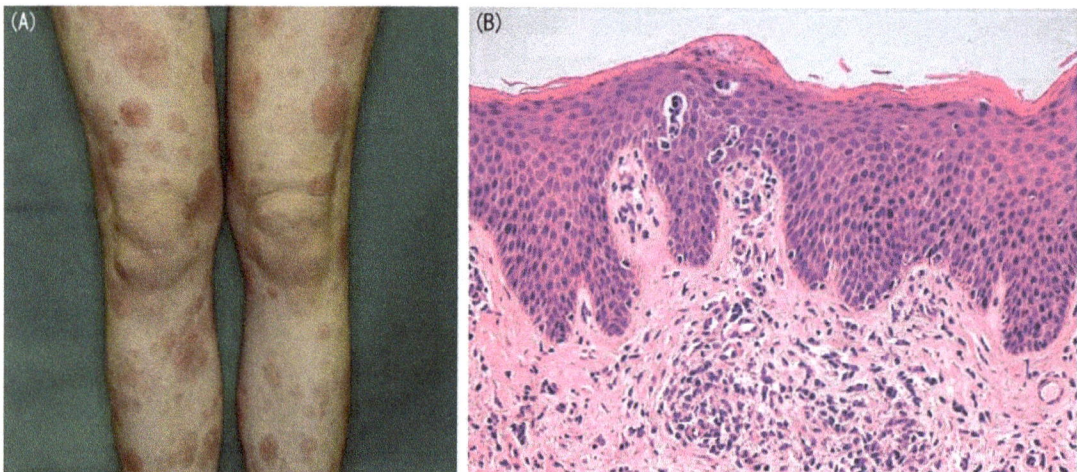

Figure 1. (**A**) Clinical presentation of classical early mycosis funogides (MF). Well-demarcated erythematous patches and plaques with occasionally poikiloderma are shown. (**B**) Pathological findings of early MF (hematoxylin-eosin, original magnification ×100). Epidermotropism of atypical lymphoid cells is shown.

Pathological analysis of the lesional skin is mandatory in the diagnosis of early MF. The pathological features in early MF are as follows: (1) the presence of atypical lymphoid cells with slight larger size than normal lymphocytes and cerebriform, hyperchromatic nuclei; (2) the distribution of lymphocytes singly or in small collections in an epidermis devoid of spongiosis, also called disproportionate epidermotropism; (3) individual haloed atypical lymphocytes within the epidermis; (4) alignment of single atypical lymphocytes along the dermal-epidermal junction; (5) fibrosis of the papillary dermis and (6) a band-like infiltrate in the dermis [12,17]. The presence of atypical lymphoid cells in the epidermis may be the most important pathological feature of early MF (Figure 1B), whereas in some MF cases, cell or nuclear atypia and epidermotropism are not remarkable. Epidermotropism-like findings or mild atypia of infiltrating lymphocytes can also be seen in BIDs. Collectively, differentiating early MF from BIDs based on pathological findings is quite difficult in some cases. Other than above findings, Dalton et al. reported that eosinophil infiltration with more than three cells per tissue section was rarely found in early MF, suggesting that eosinophil infiltration extent in lesional skin may be useful in the differential diagnosis between early MF and BIDs [18]. Anyway, repeated biopsies or multiple biopsies from various lesions may be needed for the accurate diagnosis for early MF. To enhance the pathological characteristics, topical treatment should be discontinued 2 to 4 weeks before skin biopsy.

Immunohistochemical analysis of some surface molecules may also contribute to the diagnosis of MF. The tumor cells of MF are usually positive for CD3 and CD4 and negative for CD8 [1]. The elevation of CD4/CD8 ratio greater than 4–6 may suggest the proliferation of neoplastic CD4$^+$ T cells and the diagnosis of MF (Figure 2A–C) [19]. However, it should be taken into consideration that Langerhans cells and histiocytes are also positive for CD4. The loss of pan T-cell markers, such as CD2, CD5, and CD7, in CD4$^+$ T cells in lesional skin also supports the diagnosis of MF. Among them, the loss of CD2 and CD5 is rarely found in early MF. CD2 or CD5 expression by less than 50% of infiltrating T cells is completely specific but only about 10% sensitive for MF [17]. On the other hand, diminished CD7 expression is more frequently seen in early MF (Figure 2D), whereas it can also be shown in some BID cases [17,20]. Extremely decreased CD7 expression (less than 10% infiltrating lymphocytes) was reported to be 41–80% sensitive and 93–100% specific for the diagnosis of MF [20,21]. As the number of tumor cells in the dermis is limited in early MF, the lack of such T-cell markers may be seen in only epidermis in some cases.

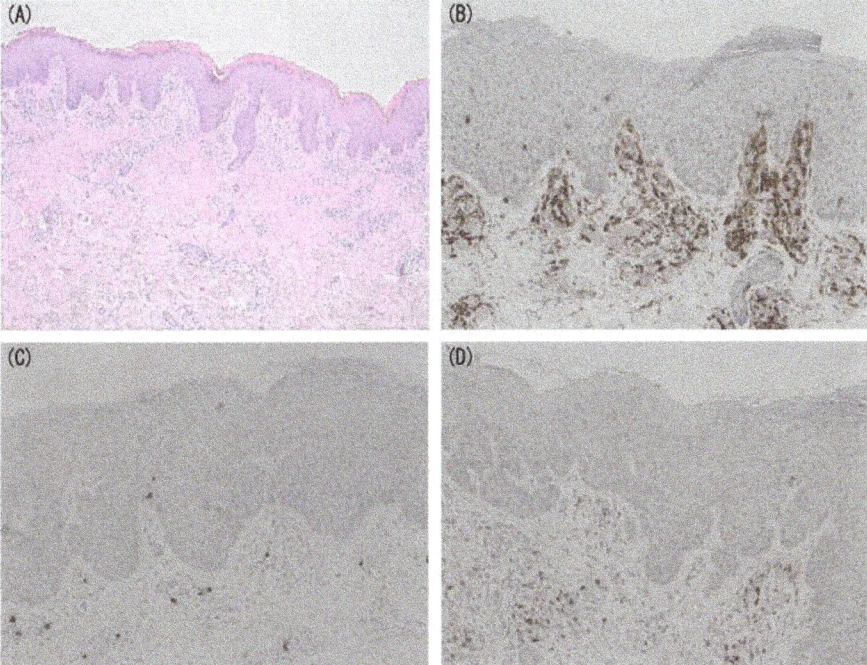

Figure 2. (**A**) Pathological findings of mycosis fungoides (MF) without epidermotropism (hematoxylin-eosin, original magnification ×40). (**B–D**) Immunohistochemical findings of CD4 (**B**), CD8 (**C**), and CD7 (**D**) in the case shown in (**A**) (original magnification ×100). The elevation of CD4/CD8 ratio and loss of CD7 are shown.

The detection of monoclonality of T-cell receptor (TCR) gene by polymerase chain reaction (PCR) or Southern blot analysis is also an important finding in MF and can be a diagnostic clue in the cases that mimic BIDs both clinically and pathologically. PCR analysis is more sensitive than Southern blot analysis [22]. Southern blot analysis could fail to detect monoclonality in many early MF cases [23] and thus, PCR analysis is more frequently used in the diagnosis of early MF. The recent report showed that clonal TCR gene rearrangement was demonstrated in 83% of early MF cases by PCR analysis [24]. However, due to high sensitivity, the presence of monoclonality by PCR can be seen in some BID cases, because not monoclonal but oligoclonal accumulation of T cells occurs in BIDs [25–27]. Detection of identical clones from two different sites was reported to be highly specific for MF [28].

3. Algorithm for Diagnosis of Early Mycosis Fungoides

The diagnosis of early MF is made comprehensively based on combined findings described above. In 2005, the International Society for Cutaneous Lymphoma proposed the algorithm for diagnosis of early classical MF (Table 1) [17]. When a sum total of four or more points is achieved, the diagnosis of MF is made. Compared to immunohistochemical and molecular findings, clinical and pathological findings are regarded as more important. If the patient meets the basic and two or more additional criteria of clinical and pathological findings, the diagnosis of early MF can be made without immunohistochemical and molecular analyses. On the other hand, even if the patient meets the immunohistochemical and molecular criteria, additional clinical and/or pathological findings are needed.

Table 1. Algorithm for diagnosis of early mycosis fungoides by Pimpinelli N et al. [17].

Criteria	Scoring System
Clinical	
Basic	
Persistent and/or progressive patches/thin plaques	2 points for basic criteria and 2 additional criteria
Additional	1 point for basic criteria and 1 additional criterion
(1) Non-sun-exposed location	
(2) Size/shape variation	
(3) Poikiloderma	
Histopathological	
Basic	2 points for basic criteria and 2 additional criteria
Superficial lymphoid infiltrate	
Additional	1 point for basic criteria and 1 additional criterion
(1) Epidermotropism without spongiosis	
(2) Lymphocytic atypia	
Molecular biology	1 point for clonality
(1) Clonal T-cell receptor rearrangement	
Immunopathological (Immunohistochemical)	
(1) <50% CD2+, CD3+, and/or CD5+ T cells	
(2) <10% CD7+ T cells	
(3) Epidermal/dermal discordance of CD2, CD3, CD5, or CD7 (T-cell antigen deficiency confined to the epidermis)	1 point for one or more criteria

The validity of the algorithm was first evaluated by Vandergriff et al. in 2015 [29]. They retrospectively applied the algorithm to 24 early MF patients and 10 patients with skin diseases mimicking MF, such as eczema, drug eruption, and psoriasis. Twenty-one out of 24 early MF patients met or exceeded the four-point threshold, while four points were achieved only in four MF mimics, and none achieved five or six points. The sensitivity and specificity were 87.5% and 60% respectively and the algorithm was found to be a statistically valid for distinguishing MF from its mimics. As the analysis of TCR clonality is unavailable in some facilities and detection rates depend on the methods, some group assessed the validity of the algorithm excluding the molecular biological criteria. Amorim et al. retrospectively reviewed 67 early MF patients clinically, pathologically, and immunohistochemically [30]. They found that 43 of 67 patients (64%) met the basic and two or more additional criteria of clinical and pathological findings and the diagnosis of early MF could be made by those findings. Moreover, when immunohistochemical analysis was added, 61 of 67 patients (91%) met the criteria for the diagnosis of early MF. Similarly, the other group also showed that the sensitivity of the algorithm excluding biological molecular criteria was 93%, while the algorithm including the criteria achieved 100% sensitivity [31]. Collectively, the algorithm is highly sensitive and most early MF cases can be diagnosed accurately, but the specificity has not yet been validated sufficiently. The modification of the algorithm to improve the specificity and sensitivity may be desirable.

4. Novel Diagnostic Markers of Early MF

The difficulty in differential diagnosis between early MF and BIDs may be partially caused by the lack of tumor cell-specific markers. Thymocyte selection-associated high mobility group box factor (TOX), belonging to DNA-binding factors, has the capacity to regulate the double dull to $CD4^+CD8^{low}$ transition during positive selection of T cells [32]. After positive selection, TOX expression disappears from $CD4^+$ T cells before they exit the thymus [32]. Early studies reported TOX to be a tumor cell-specific marker of CTCLs including early MF based on immunohistochemical findings that TOX was expressed in tumor cells of CTCLs but hardly in inflammatory infiltrates of BIDs [33,34]. However, more recent reports found that TOX was also expressed in infiltrating lymphocytes in BIDs, although the frequency was not high [35–37]. Positive TOX expression was identified in 74% of MF cases and in 32% of BID cases and normal skin [37]. Other group reported that TOX was expressed by more than 50% of tumor cells in 83% of MF cases, whereas only 2% of inflammatory dermatoses cases showed TOX expression in more than 50% infiltrating lymphocytes [36]. More recently, the report from Egypt revealed that TOX can be a potential diagnostic marker differentiating hypopigmented MF from early active vitiligo [38]. TOX expression was found in 93% of hypopigmented MF, while only 7% of vitiligo was weakly positive for TOX. Unfortunately, TOX is not considered as a tumor cell-specific marker, but TOX expression can be an adjunctive diagnostic marker, similar to loss of pan T-cell markers, and might be added in the diagnostic algorithm for early MF.

Cell adhesion molecule 1 (CADM1), one of adhesion molecules, is a well-known tumor suppressor gene in a variety of human cancers [39]. On the other hand, interestingly, CADM1 is overexpressed in tumor cells of adult T-cell leukemia/lymphoma (ATLL) and involved in oncogenesis [40]. As CADM1 is not expressed on normal T cells, it can be a diagnostic marker for ATLL [41]. Recently, CADM1 was reported to be a potential diagnostic marker also in MF. Yuki et al. revealed that 55 of 58 MF cases including 34 early cases showed CADM1 expression in more than 5% of infiltrating lymphocytes, while CADM1 expression was found in less than 5% of infiltrating lymphocytes in all 50 BID cases [42]. Although further validation from other groups is required, CADM1 can be a potential diagnostic marker for early MF.

5. Next-Generation High-Throughput Sequencing

The assessment of TCR clonality by PCR relies on length determination of the most abundant PCR product assumed to represent the predominant TCR clone. TCR clonality by PCR can be detected in a small number of BID patients, while some early MF patients who have limited number of malignant cells do not present the clonality as described above. This lack in the test's sensitivity and specificity for the detection of clonality of tumor cells also makes it difficult to differentiate early MF from BIDs. Recently, the application of next-generation high-throughput sequencing (NGS) to the detection of malignant clones in CTCL has been introduced by multiple groups. By sequencing the third complementarity determining regions (CDR3) of TCRβ and TCRγ genes, the total amount and frequencies of the individual T-cell clones can be quantified and the unique nucleotide sequences of each clone's CDR3 regions can be detected [43,44]. Based on the presence of a dominant CDR3 sequence, malignant proliferation of the clone can be identified. Dominant malignant clones were detected in 100% of MF and SS patients without the frequency criteria [45,46].

When the cases with the most frequent two TCR sequences were accounted for, over 5% of the total reads were regarded as clonal and 85% of the MF cases showed clonality [44]. The sensitivity of the NGS method is superior to that of the PCR method. On the other hand, due to its high sensitivity, expanded T cell clones were also detected in BIDs, similar to the PCR method. Although the specificity of the NGS method was also reported to be better than the PCR method [47], Kirsch et al. showed that the top clone frequency with respect to the remaining T cell population without the threshold criteria failed to distinguish CTCL from BIDs [45]. They suggested using the absolute number of clonal T cells in a particular unit of skin evaluated by the frequency of top T cell clone among total nucleated cells as a distinguishing parameter. The parameter was reported to discriminate CTCL clearly from BIDs. However, calculating this parameter is very complicated and more easier criteria may be required. Quite recently, Zimmermann et al. sought to define the optimal criteria for T-cell clonality by NGS using 101 CTCL samples including 47 early MF samples and 43 BID samples [48]. With 5% and 25% top clone frequency thresholds, the specificities for CTCL diagnosis were 95% and 100%, and sensitivity 89% and 50%, respectively. They concluded that 5% top clone frequency threshold may be useful for diagnosis of CTCL including early MF. It will take a long time to generalize NGS in multiple clinical facilities, but NGS can be an important tool in the diagnosis of early MF in the future.

6. MicroRNA for the Diagnosis of Early MF

MicroRNA (miR) profiles have been widely studied in CTCL and dysregulated expression of various miRs have been reported [49]. Given that miR profiles are varied and unique depending on the diseases including BIDs and various cancers, aberrant miR expression in CTCL may contribute to the differential diagnosis from BIDs. The potential differential diagnostic utility of miR profiles between CTCL and BIDs was first reported in 2011 [50]. Ralfkier et al. found that miR-326, miR-663b, and miR-711 were highly induced in CTCL and that miR-203 and miR-205 were repressed by microarrays. The expression levels of these five miRs could distinguish CTCL from BIDs with >90% accuracy. As microarrays can be performed only in limited facilities, they also assessed miR expression by quantitative RT-PCR. Among several miRs with dysregulated expression, they identified miR-155 (increased in CTCL), miR-203 (decreased in CTCL), and miR-205 (decreased in CTCL) as the most discriminative set of miRs. Based on their expression levels, CTCL could be differentiated from BIDs with 91% sensitivity and 97% specificity and all MF cases irrelevant to their stages were accurately diagnosed. Afterwards, the result was validated using the other cohorts [51]. Moreover, Ralfkier et al. focused on the different miR profiles between early MF and AD and found 38 differentially expressed miRs [52]. Similar to the previous report, miR-155 was upregulated and miR-203 and miR-205 were downregulated in early MF compared to AD. Recently, plasma miR-155, miR-203, and miR-205 were also reported to be potential diagnostic tools for the diagnosis of MF and Sézary syndrome (SS) [53]. In 2018, Shen et al. proposed the other miR sets to distinguish CTCL including various subtypes from BIDs [54]. The sets included miR-155 (increased in CTCL), miR-200b (decreased in CTCL), miR-203 (decreased in CTCL), miR-142-3p (increased in CTCL), and miR-130b (increased in CTCL) and the classifier achieved 96% sensitivity and 72% specificity in the diagnosis of CTCL. However, based on their data, in early MF cases, miR-200b expression was not decreased and miR-130b expression was not increased. Thus, there may be a more suitable classifier for the differential diagnosis between early MF and BIDs. Collectively, miR analysis may help the diagnosis of early MF and can be widely used in the future, although quantitative RT-PCR cannot be performed in daily clinical practice in most facilities currently and a more suitable criteria for early MF diagnosis may be needed.

7. Conclusions

In this article, general methods and novel tools for diagnosis of early MF were summarized. The current diagnostic algorithm shows high sensitivity and specificity to some extent. However, there are still many cases difficult to distinguish between early MF and

BIDs in daily clinical practice. In such cases, the detection of some molecules including TOX and CADM1, clonality analysis by NGS, and examination of miR expression might contribute to the diagnosis. There has been gradual increase in transcriptomic studies of MF [55]. Although skin samples of MF used in transcriptomic studies include many non-tumor cells, the exploration of the genome-wide expression of individual genes in skin samples may be useful in elucidating the pathogenesis and improving the diagnosis of MF. Litvinov et al. determined 17 gene sets that can distinguish MF and SS from BIDs [56]. The criteria have not been established yet, while such differentially expressed genes between early MF and BIDs may also help the diagnosis of early MF in the future. Having said that, those analysis cannot be usually conducted in many clinical facilities. Thus, repeated skin biopsy and gene analysis will be needed for the diagnosis of early MF in some cases. The most important point is that inappropriate systemic drugs, such as immunosuppressants and dupilumab, should not be started in cases suspected of CTCL. The establishment of more accurate and easier diagnostic methods and the dissemination of novel technologies are required to improve the management of patients suspected of early MF.

Funding: This work was supported by grants from the Ministry of Education, Culture, Sports, Science and Technology in Japan (20K08683).

Conflicts of Interest: The author declares no conflict of interest.

References

1. Willemze, R.; Jaffe, E.S.; Burg, G.; Cerroni, L.; Berti, E.; Swerdlow, S.H.; Ralfkiaer, E.; Chimenti, S.; Diaz-Perez, J.L.; Duncan, L.M.; et al. WHO-EORTC classification for cutaneous lymphomas. *Blood* **2005**, *105*, 3768–3785. [CrossRef]
2. Fujii, K.; Hamada, T.; Shimauchi, T.; Asai, J.; Fujisawa, Y.; Ihn, H.; Katoh, N. Cutaneous lymphoma in Japan, 2012–2017: A nationwide study. *J. Dermatol. Sci.* **2020**, *97*, 187–193. [CrossRef]
3. Ohtsuka, M.; Hamada, T.; Miyagaki, T.; Shimauchi, T.; Yonekura, K.; Kiyohara, E.; Fujita, H.; Izutsu, K.; Okuma, K.; Kawai, K.; et al. Outlines of the Japanese guidelines for the management of primary cutaneous lymphomas. *J. Dermatol.* **2021**, *48*, e49–e71. [CrossRef]
4. Willemze, R.; Cerroni, L.; Kempf, W.; Berti, E.; Facchetti, F.; Swerdlow, S.H.; Jaffe, E.S. The 2018 update of the WHO-EORTC classification for primary cutaneous lymphomas. *Blood* **2019**, *133*, 1703–1714. [CrossRef] [PubMed]
5. Agar, N.S.; Wedgeworth, E.; Crichton, S.; Mitchell, T.; Cox, M.; Ferreira, S.; Robson, A.; Calonje, E.; Stefanato, C.M.; Wain, E.M.; et al. Survival Outcomes and Prognostic Factors in Mycosis Fungoides/Sézary Syndrome: Validation of the Revised International Society for Cutaneous Lymphomas/European Organisation for Research and Treatment of Cancer Staging Proposal. *J. Clin. Oncol.* **2010**, *28*, 4730–4739. [CrossRef] [PubMed]
6. Quaglino, P.; Pimpinelli, N.; Berti, E.; Calzavara-Pinton, P.; Alfonso Lombardo, G.; Rupoli, S.; Alaibac, M.; Bottoni, U.; Carbone, A.; Fava, P.; et al. Time course, clinical pathways, and long-term hazards risk trends of disease progression in patients with classic mycosis fungoides: A multicenter, retrospective follow-up study from the Italian Group of Cutaneous Lymphomas. *Cancer* **2012**, *118*, 5830–5839. [CrossRef] [PubMed]
7. Gilson, D.; Whittaker, S.; Child, F.; Scarisbrick, J.; Illidge, T.; Parry, E.; Mustapa, M.M.; Exton, L.; Kanfer, E.; Rezvani, K.; et al. British Association of Dermatologists and U.K. Cutaneous Lymphoma Group guidelines for the management of primary cutaneous lymphomas. *Br. J. Dermatol.* **2019**, *180*, 496–526. [CrossRef]
8. Willemze, R.; Hodak, E.; Zinzani, P.L.; Specht, L.; Ladetto, M. Primary cutaneous lymphomas: ESMO Clinical Practice Guidelines for diagnosis, treatment and follow-up. *Ann. Oncol.* **2013**, *24*, iv149–iv154. [CrossRef]
9. Mehta-Shah, N.; Horwitz, S.M.; Ansell, S.; Ai, W.Z.; Barnes, J.; Barta, S.K.; Clemens, M.W.; Dogan, A.; Fisher, K.; Goodman, A.M.; et al. NCCN Guidelines Insights: Primary Cutaneous Lymphomas, Version 2.2020: Featured Updates to the NCCN Guidelines. *J. Natl. Compr. Cancer Netw.* **2020**, *18*, 522–536. [CrossRef]
10. Zackheim, H.S.; Koo, J.; LeBoit, P.E.; McCalmont, T.H.; Bowman, P.H.; Kashani-Sabet, M.; Jones, C.; Zehnder, J. Psoriasiform mycosis fungoides with fatal outcome after treatment with cyclosporine. *J. Am. Acad. Dermatol.* **2002**, *47*, 155–157. [CrossRef]
11. Sugaya, M. Is blocking IL-4 receptor alpha beneficial for patients with mycosis fungoides or Sézary syndrome? *J. Dermatol.* **2021**, *48*, e225–e226. [CrossRef]
12. Torres-Cabala, C.A. Diagnosis of T-cell lymphoid proliferations of the skin: Putting all the pieces together. *Mod. Pathol.* **2020**, *33*, 83–95. [CrossRef]
13. Guglielmo, A.; Patrizi, A.; Bardazzi, F.; Pileri, A. Erythroderma: Psoriasis or lymphoma? A diagnostic challenge and therapeutic pitfall. *Ital. J. Dermatol. Venereol.* **2021**. [CrossRef]
14. Hodak, E.; Amitay-Laish, I. Mycosis fungoides: A great imitator. *Clin. Dermatol.* **2019**, *37*, 255–267. [CrossRef]
15. Mitteldorf, C.; Stadler, R.; Sander, C.A.; Kempf, W. Folliculotropic mycosis fungoides. *JDDG J. Der Dtsch. Dermatol. Ges.* **2018**, *16*, 543–557. [CrossRef] [PubMed]

16. Zackheim, H.S.; Kashani-Sabet, M.; Amin, S. Topical Corticosteroids for Mycosis Fungoides. *Arch. Dermatol.* **1998**, *134*, 949–954. [CrossRef] [PubMed]
17. Pimpinelli, N.; Olsen, E.A.; Santucci, M.; Vonderheid, E.; Haeffner, A.C.; Stevens, S.; Burg, G.; Cerroni, L.; Dreno, B.; Glusac, E.; et al. Defining early mycosis fungoides. *J. Am. Acad. Dermatol.* **2005**, *53*, 1053–1063. [CrossRef] [PubMed]
18. Dalton, S.R.; Chandler, W.M.; Abuzeid, M.; Hossler, E.W.; Ferringer, T.; Elston, D.M.; LeBoit, P.E. Eosinophils in mycosis fungoides: An uncommon finding in the patch and plaque stages. *Am. J. Dermatopathol.* **2012**, *34*, 586–591. [CrossRef]
19. Nuckols, J.D.; Shea, C.R.; Horenstein, M.G.; Burchette, J.L.; Prieto, V.G. Quantitation of intraepidermal T-cell subsets in formalin-fixed, paraffin-embedded tissue helps in the diagnosis of mycosis fungoides. *J. Cutan. Pathol.* **1999**, *26*, 169–175. [CrossRef]
20. Murphy, M.; Fullen, D.; Carlson, J.A. Low CD7 expression in benign and malignant cutaneous lymphocytic infiltrates: Experience with an antibody reactive with paraffin-embedded tissue. *Am. J. Dermatopathol.* **2002**, *24*, 6–16. [CrossRef]
21. Wood, G.S.; Hong, S.R.; Sasaki, D.T.; Abel, E.A.; Hoppe, R.T.; Warnke, R.A.; Morhenn, V.B. Leu-8/CD7 antigen expression by CD3+ T cells: Comparative analysis of skin and blood in mycosis fungoides/Sézary syndrome relative to normal blood values. *J. Am. Acad. Dermatol.* **1990**, *22*, 602–607. [CrossRef]
22. Curcó, N.; Servitje, O.; Llucià, M.; Bertran, J.; Limón, A.; Carmona, M.; Romagosa, V.; Peyrí, J. Genotypic analysis of cutaneous T-cell lymphoma: A comparative study of Southern blot analysis with polymerase chain reaction amplification of the T-cell receptor-gamma gene. *Br. J. Dermatol.* **1997**, *137*, 673–679. [CrossRef] [PubMed]
23. Wood, G.S. Analysis of clonality in cutaneous T cell lymphoma and associated diseases. *Ann. N. Y. Acad. Sci.* **2001**, *941*, 26–30. [CrossRef] [PubMed]
24. Schachter, O.; Tabibian-Keissar, H.; Debby, A.; Segal, O.; Baum, S.; Barzilai, A. Evaluation of the polymerase chain reaction–based T-cell receptor β clonality test in the diagnosis of early mycosis fungoides. *J. Am. Acad. Dermatol.* **2020**, *83*, 1400–1405. [CrossRef] [PubMed]
25. Holm, N.; Flaig, M.J.; Yazdi, A.S.; Sander, C.A. The value of molecular analysis by PCR in the diagnosis of cutaneous lymphocytic infiltrates. *J. Cutan. Pathol.* **2002**, *29*, 447–452. [CrossRef]
26. Tanaka, A.; Takahama, H.; Kato, T.; Kubota, Y.; Kurokawa, K.; Nishioka, K.; Mizoguchi, M.; Yamamoto, K. Clonotypic Analysis of T Cells Infiltrating the Skin of Patients with Atopic Dermatitis: Evidence for Antigen-Driven Accumulation of T Cells. *Hum. Immunol.* **1996**, *48*, 107–113. [CrossRef]
27. Guitart, J.; Magro, C. Cutaneous T-cell lymphoid dyscrasia: A unifying term for idiopathic chronic dermatoses with persistent T-cell clones. *Arch. Dermatol.* **2007**, *143*, 921–932. [CrossRef]
28. Thurber, S.E.; Zhang, B.; Kim, Y.H.; Schrijver, I.; Zehnder, J.; Kohler, S. T-cell clonality analysis in biopsy specimens from two different skin sites shows high specificity in the diagnosis of patients with suggested mycosis fungoides. *J. Am. Acad. Dermatol.* **2007**, *57*, 782–790. [CrossRef]
29. Vandergriff, T.; Nezafati, K.A.; Susa, J.; Karai, L.; Sanguinetti, A.; Hynan, L.; Ambruzs, J.M.; Oliver, D.H.; Pandya, A.G. Defining early mycosis fungoides: Validation of a diagnostic algorithm proposed by the International Society for Cutaneous Lymphomas. *J. Cutan. Pathol.* **2015**, *42*, 318–328. [CrossRef]
30. Amorim, G.M.; Quintella, D.C.; Niemeyer-Corbellini, J.P.; Ferreira, L.C.; Ramos-E-Silva, M.; Cuzzi, T. Validation of an algorithm based on clinical, histopathological and immunohistochemical data for the diagnosis of early-stage mycosis fungoides. *An. Bras. Dermatol.* **2020**, *95*, 326–331. [CrossRef]
31. Kuraitis, D.; McBurney, E.; Boh, E. Utility of clonal T-cell rearrangement study in the diagnosis of early mycosis fungoides. *J. Am. Acad. Dermatol.* **2021**, *85*, 1040–1042. [CrossRef] [PubMed]
32. He, X.; He, X.; Dave, V.P.; Zhang, Y.; Hua, X.; Nicolas, E.; Xu, W.; Roe, B.A.; Kappes, D.J. The zinc finger transcription factor Th-POK regulates CD4 versus CD8 T-cell lineage commitment. *Nat. Cell Biol.* **2005**, *433*, 826–833. [CrossRef]
33. Zhang, Y.; Wang, Y.; Yu, R.; Huang, Y.; Su, M.; Xiao, C.; Martinka, M.; Dutz, J.P.; Zhang, X.; Zheng, Z.; et al. Molecular markers of early-stage mycosis fungoides. *J. Investig. Dermatol.* **2012**, *132*, 1698–1706. [CrossRef] [PubMed]
34. Morimura, S.; Sugaya, M.; Suga, H.; Miyagaki, T.; Ohmatsu, H.; Fujita, H.; Asano, Y.; Tada, Y.; Kadono, T.; Sato, S. TOX expression in different subtypes of cutaneous lymphoma. *Arch. Dermatol. Res.* **2014**, *306*, 843–849. [CrossRef]
35. Yu, X.; Luo, Y.; Liu, J.; Liu, Y.; Sun, Q. TOX Acts an Oncological Role in Mycosis Fungoides. *PLoS ONE* **2015**, *10*, e0117479. [CrossRef]
36. Schrader, A.M.; Jansen, P.M.; Willemze, R. TOX expression in cutaneous T-cell lymphomas: An adjunctive diagnostic marker that is not tumour-specific and not restricted to the CD4(+) CD8(−) phenotype. *Br. J. Dermatol.* **2016**, *175*, 382–386. [CrossRef] [PubMed]
37. McGirt, L.; Degesys, C.; Johnson, V.; Zic, J.; Zwerner, J.; Eischen, C. TOX expression and role in CTCL. *J. Eur. Acad. Dermatol. Venereol.* **2016**, *30*, 1497–1502. [CrossRef] [PubMed]
38. Ibrahim, M.A.-H.; Mohamed, A.; Soltan, M. Thymocyte selection–associated high-mobility group box as a potential diagnostic marker differentiating hypopigmented mycosis fungoides from early vitiligo: A pilot study. *Indian J. Dermatol. Venereol. Leprol.* **2019**. [CrossRef]
39. Sawada, Y.; Mashima, E.; Saito-Sasaki, N.; Nakamura, M. The Role of Cell Adhesion Molecule 1 (CADM1) in Cutaneous Malignancies. *Int. J. Mol. Sci.* **2020**, *21*, 9732. [CrossRef]

40. Sasaki, H.; Nishikata, I.; Shiraga, T.; Akamatsu, E.; Fukami, T.; Hidaka, T.; Kubuki, Y.; Okayama, A.; Hamada, K.; Okabe, H.; et al. Overexpression of a cell adhesion molecule, TSLC1, as a possible molecular marker for acute-type adult T-cell leukemia. *Blood* **2004**, *105*, 1204–1213. [CrossRef]
41. Nakahata, S.; Morishita, K. CADM1/TSLC1 is a novel cell surface marker for adult T-cell leukemia/lymphoma. *J. Clin. Exp. Hematop.* **2012**, *52*, 17–22. [CrossRef]
42. Yuki, A.; Shinkuma, S.; Hayashi, R.; Fujikawa, H.; Kato, T.; Homma, E.; Hamade, Y.; Onodera, O.; Matsuoka, M.; Shimizu, H.; et al. CADM1 is a diagnostic marker in early-stage mycosis fungoides: Multicenter study of 58 cases. *J. Am. Acad. Dermatol.* **2018**, *79*, 1039–1046. [CrossRef]
43. Weng, W.-K.; Armstrong, R.; Arai, S.; Desmarais, C.; Hoppe, R.; Kim, Y.H. Minimal Residual Disease Monitoring with High-Throughput Sequencing of T Cell Receptors in Cutaneous T Cell Lymphoma. *Sci. Transl. Med.* **2013**, *5*, 214ra171. [CrossRef] [PubMed]
44. Sufficool, K.E.; Lockwood, C.M.; Abel, H.J.; Hagemann, I.S.; Schumacher, J.A.; Kelley, T.W.; Duncavage, E.J. T-cell clonality assessment by next-generation sequencing improves detection sensitivity in mycosis fungoides. *J. Am. Acad. Dermatol.* **2015**, *73*, 228–236. [CrossRef] [PubMed]
45. Kirsch, I.R.; Watanabe, R.; O'Malley, J.T.; Williamson, D.W.; Scott, L.-L.; Elco, C.P.; Teague, J.E.; Gehad, A.; Lowry, E.L.; LeBoeuf, N.R.; et al. TCR sequencing facilitates diagnosis and identifies mature T cells as the cell of origin in CTCL. *Sci. Transl. Med.* **2015**, *7*, 308ra158. [CrossRef] [PubMed]
46. De Masson, A.; O'Malley, J.T.; Elco, C.P.; Garcia, S.S.; DiVito, S.J.; Lowry, E.L.; Tawa, M.; Fisher, D.C.; Devlin, P.M.; Teague, J.E.; et al. High-throughput sequencing of the T cell receptor β gene identifies aggressive early-stage mycosis fungoides. *Sci. Transl. Med.* **2018**, *10*, eaar5894. [CrossRef] [PubMed]
47. Rea, B.; Haun, P.; Emerson, R.; Vignali, M.; Farooqi, M.; Samimi, S.; Elenitsas, R.; Kirsch, I.; Bagg, A. Role of high-throughput sequencing in the diagnosis of cutaneous T-cell lymphoma. *J. Clin. Pathol.* **2018**, *71*, 814–820. [CrossRef] [PubMed]
48. Zimmermann, C.; Boisson, M.; Ram-Wolff, C.; Sadoux, A.; Louveau, B.; Vignon-Pennamen, M.; Rivet, J.; Cayuela, J.; Dobos, G.; Moins-Teisserenc, H.; et al. Diagnostic performance of high-throughput sequencing of the T-cell receptor beta gene for the diagnosis of cutaneous T-cell lymphoma. *Br. J. Dermatol.* **2021**, *185*, 679–680. [CrossRef]
49. Gluud, M.; Willerslev-Olsen, A.; Gjerdrum, L.M.R.; Lindahl, L.M.; Buus, T.B.; Andersen, M.H.; Bonefeld, C.M.; Krejsgaard, T.; Litvinov, I.V.; Iversen, L.; et al. MicroRNAs in the Pathogenesis, Diagnosis, Prognosis and Targeted Treatment of Cutaneous T-Cell Lymphomas. *Cancers* **2020**, *12*, 1229. [CrossRef]
50. Ralfkiaer, U.; Hagedorn, P.H.; Bangsgaard, N.; Løvendorf, M.; Ahler, C.B.; Svensson, L.; Kopp, K.L.; Vennegaard, M.T.; Lauenborg, B.; Zibert, J.R.; et al. Diagnostic microRNA profiling in cutaneous T-cell lymphoma (CTCL). *Blood* **2011**, *118*, 5891–5900. [CrossRef]
51. Marstrand, T.; Ahler, C.B.; Ralfkiaer, U.; Clemmensen, A.; Kopp, K.L.; Sibbesen, N.A.; Krejsgaard, T.; Litman, T.; Wasik, M.A.; Bonefeld, C.M.; et al. Validation of a diagnostic microRNA classifier in cutaneous T-cell lymphomas. *Leuk. Lymphoma* **2013**, *55*, 957–958. [CrossRef]
52. Ralfkiaer, U.; Lindahl, L.M.; Lindal, L.; Litman, T.; Gjerdrum, L.M.R.; Ahler, C.B.; Gniadecki, R.; Marstrand, T.; Fredholm, S.; Iversen, L.; et al. MicroRNA expression in early mycosis fungoides is distinctly different from atopic dermatitis and advanced cutaneous T-cell lymphoma. *Anticancer Res.* **2014**, *34*, 7207–7217. [PubMed]
53. Dusílková, N.; Bašová, P.; Polívka, J.; Kodet, O.; Kulvait, V.; Pešta, M.; Trněný, M.; Stopka, T. Plasma miR-155, miR-203, and miR-205 are Biomarkers for Monitoring of Primary Cutaneous T-Cell Lymphomas. *Int. J. Mol. Sci.* **2017**, *18*, 2136. [CrossRef] [PubMed]
54. Shen, X.; Wang, B.; Li, K.; Wang, L.; Zhao, X.; Xue, F.; Shi, R.; Zheng, J. MicroRNA Signatures in Diagnosis and Prognosis of Cutaneous T-Cell Lymphoma. *J. Investig. Dermatol.* **2018**, *138*, 2024–2032. [CrossRef] [PubMed]
55. Motamedi, M.; Xiao, M.; Iyer, A.; Gniadecki, R. Patterns of Gene Expression in Cutaneous T-Cell Lymphoma: Systematic Review of Transcriptomic Studies in Mycosis Fungoides. *Cells* **2021**, *10*, 1409. [CrossRef]
56. Litvinov, I.; Netchiporouk, E.; Cordeiro, B.; Doré, M.-A.; Moreau, L.; Pehr, K.; Gilbert, M.; Zhou, Y.; Sasseville, D.; Kupper, T.S. The Use of Transcriptional Profiling to Improve Personalized Diagnosis and Management of Cutaneous T-cell Lymphoma (CTCL). *Clin. Cancer Res.* **2015**, *21*, 2820–2829. [CrossRef]

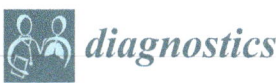

Review

The Pathology of Type 2 Inflammation-Associated Itch in Atopic Dermatitis

Catharina Sagita Moniaga [1], Mitsutoshi Tominaga [1,2,*] and Kenji Takamori [1,2,3]

[1] Juntendo Itch Research Center (JIRC), Institute for Environmental and Gender-Specific Medicine, Graduate School of Medicine, Juntendo University, 2-1-1 Tomioka, Urayasu 279-0021, Japan; m-catharina@juntendo.ac.jp (C.S.M.); ktakamor@juntendo.ac.jp (K.T.)
[2] Anti-Aging Skin Research Laboratory, Graduate School of Medicine, Juntendo University, 2-1-1 Tomioka, Urayasu 279-0021, Japan
[3] Department of Dermatology, Juntendo University Urayasu Hospital, 2-1-1 Tomioka, Urayasu 279-0021, Japan
* Correspondence: tominaga@juntendo.ac.jp; Tel./Fax: +81-47-353-3171

Abstract: Accumulated evidence on type 2 inflammation-associated itch in atopic dermatitis has recently been reported. Crosstalk between the immune and nervous systems (neuroimmune interactions) is prominent in atopic dermatitis research, particularly regarding itch and inflammation. A comprehensive understanding of bidirectional neuroimmune interactions will provide insights into the pathogenesis of itch and its treatment. There is currently no agreed cure for itch in atopic dermatitis; however, increasing numbers of novel and targeted biologic agents have potential for its management and are in the advanced stages of clinical trials. In this review, we summarize and discuss advances in our understanding of type 2 inflammation-associated itch and implications for its management and treatment in patients with atopic dermatitis.

Keywords: atopic dermatitis; biologic agents; neuroimmune interactions; type 2 inflammation

1. Introduction

Atopic dermatitis (AD) is a common chronic inflammatory skin disorder with a complex pathophysiology and clinical heterogeneity in the age of its onset, morphology, and the distribution and severity of lesions [1,2]. The prevalence of AD is approximately 4% in adults and 10% in children, with 50% developing persistent skin disease as adults [3]. The pathophysiology of AD involves complex interactions between epidermal barrier disruption, skin microbiome dysbiosis, and altered type 2 immune responses [2,4].

One of the most common symptoms in dermatology clinics is itch, which is generally intractable despite the administration of medication [5]. Hawro et al. reported itch in 90% of patients with chronic skin diseases, and showed that itch intensity was associated with the disruption of sleep quality, work productivity, and mental health [6]. Several itch-related mediators and receptors are differently expressed in pruritic skin, suggesting an "itchscriptome" for each disease. As an example, AD and psoriasis with itch showed elevated gene transcript levels of interleukin (IL)-17A, IL-23A, and IL-31. However, the gene expression of transient receptor potential (TRP) vanilloid 2, TRP ankyrin 1, protease-activated receptor (PAR) 2, PAR 4, and IL-10 was up-regulated in pruritic AD skin only, while that of TRP melastatin 8, TRP vanilloid 3, phospholipase C, and IL-36a/g in psoriatic skin only. Specific "itchscriptomes" may provide a more detailed understanding of the molecular mechanisms underlying itch and its treatment targets [7].

Despite its heterogeneity, AD is generally managed by a "one-size-fits-all" therapeutic approach, rather than precise personalized, endotype, or ethnicity-driven therapeutic strategies [2,8]. A precise medical approach to the management of AD will rely on the discovery and validation of biomarkers that facilitate tailored management, including prevention strategies, and the treatment of patients with severe disease by targeted therapies [3,8]. In

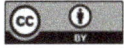

this review, we summarize the current status of the precision treatment of itch in patients with AD.

2. Disease Burden of AD

AD is ubiquitous with high morbidity and healthcare costs [4]. Moreover, it has a negative impact on the quality of life (QoL) of not only patients, but also their families and caregivers [9]. A cross-sectional study identified the most burdensome symptom as itch (54.4%), followed by excessive dryness/scaling (19.6%), and red/inflamed skin (7.2%). Severe itch has been associated with poor mental health [10]. Previous studies also revealed a correlation between suicidal ideation and AD in both girls and boys [11], which was also highly prevalent in patients with chronic pruritus [6]. Moreover, pruritus impairs sleep quality [12]. The pathophysiology of this impairment is complex and may involve inter-relatedness between sleep, the circadian rhythm, immune system, and environment [13].

Besides its psychosocial impact, AD causes major economic burdens [14], with the associated economic burden of severe AD being significant [15]. Luk et al. reported that the median annual cost of chronic pruritus was US$1067 per patient [16]. The economic burden of childhood AD in Australia, South Korea, and Singapore was USD 1000–6000 per patient annually [17]. Economic costs generally include both direct costs (e.g., the costs of medical visits, including tests, procedures, and medications) and indirect costs (e.g., the loss of earnings by patients or caregivers, productivity loss, informal caregiving, and transportation costs) [15]. Previous studies identified the most prominent costs as informal caregiving (46%) for childhood AD in Singapore [18], and productivity loss in AD patients receiving systemic immunosuppressive treatment [14].

3. Type 2 Inflammation and AD

Allergic diseases are mostly mediated by systemic type 2 helper T cell (Th2)–driven inflammation [19], which is characterized by $CD4^+$ T cells and immunoglobulin E (IgE) of B cells. Type 2 immunity involves immune responses by innate and adaptive immune systems. Group 2 lymphoid cells (ILC2), eosinophils, basophils, mast cells, and IL-4- and/or IL-13-activated macrophages play roles in the innate immune system [20]. The activation of Th2 and ILC2 pathways may be at the core of type 2 inflammation, which involves IL-4, IL-5, IL-9, IL-13, and IL-31 as Th2 cytokines and IL-5, IL-9, and IL-13 as the essential type 2 cytokines of ILC2 [21,22].

The inflammatory cascade is triggered in response to allergens, leading to allergic diseases [20]. Although not limited to type 2 immune responses, epithelial-derived cytokines, e.g., thymic stromal lymphopoietin (TSLP), IL-25, and IL-33, play important roles in the stimulation and enhancement of type 2 responses. Upon exposure to allergens, infectious agents, and toxins, epithelial cells as the first line of defense, release alarmins, including TSLP, IL-25, and IL-33 [23,24], and may directly induce type 2 cytokine production by ILC2 [25].

ILC2 are a subgroup of ILCs, a unique subset of lymphocytes without rearranged antigen receptors. They are present in both humans and mice, produce type 2 cytokines, and may promote inflammation and hyperresponsiveness [26–28]. Kim et al. reported resident group ILC2 in healthy human skin that multiplied in AD skin lesions [29]. Moreover, skin-derived ILC2 were shown to express the IL-33 receptor ST2, which was up-regulated during activation, such as in an AD mouse model [30]. The IL-33-ILC2 axis has recently been proposed as the central mediator in human AD [31]. IL-33 induces IL-31 and may trigger pruritus and scratching bouts [31], suggesting a role for ILC2 in the pathogenesis of itch in AD.

Evidence has been obtained that supports the systemic involvement of type 2 inflammation either in acute and chronic skin lesions or in the extrinsic and intrinsic classification of AD [32]. The initiation of acute lesions is accompanied by marked increases in antimicrobial peptide (AMP) levels (S100A7/S100A8/S100A9) and the up-regulation of Th2 and Th22 cytokines. The weaker induction of IL-17 was also observed in acute lesions.

The intensification of the Th2 and Th22 cytokine axes with disease chronicity has been demonstrated, with significant increases being observed in Th1 markers in patients with chronic AD [33].

The circulating immune phenotype was defined in adults and young children with early AD. Czarnowicki et al. showed that a decreased Th1/Th2 ratio characterized the AD phenotype across all age groups, while IL-9, IL-22, and regulatory T cells were detected in patients other than infants. Differences in immune events between pediatric and adult AD patients suggest the need for age-specific, rather than uniform, therapeutic interventions [34].

Recent advances in our understanding of the pathophysiology of AD have implied that systemic type 2 inflammation is one of the underlying disease characteristics of AD, as evidenced by the activation of the Th2 pathway in the non-lesional skin of AD [35] as well as eosinophilia in the blood of AD patients [36]. Furthermore, the serum level of thymus and activation-regulated chemokine (TARC), an IL-4- and IL-13-induced chemokine that functions as a selective chemoattractant for T cells, was enhanced in AD patients compared with normal controls [37,38]. Furthermore, IL-4 has been shown to induce Th2 cell differentiation and isotype switching to IgE production in B cells [39], while IL-13 regulates the proliferation of IgE-producing B cells and disrupts the epithelial tight junction barrier [40,41].

In addition, a bacterial artificial chromosome (BAC) transgenic mouse model that overexpresses the type 2 cytokines, IL-4, IL-5, and IL-13, spontaneously developed AD-like skin lesions due to an exaggerated type 2 response, e.g., high serum IgE levels, excessive immune cell infiltration (including eosinophils and lymphocytes) in the skin, and dermal thickening [42].

Collectively, these findings demonstrate that AD is characterized by the potent activation of Th2 cells and ILC2, with the excessive production of type 2 cytokines, particularly IL-4 and IL-13. While the activation of type 2 immune responses is common in all patients with AD, the variable activation of epithelial-derived cytokines also disseminates this response [20,43].

4. Neuroimmune Interactions Associated with Type 2 Inflammation in Pruritic AD

Interactions between the nervous and immune systems are essential for sensing potential pathogens and activating protective mechanisms in the host [44,45]. Intensive crosstalk has been reported between these systems at multiple barrier surfaces, including the gut [46], lungs [47], and skin [48]. Various responses are induced by interactions involving neurophysiological reflexes, e.g., scratching to expel invading pathogens and noxious environmental stimuli [45,49].

The itch–scratch cycle is a prominent feature of AD, starting from the sensation of itch, which evokes scratching behavior, thereby causing more damage to the defective skin barrier, which allows for the permeation of allergens and irritants, and the activation of alarm signals [50]. Previous studies demonstrated that itch was induced by multifaced pruritogens, including type 2 cytokines [51] (Figure 1).

4.1. IL-4 and IL-13

The presence of IL-4 receptor subunit α (IL-4Rα) on afferent neurons reinforces the potential of a relationship between the type 2 response and neural itch control. Oetjen et al. reported that the dorsal root ganglion (DRG) in mice and humans expressed IL-4Rα and IL-13Rα, and that IL-4 and IL-13 can directly activate sensory neurons. An injection of IL-4 enhanced the responsiveness of sensory neurons to many different pruritogens, such as histamine, chloroquine, and IL-31 via a signaling pathway that was dependent on IL-4Rα-Janus kinase (JAK), which led to the amplification of scratching behavior. Moreover, a treatment with a JAK inhibitor significantly attenuated recalcitrant chronic itch that was resistant to other immunosuppressive therapies [52]. The findings of clinical trials also supported the type 2 neuroimmune interaction by showing the responsiveness of itch to the inhibition of IL-4Rα by dupilumab and downstream JAK inhibition [53,54].

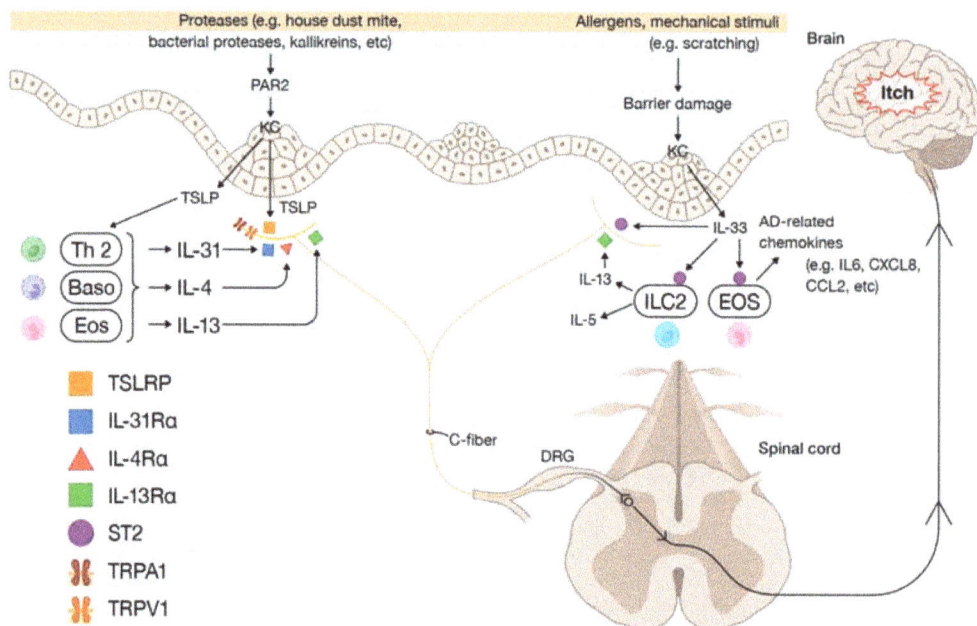

Figure 1. Neuroimmune crosstalk between keratinocytes, primary sensory neurons, and type 2 immune cells in AD skin. Epithelial barrier disruption during exposure to various allergens or triggers, e.g., proteases or scratching, induces keratinocytes to secrete alarmins, such as TSLP and IL-33. TSLP and IL-33 initiate allergic responses by activating ILC2, Th2 cells, and other immune cells, for the production of large amounts of type 2 cytokines, including IL-4, IL-5, IL-13, and IL-31. Alarmins and type 2 cytokines directly activate sensory neurons via their receptors, which signal to the somatosensory cortex in the brain triggering itch or itch sensitization in AD.

Previous studies reported prominent roles for IL-13 in AD, e.g., inflammation, skin barrier disruption, infection, itch, and epidermal thickening [2,55]. Elevated levels of IL-13 mRNA have been detected in both the lesional and non-lesional skin of AD patients [56], in addition to increases in the number of IL-13-producing circulating T cells [57], which were both closely associated with disease severity [55–57]. IL-13 has been suggested to drive inflammation in the periphery [55] and is considered to be pruritogenic on sensory neurons [52]. A low-dose (1 µg) intradermal injection of IL-13 induced scratching behavior in mice, while a combined exposure to IL-13 and IL-4 increased the frequency of scratching bouts, implicating IL-13 as the predominant acute pruritogen on peripheral sensory nerves [58]. On the other hand, Oetjen et al. demonstrated that a high-dose (2.5 µg) intradermal injection of IL-13 did not elicit acute itch in mice, suggesting that differences in IL-13 concentrations affect the scratching behavior in mice [52].

4.2. IL-31

Since the initial identification of the T cell-derived cytokine IL-31 in 2004 [59], AD patients were found to have elevated expression levels of IL-31 in skin-infiltrating cells (e.g., mononuclear cells) and IL-31 receptor subunit α (IL-31Rα) in keratinocytes and nerve fibers in the dermis [60]. IL-31Rα is mainly expressed in small- to medium-sized human DRG neurons, and is exclusively expressed by a subpopulation of TRPV1$^+$/TRPA1$^+$ DRG neurons [61]. In addition, several type 2 immune cells release IL-31 and induce itch through the direct stimulation of IL-31Rα [61].

Prolonged itch may be initiated by the overexpression of IL-31 and promotion of sensory neuronal outgrowth [62] and stimulation [63]. Transgenic IL-31 overexpression and subcutaneously administered IL-31 increased cutaneous nerve fiber density in lesional skin in vivo [62]. These findings suggest that the IL-31 axis plays an important role in the neuroimmune link between IL-31-expressing T cells and IL-31Rα-expressing sensory neurons [60,64], and may partly explain increased epidermal sensory nerve fiber density in AD patients [65–67] in the supreme "skin sensitivity" to minimal stimuli in AD patients.

However, the sequential in vivo imaging of peripheral sensory nerves and blood vessels in a mouse model of AD revealed that neural sprouting preceded vascularization, immune cell infiltration, and vascular permeability, suggesting that an allergic stimulation in chronic eczema requires neural recruitment and activation early in the process of the inflammatory cascade [65]. The development of early neuronal imprinting is followed by the recruitment of IL-31$^+$ T cells to neuronal IL-31Rα$^+$, and neuroimmune interactions may induce increases in epidermal nerve fiber density, inflammation, and itch [68].

Collectively, these findings indicate that IL-31 plays a central role in neuroimmune communication between Th2 cells (the main source of IL-31), sensory nerves, and keratinocytes, which are, in turn, involved in the pathophysiology of AD, including inflammation, epithelial disruption, and itch [68]. Furthermore, the attenuation of itch by nemolizumab, a humanized monoclonal anti-IL-31Rα antibody, supports the key role of IL-31 in AD-related itch [69].

4.3. IL-33

IL-33 is a member of the IL-1 cytokine family and is constitutively expressed in structural and lining cells exposed to the environment, including fibroblasts, the endothelium, keratinocytes, the gastrointestinal tract, and lungs. IL-33 activates allergic inflammation-related immune cells, such as basophils, mast cells, and macrophages as well as eosinophils and ILC2 (through its receptor ST2). Therefore, IL-33 plays a role in the mediation of type 2 immune responses [70–75].

IL-33 is one of the main mediators frequently associated with other cytokines. A stimulation with IL-33 was previously shown to augment the production of IL-5 and IL-13, which are constitutively expressed by fibrocytes [76]. In addition, the stimulation of human mast cells with IL-33 induced the expression of IL-31, which was augmented by neuropeptide substance P or IgE, in the presence or absence of IL-4 [77]. These findings suggest that neuroimmune interconnections between IL-33 and other cytokines may arise under allergic or inflammatory conditions.

Liu et al. detected the expression of ST2 on small- to medium-sized DRG neurons, including neurons that innervate the skin, in an urushiol-induced allergic contact dermatitis (ACD) mouse model. In the inflamed skin of this ACD mouse model, an increased level of IL-33 was responsible for the initiation of itch in sensitized mice. TRPV1 and TRPA1 ion channels mediated the activation of neurons by IL-33. Moreover, the blockade of IL-33/ST2 signaling attenuated the itch sensation in urushiol-challenged mice [78]. Although the comprehensive role of IL-33 in itch in AD remains unclear, these findings suggest that it plays an important role.

4.4. TSLP

Numerous studies suggest that TSLP produced by keratinocytes serves as a master switch that triggers both the initiation and maintenance of AD and the atopic march [79,80]. TSLP activates dendritic cells (DCs) to produce chemokines, which attract Th2 cells to the skin, which then produce proallergic cytokines, e.g., IL-4, IL-5, and IL-13. The up-regulated expression of TSLP has been reported in the skin of AD patients [81]. Wilson et al. showed that TSLP released from epidermal keratinocytes directly acted on cutaneous sensory neurons to initiate itch. They also found that an injection of TSLP bound to its receptor via the TRPA1 cation channel, which was expressed in neurons and promoted scratching behavior in mice. Therefore, the activation of primary afferent neurons and immune cells via the calcium-dependent TSLP release by keratinocytes may initiate skin inflammatory responses and induce itch signaling [82], such as in AD.

5. Treatment for Itch in AD

Despite numerous and extensive studies of the pathophysiology of itch in AD, currently available systemic treatments have limited potency and restricted use due to safety concerns. Newly emerging biologic agents may become superior AD treatments, and their efficacy and safety are now being investigated in systematic reviews and meta-analyses. At the time of writing, dupilumab was the only biologic therapy being extensively investigated, and although other drugs were promising, available data were insufficient. Longer follow-ups and larger population studies are required to obtain reliable biologic safety profiles [83]. Recently developed biologic agents related to type 2 inflammation for the treatment of itch in AD are summarized in Table 1.

5.1. Anti-IL-4 Receptor Antibody

A well-known human monoclonal antibody (mAb), dupilumab, binds to the shared alpha subunit of IL-4 and IL-13 receptors and induces the activation of T cells via the IL-4 and IL-13 pathways. This receptor has been detected on DCs, keratinocytes, and eosinophils [107]. The beneficial effects of dupilumab include the dose-dependent enhancement of the molecular signature in AD skin in vitro, and the down-regulated mRNA expression of the genes involved in activated T cells, DCs, or eosinophils [108]. In clinical trials on dupilumab, clinical symptoms were ameliorated in adult patients with moderate-to-severe AD [53,84]. Two large phase-3 trials (SOLO1 and 2) demonstrated that in comparisons with controls, dupilumab attenuated the signs and symptoms of AD, including improvements in the Numerical Rating Scale (NRS) for itch by at least 4 points, anxiety, depression, and QoL [85,109].

The effects of dupilumab in real-world patient populations were consistent with the findings of clinical trials [110,111]. The adverse events (AEs) of dupilumab are minimal and tolerable, with ocular side effects (particularly conjunctivitis) being the most common [110–112]. Furthermore, current trial data show the minimal need for laboratory monitoring during consumption. An open-label extension study of adults with AD treated weekly with dupilumab for 72 weeks reported continuing efficacy with no additional safety effects; however, longer observations for AEs are advised [86,113]. Dupilumab was the first biologic to be approved by the US Food and Drug Administration (FDA) as the first-line treatment for moderate-to-severe AD in patients aged 6 years and older in the USA and it has also been approved for use in patients aged 12 years and older in the EU [4,107].

The mechanism of action of dupilumab does not only involve the IL-4/IL-13 pathways. Mack et al. performed the high-dimensional immune profiling of patients with AD and found deficiencies in specific subsets of natural killer (NK) cells. NK cell defects were reversed after the blockade of type 2 cytokines in patients with AD. A treatment with dupilumab was associated with the significant recovery of NK cells, as confirmed by clinical flow cytometry, together with improved clinical scores and inflammatory cytokine levels. These findings suggest that NK cells play an immunoregulatory role in type 2 inflammation in AD, possibly via the IL-4 pathway [114].

Table 1. Therapeutic potential of the biologic agent-type 2 inflammation-related regulation of itch in atopic dermatitis.

Mediator	Mechanism	Drug	Status	Clinical Effects	References
IL-4, IL-13	Anti-IL-4Rα	Dupilumab	Approved for moderate-to-severe AD (FDA)	Improvement in pruritus NRS by ≥4 points; IGA, EASI, SCORAD, DLQI	[53,84–86]
IL-13	Anti-IL-13	Lebrikizumab	Phase 2b	Improvement in pruritus NRS by ≥4 points; EASI, IGA, BSA, POEM	[87]
	Anti-IL-13	Tralokinumab	Phase 3	Improvement in pruritus NRS by ≥4 points; IGA, BSA, EASI, SCORAD, POEM	[88,89]
IL-31	Anti-IL-31	BMS-981164	Phase 1	Data not yet released	https://clinicaltrials.gov/ct2/show/NCT01614756 (accessed on 15 September 2021)
	Anti-IL-31Rα	Nemolizumab	Phase 3	Improvement in pruritus VAS by 40–60%	[69,90–92]
JAK	JAK1/JAK2 inhibitor	Baricitinib	Approved for AD in Japan and the EU; undergoing phase 3 trials in other countries	Improvement in pruritus NRS by ≥4 points; IGA, EASI, SCORAD, skin pain, POEM, DLQI	[93,94] https://clinicaltrials.gov/ct2/results?cond=Atopic+Dermatitis&term=baricitinib&cntry=&state=&city=&dist= (accessed on 15 September 2021)
	JAK1, JAK2, JAK3, and a tyrosine kinase 2 inhibitor	Delgocitinib 0.5% (topical)	Approved for AD in Japan; undergoing phase 3 trials in other countries	Improvement in pruritus NRS points; IGA, EASI, BSA	[95,96] https://clinicaltrials.gov/ct2/show/NCT04949841?term=delgocitinib&cond=Atopic+Dermatitis&draw=2&rank=6 (accessed on 15 September 2021)
	JAK1/3 inhibitor	Tofacitinib 2% (topical)	Phase 2a	Improvement in ISI; EASI, PGA, BSA	[54]
	JAK1 inhibitor	Abrocitinib (oral)	Phase 3	Improvement in pruritus NRS by ≥4 points; IGA, EASI	[97,98]
	JAK1 inhibitor	Upadacitinib (oral)	Phase 3	Improvement in pruritus NRS by ≥4 points; IGA, EASI	[99–101]
PDE4	PDE4 inhibitor	Crisaborole 2% (topical)	Approved for mild-to-moderate AD (FDA)	Improvement in the severity pruritus scale & NRS points; IGA, AD signs, DLQI	[102–104]
TSLP	Anti-TSLPR	Tezepelumab	Phase 2a	Improvement in pruritus NRS points & the 5-D itch scale; EASI, IGA, SCORAD (Numerical improvement *)	[105]
#IL-33	Anti-IL-33	Etokimab	Phase 2a proof-of-concept study	Improvement in 5D itch scores; EASI, SCORAD, IGA, DLQI	[106]

* No significant difference; # Proof-of-concept study; NRS = Numerical Rating Scale; FDA = Food and Drug Administration; IGA = Investigator Global Assessment; EASI = Eczema Area and Severity Index; SCORAD= SCORing Atopic Dermatitis; DLQI= Dermatology Life Quality Index; VAS = Visual Analog Score; ISI = Itch Severity Item; BSA = Body Surface Area; POEM = Patient-Oriented Eczema Measure.

5.2. Anti-IL-13

Anti-IL-13 interrupts type 2 immune signaling by directly binding to soluble IL-13 [1,115]. Agents for anti-IL-13 activity include lebrikizumab, which selectively hinders the establishment of the IL-13Rα1/IL-4Rα heterodimer receptor signaling complex [87], and tralokinumab, which specifically binds to IL-13, thereby preventing any interplay with the IL-13 receptor and subsequent downstream IL-13 signaling [88].

A phase 2b placebo-controlled randomized clinical trial (RCT) on patients with moderate-to-severe AD demonstrated that a 16-week treatment with lebrikizumab significantly improved pruritus NRS by ≥ 4 points, clinical scores, and QoL in a dose-dependent manner with good safety [87]. In two parallel 16-week phase 3 (ECZTRA1 and 2) trials on moderate-to-severe AD adults, tralokinumab monotherapy was more effective than a control treatment after 16 weeks (improvement in pruritus NRS by ≥ 4 points, sleep interference, QoL, and clinical signs), and was tolerated well at 52 weeks [89]. An additional phase 3 (ECZTRA3) trial on these patients demonstrated that the combination of tralokinumab and topical corticosteroids (TCS) as needed was effective and achieved similar favorable outcomes and AEs to those in ECZTRA1 and 2 [88].

5.3. Anti-IL-31 Signaling

5.3.1. Anti-IL-31

An agent targeting IL-31 for clinical use (BMS-981164) was examined in a phase I study between 2012 and 2015 [116]; however, the findings obtained were not released until now (https://clinicaltrials.gov/ct2/show/NCT01614756, accessed on 15 September 2021).

5.3.2. Anti-IL-31RA

Nemolizumab is a subcutaneously administered humanized mAb against IL-31Rα, which is involved in itch in AD [116]. Among IL-31 strategies to alleviate pruritus, only nemolizumab has successfully completed late-stage clinical studies. This drug binds to IL-31Rα in cells such as neurons, blocking the binding of IL-31, which inhibits IL-31 signaling [107]. Moreover, nemolizumab has been investigated for the refinement of sleep, daily functioning, and QoL disruptions in patients with AD [90].

In an RCT, double-blind phase I/Ib study, the administration of nemolizumab as a single subcutaneous dose improved the pruritus visual analog score (VAS) score to approximately 50% by week 4, in contrast to 20% by a control treatment. It improved sleep comfort and decreased the need to use hydrocortisone butyrate. Furthermore, there were no serious AEs or discontinuation due to AEs [91].

In a phase 2 trial, nemolizumab significantly improved the pruritus VAS score (43.7%) vs. control (20.9%), which was inadequately controlled by topical treatments in moderate-to-severe AD patients. The incidence and types of AEs in the nemolizumab group were similar to those in the placebo group, except for exacerbations in AD and peripheral edema, which were more prevalent in those receiving nemolizumab [69]. In a phase 2B 24-week RCT study, nemolizumab achieved improvements in pruritus NRS by ≥ 4 points, the NRS-sleep scale, Investigator Global Assessment (IGA) response, EASI score, and SCORAD [92].

In a 16-week double-blind phase 3 trial, moderate-to-severe pruritus AD patients with an inadequate response to topical agents showed greater improvements in the pruritus VAS score with the subcutaneous administration of nemolizumab plus topical agents (42.8%) than with placebo plus topical agents (21.4%). Injection-site reactions were more common in the nemolizumab group than in the placebo group. Longer and larger trials to establish the long-lasting impact and safety of nemolizumab for AD are needed [90].

5.4. JAK Inhibitors

The JAK and signal transducer and activator of transcription (JAK-STAT) pathway is used by cytokines as an intracellular signaling pathway. The phosphorylation, dimerization, and translocation of specific STAT proteins occur in the nucleus after the activation of JAK proteins, and each JAK protein then communicates with numerous cytokine receptors involved in inflammatory diseases [117]. The JAK-STAT pathway has been reported to encompass several tyrosine kinase proteins that interact with the common γ-chain of cytokine receptors and generate cytokine-mediated responses, and is essential for T helper 2 cell differentiation [107,118].

Baricitinib, an oral selective JAK1/JAK2 inhibitor, was the first oral JAK inhibitor to progress to phase 3 clinical trials for AD [119]. In two multicenter, double-blind, phase III monotherapy trials (BREEZE-AD1 and BREEZE-AD2) on moderate-to-severe AD adults, baricitinib attenuated the clinical signs of AD within 16 weeks with the prompt amelioration of itch. AEs were similar between the baricitinib and control groups [93]. In another phase 3 RCT (BREEZE-AD7), moderate-to-severe AD adults with an inadequate response to TCS therapy who received 4 mg of baricitinib plus TCS showed significant improvements in pruritus NRS by ≥4 points, the signs and symptoms of AD, sleep, skin pain, and QoL. The safety profile was similar to that reported in previous studies on baricitinib for AD [94]. Baricitinib has been approved for AD in Japan and the EU, and is being investigated in phase 3 trials in other countries (https://clinicaltrials.gov/ct2/results?cond=Atopic+Dermatitis&term=baricitinib&cntry=&state=&city=&dist=, accessed on 15 September 2021).

Delgocitinib (formerly JTE-052) is a novel, small-molecule JAK inhibitor that is being developed in Japan. It exerts inhibitory effects on JAK1, JAK2, JAK3, and tyrosine kinase 2 [120]. In a phase 3 RCT, double-blind open-label study, 0.5% delgocitinib ointment improved pruritus NRS points (daytime and nighttime) as well as clinical signs and symptoms with good safety for up to 28 weeks in Japanese adults with moderate-to-severe AD [95]. A long-term study of the safety and efficacy of this ointment revealed that it was tolerated well and effectively improved pruritus NRS points up to 52 weeks [96]. Delgocitinib has been approved for the treatment of AD in Japan. It is being investigated in phase 3 trials elsewhere (https://clinicaltrials.gov/ct2/show/NCT04949841?term=delgocitinib&cond=Atopic+Dermatitis&draw=2&rank=6, accessed on 15 September 2021).

Tofacitinib citrate, an oral small-molecule JAK1/3 inhibitor that was initially approved to treat rheumatoid arthritis, acts by blocking Th2 cytokine signaling (IL-4, -5, and -13). Tofacitinib is presently being examined for its potential as a treatment for AD [107]. The efficacy of topical tofacitinib was evaluated in 69 adults with mild-to-moderate AD in a phase 2a, double-blind RCT. Tofacitinib 2% ointment showed significantly higher efficacy than a control treatment for improvements in the Itch Severity Item score and clinical signs, with the early onset of effects and tolerable AEs [54].

Oral selective JAK1 inhibitors, such as abrocitinib and upadacitinib, have been shown to alleviate itch and clinical manifestations in patients with moderate-to-severe AD. Two phase 3 RCTs demonstrated that abrocitinib monotherapy for 12 weeks was effective and tolerated well, e.g., improvements in pruritus NRS by ≥4 points, EASI, and IGA responses [97,98]. Upadacitinib has been approved for moderate-to-severe active rheumatoid arthritis, and may disrupt JAK1 signaling followed by the Th2 cytokines involved, thereby alleviating chronic itch [99,100]. In a phase 2B dose-ranging RCT, 30 mg of upadacitinib was shown to improve pruritus NRS by ≥4 points as well as clinical manifestations [99]. The combination of upadacitinib and TCS in a phase 3 double-blind AD study achieved similar clinical outcomes [100] and was tolerated well [101].

5.5. A Phosphodiesterase 4 (PDE4) Inhibitor

PDE4 inhibitors decrease cyclic adenosine monophosphate concentrations, which reduces the production of proinflammatory cytokines involved in AD. Crisaborole 2% ointment was the first nonsteroidal PDE4 inhibitor used to treat mild-to-moderate AD [1]. Two pivotal phase 3 28-day, double-blind RCTs of crisaborole 2% in mild-to-moderate AD adults showed the earlier achievement and greater proportion of itch improvements (measured by the severity of pruritus scale and IGA scores) [102]. Moreover, a post hoc analysis revealed the significantly earlier achievement of itch management by crisaborole than by a control treatment [103].

Another study reported that crisaborole reversed the biomarker profiles of skin inflammation (e.g., Th2 and Th17/Th22 axes) and improved barrier function (e.g., immune cell infiltration and epidermal hyperplasia/proliferation) with good clinical efficacy (pruritus NRS and clinical signs), thereby supporting the therapeutic benefits of targeting PDE4 in AD patients [104]. Crisaborole 2% ointment was approved by the FDA for the treatment of mild-to-moderate AD in infants aged 3 months and older.

5.6. Anti-TSLP

Tezepelumab (AMG 157) is a human anti-TSLP monoclonal immunoglobulin G2λ that specifically binds to human TSLP and inhibits interactions with its receptor [121]. In a double-blind, placebo-controlled study, a treatment with tezepelumab attenuated allergen-induced bronchoconstriction and indexes of airway inflammation before and after an allergen challenge in mild allergic asthma patients [121]. A phase 2 clinical trial conducted among patients receiving long-acting beta-agonists and medium-to-high doses of inhaled glucocorticoids showed lower rates of clinical asthma exacerbation by tezepelumab than by a placebo. The incidence of AEs was similar among trial groups [122].

A phase 2a study on tezepelumab- or placebo plus TCS-treated moderate-to-severe AD adults reported slight improvements (clinical signs and pruritus) from the control following 12 weeks of treatment, and greater responses at 16 weeks. In tezepelumab vs. placebo groups, pruritus NRS were 33.54 vs. 25.41 ($p = 0.258$), EASI50 responses were 64.7% vs. 48.2% ($p = 0.091$), and SCORAD50 were 41% vs. 29.4% ($p = 0.219$), respectively [105]. Overall, these findings suggest that targeting TSLP is beneficial for the treatment of asthma, but may not be as effective at attenuating dermatitis-related itch.

5.7. Anti-IL-33

A previous study evaluated the efficacy of vaccination against IL-33 in a house dust mite (HDM)-induced airway inflammation mouse model. The inhibition of HDM-induced airway hyperresponsiveness and inflammation and the production of inflammatory cytokines were observed after the vaccination against IL-33 [123]. In a 6-week placebo-controlled phase 2a study, a single dose of etokimab, an anti–IL-33 biologic, was administered to desensitize peanut-allergic adults. The findings obtained revealed the safety of etokimab, and that a single dose of etokimab may desensitize peanut-allergic individuals and attenuate atopy-related AEs [124]. Chen et al. investigated the efficacy of etokimab in a proof-of-concept clinical study among moderate-to-severe AD. A single intravenous dose of 300 mg of etokimab achieved improvements in 5D itch scores, EASI, SCORAD, IGA, and DLQI 29 days after drug administration and was generally tolerated [106]. The inhibition of IL-33 appears to be effective for alleviating allergic disease symptoms, including AD; however, further studies on its efficacy are needed.

6. Conclusions

The pathogenesis of AD encompasses various immune pathways. Recent studies revealed that type 2 immune inflammation is the dominant pathway involved, driven by innate type 2 ILC and Th2 cells as well as their cytokines, such as IL-4 and IL-13. Itch is a sensation associated with AD. Previous studies revealed that neuroimmune communication is a key player in the development of itch in inflammatory skin diseases, such as AD. Therefore, targeting type 2 pathways in the neuroimmune interaction appears to be a reasonable therapeutic strategy for itch in AD. Recently developed biologic agents targeting type 2-associated cytokines have achieved promising outcomes. The mAb anti-IL-4Rα (dupilumab) and topical PDE4 inhibitor (crisaborole) have been approved by the FDA for moderate-to-severe and mild-to-moderate AD, while JAK inhibitors (baricitinib and delgocitinib) have been approved for AD in Japan. Based on the findings of recent clinical trials on the treatment of itch in AD, dupilumab appears to be the best option for moderate-to-severe AD, and crisaborole 2% for mild-to moderate AD. Further studies on other agents will offer novel insights into the underlying pathogeneses and new targeted treatment alternatives for itch in AD.

Funding: This work was funded by the Foundation of Strategic Research Projects in Private Universities (Grant-in-Aid S1311011) and JSPS KAKENHI (Grant Numbers 18K07396 and 20H03568) from the Ministry of Education, Culture, Sports, Science, and Technology, Japan; and a grant from the Lydia O'Leary Memorial Pias Dermatological Foundation (2021).

Conflicts of Interest: The authors declare no conflict of interest.

References

1. Puar, N.; Chovatiya, R.; Paller, A.S. New treatments in atopic dermatitis. *Ann. Allergy Asthma Immunol.* **2021**, *126*, 21–31. [CrossRef] [PubMed]
2. Czarnowicki, T.; He, H.; Krueger, J.G.; Guttman-Yassky, E. Atopic dermatitis endotypes and implications for targeted therapeutics. *J. Allergy Clin. Immunol.* **2019**, *143*, 1–11. [CrossRef] [PubMed]
3. Leung, D.Y.; Guttman-Yassky, E. Assessing the current treatment of atopic dermatitis: Unmet needs. *J. Allergy Clin. Immunol.* **2017**, *139*, S47–S48. [CrossRef] [PubMed]
4. Langan, S.M.; Irvine, A.D.; Weidinger, S. Atopic dermatitis. *Lancet* **2020**, *396*, 345–360. [CrossRef]
5. Wong, L.S.; Wu, T.; Lee, C.H. Inflammatory and Noninflammatory Itch: Implications in Pathophysiology-Directed Treatments. *Int. J. Mol. Sci.* **2017**, *18*, 1485. [CrossRef]
6. Hawro, T.; Przybylowicz, K.; Spindler, M.; Hawro, M.; Stec, M.; Altrichter, S.; Weller, K.; Magerl, M.; Reidel, U.; Alarbeed, E.; et al. The characteristics and impact of pruritus in adult dermatology patients: A prospective, cross-sectional study. *J. Am. Acad. Dermatol.* **2021**, *84*, 691–700. [CrossRef]
7. Nattkemper, L.A.; Tey, H.L.; Valdes-Rodriguez, R.; Lee, H.; Mollanazar, N.K.; Albornoz, C.; Sanders, K.M.; Yosipovitch, G. The Genetics of Chronic Itch: Gene Expression in the Skin of Patients with Atopic Dermatitis and Psoriasis with Severe Itch. *J. Investig. Dermatol.* **2018**, *138*, 1311–1317. [CrossRef]
8. Bieber, T.; D'Erme, A.M.; Akdis, C.A.; Traidl-Hoffmann, C.; Lauener, R.; Schappi, G.; Schmid-Grendelmeier, P. Clinical phenotypes and endophenotypes of atopic dermatitis: Where are we, and where should we go? *J. Allergy Clin. Immunol.* **2017**, *139*, S58–S64. [CrossRef]
9. Drucker, A.M.; Wang, A.R.; Li, W.Q.; Sevetson, E.; Block, J.K.; Qureshi, A.A. The Burden of Atopic Dermatitis: Summary of a Report for the National Eczema Association. *J. Investig. Dermatol.* **2017**, *137*, 26–30. [CrossRef]
10. Silverberg, J.I.; Gelfand, J.M.; Margolis, D.J.; Boguniewicz, M.; Fonacier, L.; Grayson, M.H.; Simpson, E.L.; Ong, P.Y.; Chiesa Fuxench, Z.C. Patient burden and quality of life in atopic dermatitis in US adults: A population-based cross-sectional study. *Ann. Allergy Asthma Immunol.* **2018**, *121*, 340–347. [CrossRef]
11. Halvorsen, J.A.; Lien, L.; Dalgard, F.; Bjertness, E.; Stern, R.S. Suicidal ideation, mental health problems, and social function in adolescents with eczema: A population-based study. *J. Investig. Dermatol.* **2014**, *134*, 1847–1854. [CrossRef]
12. Xerfan, E.M.S.; Tomimori, J.; Andersen, M.L.; Tufik, S.; Facina, A.S. Sleep disturbance and atopic dermatitis: A bidirectional relationship? *Med. Hypotheses* **2020**, *140*, 109637. [CrossRef]
13. Chang, Y.S.; Chiang, B.L. Mechanism of Sleep Disturbance in Children with Atopic Dermatitis and the Role of the Circadian Rhythm and Melatonin. *Int. J. Mol. Sci.* **2016**, *17*, 462. [CrossRef] [PubMed]
14. Ariens, L.F.M.; van Nimwegen, K.J.M.; Shams, M.; de Bruin, D.T.; van der Schaft, J.; van Os-Medendorp, H.; De Bruin-Weller, M. Economic Burden of Adult Patients with Moderate to Severe Atopic Dermatitis Indicated for Systemic Treatment. *Acta Derm.-Venereol.* **2019**, *99*, 762–768. [CrossRef] [PubMed]
15. Tsai, T.F.; Rajagopalan, M.; Chu, C.Y.; Encarnacion, L.; Gerber, R.A.; Santos-Estrella, P.; Llamado, L.J.Q.; Tallman, A.M. Burden of atopic dermatitis in Asia. *J. Dermatol.* **2019**, *46*, 825–834. [CrossRef] [PubMed]
16. Luk, K.M.; Shaw, F.M.; Zhang, C.; Culler, S.D.; Chen, S.C. The Annual Direct and Indirect Health Care Costs for Patients with Chronic Pruritus and their Determining Factors. *J. Investig. Dermatol.* **2020**, *140*, 699–701.e5. [CrossRef]
17. Lee, B.W.; Detzel, P.R. Treatment of childhood atopic dermatitis and economic burden of illness in Asia Pacific countries. *Ann. Nutr. Metab.* **2015**, *66* (Suppl. 1), 18–24. [CrossRef]
18. Olsson, M.; Bajpai, R.; Wee, L.W.Y.; Yew, Y.W.; Koh, M.J.A.; Thng, S.; Car, J.; Jarbrink, K. The cost of childhood atopic dermatitis in a multi-ethnic Asian population: A cost-of-illness study. *Br. J. Dermatol.* **2020**, *182*, 1245–1252. [CrossRef]
19. Matsunaga, K.; Katoh, N.; Fujieda, S.; Izuhara, K.; Oishi, K. Dupilumab: Basic aspects and applications to allergic diseases. *Allergol. Int. Off. J. Jpn. Soc. Allergol.* **2020**, *69*, 187–196. [CrossRef]
20. Gandhi, N.A.; Bennett, B.L.; Graham, N.M.; Pirozzi, G.; Stahl, N.; Yancopoulos, G.D. Targeting key proximal drivers of type 2 inflammation in disease. *Nat. Rev. Drug Discov.* **2016**, *15*, 35–50. [CrossRef]
21. Tojima, I.; Matsumoto, K.; Kikuoka, H.; Hara, S.; Yamamoto, S.; Shimizu, S.; Kouzaki, H.; Shimizu, T. Evidence for the induction of Th2 inflammation by group 2 innate lymphoid cells in response to prostaglandin D2 and cysteinyl leukotrienes in allergic rhinitis. *Allergy* **2019**, *74*, 2417–2426. [CrossRef] [PubMed]

22. Li, S.; Morita, H.; Sokolowska, M.; Tan, G.; Boonpiyathad, T.; Opitz, L.; Orimo, K.; Archer, S.K.; Jansen, K.; Tang, M.L.K.; et al. Gene expression signatures of circulating human type 1, 2, and 3 innate lymphoid cells. *J. Allergy Clin. Immunol.* **2019**, *143*, 2321–2325. [CrossRef] [PubMed]
23. Toki, S.; Goleniewska, K.; Zhang, J.; Zhou, W.; Newcomb, D.C.; Zhou, B.; Kita, H.; Boyd, K.L.; Peebles, R.S., Jr. TSLP and IL-33 reciprocally promote each other's lung protein expression and ILC2 receptor expression to enhance innate type-2 airway inflammation. *Allergy* **2020**, *75*, 1606–1617. [CrossRef] [PubMed]
24. Xiong, Y.; Cui, X.; Li, W.; Lv, J.; Du, L.; Mi, W.; Li, H.; Chen, Z.; Leng, Q.; Zhou, H.; et al. BLT1 signaling in epithelial cells mediates allergic sensitization via promotion of IL-33 production. *Allergy* **2019**, *74*, 495–506. [CrossRef]
25. Ro, M.; Lee, A.J.; Kim, J.H. 5-/12-Lipoxygenase-linked cascade contributes to the IL-33-induced synthesis of IL-13 in mast cells, thus promoting asthma development. *Allergy* **2018**, *73*, 350–360. [CrossRef]
26. Pasha, M.A.; Patel, G.; Hopp, R.; Yang, Q. Role of innate lymphoid cells in allergic diseases. *Allergy Asthma Proc.* **2019**, *40*, 138–145. [CrossRef]
27. von Moltke, J.; O'Leary, C.E.; Barrett, N.A.; Kanaoka, Y.; Austen, K.F.; Locksley, R.M. Leukotrienes provide an NFAT-dependent signal that synergizes with IL-33 to activate ILC2s. *J. Exp. Med.* **2017**, *214*, 27–37. [CrossRef]
28. Neill, D.R.; Wong, S.H.; Bellosi, A.; Flynn, R.J.; Daly, M.; Langford, T.K.; Bucks, C.; Kane, C.M.; Fallon, P.G.; Pannell, R.; et al. Nuocytes represent a new innate effector leukocyte that mediates type-2 immunity. *Nature* **2010**, *464*, 1367–1370. [CrossRef]
29. Kim, B.S.; Siracusa, M.C.; Saenz, S.A.; Noti, M.; Monticelli, L.A.; Sonnenberg, G.F.; Hepworth, M.R.; Van Voorhees, A.S.; Comeau, M.R.; Artis, D. TSLP elicits IL-33-independent innate lymphoid cell responses to promote skin inflammation. *Sci. Transl. Med.* **2013**, *5*, 170ra116. [CrossRef]
30. Salimi, M.; Barlow, J.L.; Saunders, S.P.; Xue, L.; Gutowska-Owsiak, D.; Wang, X.; Huang, L.C.; Johnson, D.; Scanlon, S.T.; McKenzie, A.N.; et al. A role for IL-25 and IL-33-driven type-2 innate lymphoid cells in atopic dermatitis. *J. Exp. Med.* **2013**, *210*, 2939–2950. [CrossRef]
31. Imai, Y. Interleukin-33 in atopic dermatitis. *J. Dermatol. Sci.* **2019**, *96*, 2–7. [CrossRef] [PubMed]
32. Suarez-Farinas, M.; Dhingra, N.; Gittler, J.; Shemer, A.; Cardinale, I.; de Guzman Strong, C.; Krueger, J.G.; Guttman-Yassky, E. Intrinsic atopic dermatitis shows similar TH2 and higher TH17 immune activation compared with extrinsic atopic dermatitis. *J. Allergy Clin. Immunol.* **2013**, *132*, 361–370. [CrossRef] [PubMed]
33. Gittler, J.K.; Shemer, A.; Suarez-Farinas, M.; Fuentes-Duculan, J.; Gulewicz, K.J.; Wang, C.Q.; Mitsui, H.; Cardinale, I.; de Guzman Strong, C.; Krueger, J.G.; et al. Progressive activation of T(H)2/T(H)22 cytokines and selective epidermal proteins characterizes acute and chronic atopic dermatitis. *J. Allergy Clin. Immunol.* **2012**, *130*, 1344–1354. [CrossRef]
34. Czarnowicki, T.; He, H.; Canter, T.; Han, J.; Lefferdink, R.; Erickson, T.; Rangel, S.; Kameyama, N.; Kim, H.J.; Pavel, A.B.; et al. Evolution of pathologic T-cell subsets in patients with atopic dermatitis from infancy to adulthood. *J. Allergy Clin. Immunol.* **2020**, *145*, 215–228. [CrossRef] [PubMed]
35. Suarez-Farinas, M.; Tintle, S.J.; Shemer, A.; Chiricozzi, A.; Nograles, K.; Cardinale, I.; Duan, S.; Bowcock, A.M.; Krueger, J.G.; Guttman-Yassky, E. Nonlesional atopic dermatitis skin is characterized by broad terminal differentiation defects and variable immune abnormalities. *J. Allergy Clin. Immunol.* **2011**, *127*, 954–964.e4. [CrossRef]
36. Pacor, M.L.; Di Lorenzo, G.; Martinelli, N.; Mansueto, P.; Rini, G.B.; Corrocher, R. Comparing tacrolimus ointment and oral cyclosporine in adult patients affected by atopic dermatitis: A randomized study. *Clin. Exp. Allergy J. Br. Soc. Allergy Clin. Immunol.* **2004**, *34*, 639–645. [CrossRef]
37. Hijnen, D.; De Bruin-Weller, M.; Oosting, B.; Lebre, C.; De Jong, E.; Bruijnzeel-Koomen, C.; Knol, E. Serum thymus and activation-regulated chemokine (TARC) and cutaneous T cell-attracting chemokine (CTACK) levels in allergic diseases: TARC and CTACK are disease-specific markers for atopic dermatitis. *J. Allergy Clin. Immunol.* **2004**, *113*, 334–340. [CrossRef] [PubMed]
38. Jahnz-Rozyk, K.; Targowski, T.; Paluchowska, E.; Owczarek, W.; Kucharczyk, A. Serum thymus and activation-regulated chemokine, macrophage-derived chemokine and eotaxin as markers of severity of atopic dermatitis. *Allergy* **2005**, *60*, 685–688. [CrossRef]
39. Meng, Y.; Wang, C.; Zhang, L. Recent developments and highlights in allergic rhinitis. *Allergy* **2019**, *74*, 2320–2328. [CrossRef]
40. Sugita, K.; Altunbulakli, C.; Morita, H.; Sugita, A.; Kubo, T.; Kimura, R.; Goto, H.; Yamamoto, O.; Ruckert, B.; Akdis, M.; et al. Human type 2 innate lymphoid cells disrupt skin keratinocyte tight junction barrier by IL-13. *Allergy* **2019**, *74*, 2534–2537. [CrossRef]
41. Sugita, K.; Steer, C.A.; Martinez-Gonzalez, I.; Altunbulakli, C.; Morita, H.; Castro-Giner, F.; Kubo, T.; Wawrzyniak, P.; Ruckert, B.; Sudo, K.; et al. Type 2 innate lymphoid cells disrupt bronchial epithelial barrier integrity by targeting tight junctions through IL-13 in asthmatic patients. *J. Allergy Clin. Immunol.* **2018**, *141*, 300–310.e11. [CrossRef]
42. Lee, G.R.; Flavell, R.A. Transgenic mice which overproduce Th2 cytokines develop spontaneous atopic dermatitis and asthma. *Int. Immunol.* **2004**, *16*, 1155–1160. [CrossRef] [PubMed]
43. Moyle, M.; Cevikbas, F.; Harden, J.L.; Guttman-Yassky, E. Understanding the immune landscape in atopic dermatitis: The era of biologics and emerging therapeutic approaches. *Exp. Dermatol.* **2019**, *28*, 756–768. [CrossRef] [PubMed]
44. Ordovas-Montanes, J.; Rakoff-Nahoum, S.; Huang, S.; Riol-Blanco, L.; Barreiro, O.; von Andrian, U.H. The Regulation of Immunological Processes by Peripheral Neurons in Homeostasis and Disease. *Trends Immunol.* **2015**, *36*, 578–604. [CrossRef]
45. Veiga-Fernandes, H.; Mucida, D. Neuro-Immune Interactions at Barrier Surfaces. *Cell* **2016**, *165*, 801–811. [CrossRef]
46. Gabanyi, I.; Muller, P.A.; Feighery, L.; Oliveira, T.Y.; Costa-Pinto, F.A.; Mucida, D. Neuro-immune Interactions Drive Tissue Programming in Intestinal Macrophages. *Cell* **2016**, *164*, 378–391. [CrossRef] [PubMed]

47. Talbot, S.; Abdulnour, R.E.; Burkett, P.R.; Lee, S.; Cronin, S.J.; Pascal, M.A.; Laedermann, C.; Foster, S.L.; Tran, J.V.; Lai, N.; et al. Silencing Nociceptor Neurons Reduces Allergic Airway Inflammation. *Neuron* **2015**, *87*, 341–354. [CrossRef] [PubMed]
48. Kashem, S.W.; Riedl, M.S.; Yao, C.; Honda, C.N.; Vulchanova, L.; Kaplan, D.H. Nociceptive Sensory Fibers Drive Interleukin-23 Production from CD301b+ Dermal Dendritic Cells and Drive Protective Cutaneous Immunity. *Immunity* **2015**, *43*, 515–526. [CrossRef] [PubMed]
49. Bautista, D.M.; Wilson, S.R.; Hoon, M.A. Why we scratch an itch: The molecules, cells and circuits of itch. *Nat. Neurosci.* **2014**, *17*, 175–182. [CrossRef] [PubMed]
50. Mack, M.R.; Kim, B.S. The Itch-Scratch Cycle: A Neuroimmune Perspective. *Trends Immunol.* **2018**, *39*, 980–991. [CrossRef] [PubMed]
51. Yang, T.B.; Kim, B.S. Pruritus in allergy and immunology. *J. Allergy Clin. Immunol.* **2019**, *144*, 353–360. [CrossRef]
52. Oetjen, L.K.; Mack, M.R.; Feng, J.; Whelan, T.M.; Niu, H.; Guo, C.J.; Chen, S.; Trier, A.M.; Xu, A.Z.; Tripathi, S.V.; et al. Sensory Neurons Co-opt Classical Immune Signaling Pathways to Mediate Chronic Itch. *Cell* **2017**, *171*, 217–228.e213. [CrossRef]
53. Beck, L.A.; Thaci, D.; Hamilton, J.D.; Graham, N.M.; Bieber, T.; Rocklin, R.; Ming, J.E.; Ren, H.; Kao, R.; Simpson, E.; et al. Dupilumab treatment in adults with moderate-to-severe atopic dermatitis. *N. Engl. J. Med.* **2014**, *371*, 130–139. [CrossRef] [PubMed]
54. Bissonnette, R.; Papp, K.A.; Poulin, Y.; Gooderham, M.; Raman, M.; Mallbris, L.; Wang, C.; Purohit, V.; Mamolo, C.; Papacharalambous, J.; et al. Topical tofacitinib for atopic dermatitis: A phase IIa randomized trial. *Br. J. Dermatol.* **2016**, *175*, 902–911. [CrossRef]
55. Bieber, T. Interleukin-13: Targeting an underestimated cytokine in atopic dermatitis. *Allergy* **2020**, *75*, 54–62. [CrossRef] [PubMed]
56. Tsoi, L.C.; Rodriguez, E.; Degenhardt, F.; Baurecht, H.; Wehkamp, U.; Volks, N.; Szymczak, S.; Swindell, W.R.; Sarkar, M.K.; Raja, K.; et al. Atopic Dermatitis Is an IL-13-Dominant Disease with Greater Molecular Heterogeneity Compared to Psoriasis. *J. Investig. Dermatol.* **2019**, *139*, 1480–1489. [CrossRef]
57. Czarnowicki, T.; Gonzalez, J.; Shemer, A.; Malajian, D.; Xu, H.; Zheng, X.; Khattri, S.; Gilleaudeau, P.; Sullivan-Whalen, M.; Suarez-Farinas, M.; et al. Severe atopic dermatitis is characterized by selective expansion of circulating TH2/TC2 and TH22/TC22, but not TH17/TC17, cells within the skin-homing T-cell population. *J. Allergy Clin. Immunol.* **2015**, *136*, 104–115.e7. [CrossRef]
58. Campion, M.; Smith, L.; Gatault, S.; Metais, C.; Buddenkotte, J.; Steinhoff, M. Interleukin-4 and interleukin-13 evoke scratching behaviour in mice. *Exp. Dermatol.* **2019**, *28*, 1501–1504. [CrossRef] [PubMed]
59. Dillon, S.R.; Sprecher, C.; Hammond, A.; Bilsborough, J.; Rosenfeld-Franklin, M.; Presnell, S.R.; Haugen, H.S.; Maurer, M.; Harder, B.; Johnston, J.; et al. Interleukin 31, a cytokine produced by activated T cells, induces dermatitis in mice. *Nat. Immunol.* **2004**, *5*, 752–760. [CrossRef]
60. Kato, A.; Fujii, E.; Watanabe, T.; Takashima, Y.; Matsushita, H.; Furuhashi, T.; Morita, A. Distribution of IL-31 and its receptor expressing cells in skin of atopic dermatitis. *J. Dermatol. Sci.* **2014**, *74*, 229–235. [CrossRef] [PubMed]
61. Cevikbas, F.; Wang, X.; Akiyama, T.; Kempkes, C.; Savinko, T.; Antal, A.; Kukova, G.; Buhl, T.; Ikoma, A.; Buddenkotte, J.; et al. A sensory neuron-expressed IL-31 receptor mediates T helper cell-dependent itch: Involvement of TRPV1 and TRPA1. *J. Allergy Clin. Immunol.* **2014**, *133*, 448–460. [CrossRef]
62. Feld, M.; Garcia, R.; Buddenkotte, J.; Katayama, S.; Lewis, K.; Muirhead, G.; Hevezi, P.; Plesser, K.; Schrumpf, H.; Krjutskov, K.; et al. The pruritus- and TH2-associated cytokine IL-31 promotes growth of sensory nerves. *J. Allergy Clin. Immunol.* **2016**, *138*, 500–508.e24. [CrossRef]
63. Furue, M.; Ulzii, D.; Vu, Y.H.; Tsuji, G.; Kido-Nakahara, M.; Nakahara, T. Pathogenesis of Atopic Dermatitis: Current Paradigm. *Iran. J. Immunol.* **2019**, *16*, 97–107. [CrossRef]
64. Sonkoly, E.; Muller, A.; Lauerma, A.I.; Pivarcsi, A.; Soto, H.; Kemeny, L.; Alenius, H.; Dieu-Nosjean, M.C.; Meller, S.; Rieker, J.; et al. IL-31: A new link between T cells and pruritus in atopic skin inflammation. *J. Allergy Clin. Immunol.* **2006**, *117*, 411–417. [CrossRef] [PubMed]
65. Lerner, E.A. Is the Nervous System More Important Than the Immune System in Itch and Atopic Dermatitis? *J. Investig. Dermatol. Symp. Proc.* **2018**, *19*, S94. [CrossRef] [PubMed]
66. Tominaga, M.; Takamori, K. Itch and nerve fibers with special reference to atopic dermatitis: Therapeutic implications. *J. Dermatol.* **2014**, *41*, 205–212. [CrossRef]
67. Cevikbas, F.; Steinhoff, A.; Homey, B.; Steinhoff, M. Neuroimmune interactions in allergic skin diseases. *Curr. Opin. Allergy Clin. Immunol.* **2007**, *7*, 365–373. [CrossRef]
68. Datsi, A.; Steinhoff, M.; Ahmad, F.; Alam, M.; Buddenkotte, J. Interleukin-31: The "itchy" cytokine in inflammation and therapy. *Allergy* **2021**, *76*, 2982–2997. [CrossRef] [PubMed]
69. Ruzicka, T.; Hanifin, J.M.; Furue, M.; Pulka, G.; Mlynarczyk, I.; Wollenberg, A.; Galus, R.; Etoh, T.; Mihara, R.; Yoshida, H.; et al. Anti-Interleukin-31 Receptor A Antibody for Atopic Dermatitis. *N. Engl. J. Med.* **2017**, *376*, 826–835. [CrossRef]
70. Chan, B.C.L.; Lam, C.W.K.; Tam, L.S.; Wong, C.K. IL33: Roles in Allergic Inflammation and Therapeutic Perspectives. *Front. Immunol.* **2019**, *10*, 364. [CrossRef]
71. Voisin, T.; Bouvier, A.; Chiu, I.M. Neuro-immune interactions in allergic diseases: Novel targets for therapeutics. *Int. Immunol.* **2017**, *29*, 247–261. [CrossRef]
72. Cherry, W.B.; Yoon, J.; Bartemes, K.R.; Iijima, K.; Kita, H. A novel IL-1 family cytokine, IL-33, potently activates human eosinophils. *J. Allergy Clin. Immunol.* **2008**, *121*, 1484–1490. [CrossRef] [PubMed]
73. Mitchell, P.D.; Salter, B.M.; Oliveria, J.P.; El-Gammal, A.; Tworek, D.; Smith, S.G.; Sehmi, R.; Gauvreau, G.M.; PM, O.A.B. IL-33 and Its Receptor ST2 after Inhaled Allergen Challenge in Allergic Asthmatics. *Int. Arch. Allergy Immunol.* **2018**, *176*, 133–142. [CrossRef] [PubMed]

74. Rak, G.D.; Osborne, L.C.; Siracusa, M.C.; Kim, B.S.; Wang, K.; Bayat, A.; Artis, D.; Volk, S.W. IL-33-Dependent Group 2 Innate Lymphoid Cells Promote Cutaneous Wound Healing. *J. Investig. Dermatol.* **2016**, *136*, 487–496. [CrossRef] [PubMed]
75. Wallrapp, A.; Burkett, P.R.; Riesenfeld, S.J.; Kim, S.J.; Christian, E.; Abdulnour, R.E.; Thakore, P.I.; Schnell, A.; Lambden, C.; Herbst, R.H.; et al. Calcitonin Gene-Related Peptide Negatively Regulates Alarmin-Driven Type 2 Innate Lymphoid Cell Responses. *Immunity* **2019**, *51*, 709–723.e6. [CrossRef] [PubMed]
76. Hayashi, H.; Kawakita, A.; Okazaki, S.; Murai, H.; Yasutomi, M.; Ohshima, Y. IL-33 enhanced the proliferation and constitutive production of IL-13 and IL-5 by fibrocytes. *BioMed Res. Int.* **2014**, *2014*, 738625. [CrossRef]
77. Petra, A.I.; Tsilioni, I.; Taracanova, A.; Katsarou-Katsari, A.; Theoharides, T.C. Interleukin 33 and interleukin 4 regulate interleukin 31 gene expression and secretion from human laboratory of allergic diseases 2 mast cells stimulated by substance P and/or immunoglobulin E. *Allergy Asthma Proc.* **2018**, *39*, 153–160. [CrossRef] [PubMed]
78. Liu, B.; Tai, Y.; Achanta, S.; Kaelberer, M.M.; Caceres, A.I.; Shao, X.; Fang, J.; Jordt, S.E. IL-33/ST2 signaling excites sensory neurons and mediates itch response in a mouse model of poison ivy contact allergy. *Proc. Natl. Acad. Sci. USA* **2016**, *113*, E7572–E7579. [CrossRef] [PubMed]
79. Moniaga, C.S.; Jeong, S.K.; Egawa, G.; Nakajima, S.; Hara-Chikuma, M.; Jeon, J.E.; Lee, S.H.; Hibino, T.; Miyachi, Y.; Kabashima, K. Protease activity enhances production of thymic stromal lymphopoietin and basophil accumulation in flaky tail mice. *Am. J. Pathol.* **2013**, *182*, 841–851. [CrossRef]
80. Ziegler, S.F.; Roan, F.; Bell, B.D.; Stoklasek, T.A.; Kitajima, M.; Han, H. The biology of thymic stromal lymphopoietin (TSLP). *Adv. Pharmacol.* **2013**, *66*, 129–155. [CrossRef]
81. Soumelis, V.; Reche, P.A.; Kanzler, H.; Yuan, W.; Edward, G.; Homey, B.; Gilliet, M.; Ho, S.; Antonenko, S.; Lauerma, A.; et al. Human epithelial cells trigger dendritic cell mediated allergic inflammation by producing TSLP. *Nat. Immunol.* **2002**, *3*, 673–680. [CrossRef] [PubMed]
82. Wilson, S.R.; The, L.; Batia, L.M.; Beattie, K.; Katibah, G.E.; McClain, S.P.; Pellegrino, M.; Estandian, D.M.; Bautista, D.M. The epithelial cell-derived atopic dermatitis cytokine TSLP activates neurons to induce itch. *Cell* **2013**, *155*, 285–295. [CrossRef]
83. Snast, I.; Reiter, O.; Hodak, E.; Friedland, R.; Mimouni, D.; Leshem, Y.A. Are Biologics Efficacious in Atopic Dermatitis? A Systematic Review and Meta-Analysis. *Am. J. Clin. Dermatol.* **2018**, *19*, 145–165. [CrossRef]
84. Paller, A.S.; Bansal, A.; Simpson, E.L.; Boguniewicz, M.; Blauvelt, A.; Siegfried, E.C.; Guttman-Yassky, E.; Hultsch, T.; Chen, Z.; Mina-Osorio, P.; et al. Clinically Meaningful Responses to Dupilumab in Adolescents with Uncontrolled Moderate-to-Severe Atopic Dermatitis: Post-hoc Analyses from a Randomized Clinical Trial. *Am. J. Clin. Dermatol.* **2020**, *21*, 119–131. [CrossRef]
85. Simpson, E.L.; Bieber, T.; Guttman-Yassky, E.; Beck, L.A.; Blauvelt, A.; Cork, M.J.; Silverberg, J.I.; Deleuran, M.; Kataoka, Y.; Lacour, J.P.; et al. Two Phase 3 Trials of Dupilumab versus Placebo in Atopic Dermatitis. *N. Engl. J. Med.* **2016**, *375*, 2335–2348. [CrossRef]
86. Deleuran, M.; Thaci, D.; Beck, L.A.; de Bruin-Weller, M.; Blauvelt, A.; Forman, S.; Bissonnette, R.; Reich, K.; Soong, W.; Hussain, I.; et al. Dupilumab shows long-term safety and efficacy in patients with moderate to severe atopic dermatitis enrolled in a phase 3 open-label extension study. *J. Am. Acad. Dermatol.* **2020**, *82*, 377–388. [CrossRef]
87. Guttman-Yassky, E.; Blauvelt, A.; Eichenfield, L.F.; Paller, A.S.; Armstrong, A.W.; Drew, J.; Gopalan, R.; Simpson, E.L. Efficacy and Safety of Lebrikizumab, a High-Affinity Interleukin 13 Inhibitor, in Adults with Moderate to Severe Atopic Dermatitis: A Phase 2b Randomized Clinical Trial. *JAMA Dermatol.* **2020**, *156*, 411–420. [CrossRef] [PubMed]
88. Silverberg, J.I.; Toth, D.; Bieber, T.; Alexis, A.F.; Elewski, B.E.; Pink, A.E.; Hijnen, D.; Jensen, T.N.; Bang, B.; Olsen, C.K.; et al. Tralokinumab plus topical corticosteroids for the treatment of moderate-to-severe atopic dermatitis: Results from the double-blind, randomized, multicentre, placebo-controlled phase III ECZTRA 3 trial. *Br. J. Dermatol.* **2021**, *184*, 450–463. [CrossRef]
89. Wollenberg, A.; Blauvelt, A.; Guttman-Yassky, E.; Worm, M.; Lynde, C.; Lacour, J.P.; Spelman, L.; Katoh, N.; Saeki, H.; Poulin, Y.; et al. Tralokinumab for moderate-to-severe atopic dermatitis: Results from two 52-week, randomized, double-blind, multicentre, placebo-controlled phase III trials (ECZTRA 1 and ECZTRA 2). *Br. J. Dermatol.* **2021**, *184*, 437–449. [CrossRef]
90. Kabashima, K.; Matsumura, T.; Komazaki, H.; Kawashima, M.; Nemolizumab, J.P.S.G. Trial of Nemolizumab and Topical Agents for Atopic Dermatitis with Pruritus. *N. Engl. J. Med.* **2020**, *383*, 141–150. [CrossRef] [PubMed]
91. Nemoto, O.; Furue, M.; Nakagawa, H.; Shiramoto, M.; Hanada, R.; Matsuki, S.; Imayama, S.; Kato, M.; Hasebe, I.; Taira, K.; et al. The first trial of CIM331, a humanized antihuman interleukin-31 receptor A antibody, in healthy volunteers and patients with atopic dermatitis to evaluate safety, tolerability and pharmacokinetics of a single dose in a randomized, double-blind, placebo-controlled study. *Br. J. Dermatol.* **2016**, *174*, 296–304. [CrossRef]
92. Silverberg, J.I.; Pinter, A.; Pulka, G.; Poulin, Y.; Bouaziz, J.D.; Wollenberg, A.; Murrell, D.F.; Alexis, A.; Lindsey, L.; Ahmad, F.; et al. Phase 2B randomized study of nemolizumab in adults with moderate-to-severe atopic dermatitis and severe pruritus. *J. Allergy Clin. Immunol.* **2020**, *145*, 173–182. [CrossRef]
93. Simpson, E.L.; Lacour, J.P.; Spelman, L.; Galimberti, R.; Eichenfield, L.F.; Bissonnette, R.; King, B.A.; Thyssen, J.P.; Silverberg, J.I.; Bieber, T.; et al. Baricitinib in patients with moderate-to-severe atopic dermatitis and inadequate response to topical corticosteroids: Results from two randomized monotherapy phase III trials. *Br. J. Dermatol.* **2020**, *183*, 242–255. [CrossRef]
94. Reich, K.; Kabashima, K.; Peris, K.; Silverberg, J.I.; Eichenfield, L.F.; Bieber, T.; Kaszuba, A.; Kolodsick, J.; Yang, F.E.; Gamalo, M.; et al. Efficacy and Safety of Baricitinib Combined with Topical Corticosteroids for Treatment of Moderate to Severe Atopic Dermatitis: A Randomized Clinical Trial. *JAMA Dermatol.* **2020**, *156*, 1333–1343. [CrossRef]

95. Nakagawa, H.; Nemoto, O.; Igarashi, A.; Saeki, H.; Kaino, H.; Nagata, T. Delgocitinib ointment, a topical Janus kinase inhibitor, in adult patients with moderate to severe atopic dermatitis: A phase 3, randomized, double-blind, vehicle-controlled study and an open-label, long-term extension study. *J. Am. Acad. Dermatol.* **2020**, *82*, 823–831. [CrossRef] [PubMed]
96. Nakagawa, H.; Nemoto, O.; Igarashi, A.; Saeki, H.; Murata, R.; Kaino, H.; Nagata, T. Long-term safety and efficacy of delgocitinib ointment, a topical Janus kinase inhibitor, in adult patients with atopic dermatitis. *J. Dermatol.* **2020**, *47*, 114–120. [CrossRef] [PubMed]
97. Silverberg, J.I.; Simpson, E.L.; Thyssen, J.P.; Gooderham, M.; Chan, G.; Feeney, C.; Biswas, P.; Valdez, H.; DiBonaventura, M.; Nduaka, C.; et al. Efficacy and Safety of Abrocitinib in Patients with Moderate-to-Severe Atopic Dermatitis: A Randomized Clinical Trial. *JAMA Dermatol.* **2020**, *156*, 863–873. [CrossRef]
98. Simpson, E.L.; Sinclair, R.; Forman, S.; Wollenberg, A.; Aschoff, R.; Cork, M.; Bieber, T.; Thyssen, J.P.; Yosipovitch, G.; Flohr, C.; et al. Efficacy and safety of abrocitinib in adults and adolescents with moderate-to-severe atopic dermatitis (JADE MONO-1): A multi-centre, double-blind, randomised, placebo-controlled, phase 3 trial. *Lancet* **2020**, *396*, 255–266. [CrossRef]
99. Guttman-Yassky, E.; Thaci, D.; Pangan, A.L.; Hong, H.C.; Papp, K.A.; Reich, K.; Beck, L.A.; Mohamed, M.F.; Othman, A.A.; Anderson, J.K.; et al. Upadacitinib in adults with moderate to severe atopic dermatitis: 16-week results from a randomized, placebo-controlled trial. *J. Allergy Clin. Immunol.* **2020**, *145*, 877–884. [CrossRef] [PubMed]
100. Silverberg, J.I.; de Bruin-Weller, M.; Bieber, T.; Soong, W.; Kabashima, K.; Costanzo, A.; Rosmarin, D.; Lynde, C.; Liu, J.; Gamelli, A.; et al. Upadacitinib plus topical corticosteroids in atopic dermatitis: Week-52 AD Up study results. *J. Allergy Clin. Immunol.* **2021**. [CrossRef]
101. Reich, K.; Teixeira, H.D.; de Bruin-Weller, M.; Bieber, T.; Soong, W.; Kabashima, K.; Werfel, T.; Zeng, J.; Huang, X.; Hu, X.; et al. Safety and efficacy of upadacitinib in combination with topical corticosteroids in adolescents and adults with moderate-to-severe atopic dermatitis (AD Up): Results from a randomised, double-blind, placebo-controlled, phase 3 trial. *Lancet* **2021**, *397*, 2169–2181. [CrossRef]
102. Paller, A.S.; Tom, W.L.; Lebwohl, M.G.; Blumenthal, R.L.; Boguniewicz, M.; Call, R.S.; Eichenfield, L.F.; Forsha, D.W.; Rees, W.C.; Simpson, E.L.; et al. Efficacy and safety of crisaborole ointment, a novel, nonsteroidal phosphodiesterase 4 (PDE4) inhibitor for the topical treatment of atopic dermatitis (AD) in children and adults. *J. Am. Acad. Dermatol.* **2016**, *75*, 494–503.e6. [CrossRef]
103. Yosipovitch, G.; Gold, L.F.; Lebwohl, M.G.; Silverberg, J.I.; Tallman, A.M.; Zane, L.T. Early Relief of Pruritus in Atopic Dermatitis with Crisaborole Ointment, A Non-steroidal, Phosphodiesterase 4 Inhibitor. *Acta Derm.-Venereol.* **2018**, *98*, 484–489. [CrossRef]
104. Bissonnette, R.; Pavel, A.B.; Diaz, A.; Werth, J.L.; Zang, C.; Vranic, I.; Purohit, V.S.; Zielinski, M.A.; Vlahos, B.; Estrada, Y.D.; et al. Crisaborole and atopic dermatitis skin biomarkers: An intrapatient randomized trial. *J. Allergy Clin. Immunol.* **2019**, *144*, 1274–1289. [CrossRef] [PubMed]
105. Simpson, E.L.; Parnes, J.R.; She, D.; Crouch, S.; Rees, W.; Mo, M.; van der Merwe, R. Tezepelumab, an anti-thymic stromal lymphopoietin monoclonal antibody, in the treatment of moderate to severe atopic dermatitis: A randomized phase 2a clinical trial. *J. Am. Acad. Dermatol.* **2019**, *80*, 1013–1021. [CrossRef] [PubMed]
106. Chen, Y.L.; Gutowska-Owsiak, D.; Hardman, C.S.; Westmoreland, M.; MacKenzie, T.; Cifuentes, L.; Waithe, D.; Lloyd-Lavery, A.; Marquette, A.; Londei, M.; et al. Proof-of-concept clinical trial of etokimab shows a key role for IL-33 in atopic dermatitis pathogenesis. *Sci. Transl. Med.* **2019**, *11*, eaax2945. [CrossRef]
107. Cabanillas, B.; Brehler, A.C.; Novak, N. Atopic dermatitis phenotypes and the need for personalized medicine. *Curr. Opin. Allergy Clin. Immunol.* **2017**, *17*, 309–315. [CrossRef]
108. Hamilton, J.D.; Suarez-Farinas, M.; Dhingra, N.; Cardinale, I.; Li, X.; Kostic, A.; Ming, J.E.; Radin, A.R.; Krueger, J.G.; Graham, N.; et al. Dupilumab improves the molecular signature in skin of patients with moderate-to-severe atopic dermatitis. *J. Allergy Clin. Immunol.* **2014**, *134*, 1293–1300. [CrossRef]
109. Iannone, M.; Tonini, G.; Janowska, A.; Dini, V.; Romanelli, M. Definition of treatment goals in terms of clinician-reported disease severity and patient-reported outcomes in moderate-to-severe adult atopic dermatitis: A systematic review. *Curr. Med. Res. Opin.* **2021**, *37*, 1295–1301. [CrossRef] [PubMed]
110. Ariens, L.F.M.; van der Schaft, J.; Bakker, D.S.; Balak, D.; Romeijn, M.L.E.; Kouwenhoven, T.; Kamsteeg, M.; Giovannone, B.; Drylewicz, J.; van Amerongen, C.C.A.; et al. Dupilumab is very effective in a large cohort of difficult-to-treat adult atopic dermatitis patients: First clinical and biomarker results from the BioDay registry. *Allergy* **2020**, *75*, 116–126. [CrossRef]
111. Abraham, S.; Haufe, E.; Harder, I.; Heratizadeh, A.; Kleinheinz, A.; Wollenberg, A.; Weisshaar, E.; Augustin, M.; Wiemers, F.; Zink, A.; et al. Implementation of dupilumab in routine care of atopic eczema: Results from the German national registry TREATgermany. *Br. J. Dermatol.* **2020**, *183*, 382–384. [CrossRef]
112. Bansal, A.; Simpson, E.L.; Paller, A.S.; Siegfried, E.C.; Blauvelt, A.; de Bruin-Weller, M.; Corren, J.; Sher, L.; Guttman-Yassky, E.; Chen, Z.; et al. Conjunctivitis in Dupilumab Clinical Trials for Adolescents with Atopic Dermatitis or Asthma. *Am. J. Clin. Dermatol.* **2021**, *22*, 101–115. [CrossRef]
113. Wollenberg, A.; Beck, L.A.; Blauvelt, A.; Simpson, E.L.; Chen, Z.; Chen, Q.; Shumel, B.; Khokhar, F.A.; Hultsch, T.; Rizova, E.; et al. Laboratory safety of dupilumab in moderate-to-severe atopic dermatitis: Results from three phase III trials (LIBERTY AD SOLO 1, LIBERTY AD SOLO 2, LIBERTY AD CHRONOS). *Br. J. Dermatol.* **2020**, *182*, 1120–1135. [CrossRef] [PubMed]
114. Mack, M.R.; Brestoff, J.R.; Berrien-Elliott, M.M.; Trier, A.M.; Yang, T.B.; McCullen, M.; Collins, P.L.; Niu, H.; Bodet, N.D.; Wagner, J.A.; et al. Blood natural killer cell deficiency reveals an immunotherapy strategy for atopic dermatitis. *Sci. Transl. Med.* **2020**, *12*, eaay1005. [CrossRef]
115. Erickson, S.; Heul, A.V.; Kim, B.S. New and emerging treatments for inflammatory itch. *Ann. Allergy Asthma Immunol. Off. Publ. Am. Coll. Allergy Asthma Immunol.* **2021**, *126*, 13–20. [CrossRef] [PubMed]
116. Kabashima, K.; Irie, H. Interleukin-31 as a Clinical Target for Pruritus Treatment. *Front. Med.* **2021**, *8*, 638325. [CrossRef] [PubMed]

117. Damsky, W.; King, B.A. JAK inhibitors in dermatology: The promise of a new drug class. *J. Am. Acad. Dermatol.* **2017**, *76*, 736–744. [CrossRef]
118. Deleanu, D.; Nedelea, I. Biological therapies for atopic dermatitis: An update. *Exp. Ther. Med.* **2019**, *17*, 1061–1067. [CrossRef] [PubMed]
119. Schwartz, D.M.; Kanno, Y.; Villarino, A.; Ward, M.; Gadina, M.; O'Shea, J.J. JAK inhibition as a therapeutic strategy for immune and inflammatory diseases. *Nat. Rev. Drug Discov.* **2017**, *17*, 78. [CrossRef]
120. Tanimoto, A.; Ogawa, Y.; Oki, C.; Kimoto, Y.; Nozawa, K.; Amano, W.; Noji, S.; Shiozaki, M.; Matsuo, A.; Shinozaki, Y.; et al. Pharmacological properties of JTE-052: A novel potent JAK inhibitor that suppresses various inflammatory responses in vitro and in vivo. *Inflamm. Res. Off. J. Eur. Histamine Res. Soc.* **2015**, *64*, 41–51. [CrossRef]
121. Gauvreau, G.M.; O'Byrne, P.M.; Boulet, L.P.; Wang, Y.; Cockcroft, D.; Bigler, J.; FitzGerald, J.M.; Boedigheimer, M.; Davis, B.E.; Dias, C.; et al. Effects of an anti-TSLP antibody on allergen-induced asthmatic responses. *N. Engl. J. Med.* **2014**, *370*, 2102–2110. [CrossRef] [PubMed]
122. Corren, J.; Parnes, J.R.; Wang, L.; Mo, M.; Roseti, S.L.; Griffiths, J.M.; van der Merwe, R. Tezepelumab in Adults with Uncontrolled Asthma. *N. Engl. J. Med.* **2017**, *377*, 936–946. [CrossRef] [PubMed]
123. Lei, Y.; Boinapally, V.; Zoltowska, A.; Adner, M.; Hellman, L.; Nilsson, G. Vaccination against IL-33 Inhibits Airway Hyperresponsiveness and Inflammation in a House Dust Mite Model of Asthma. *PLoS ONE* **2015**, *10*, e0133774. [CrossRef] [PubMed]
124. Chinthrajah, S.; Cao, S.; Liu, C.; Lyu, S.C.; Sindher, S.B.; Long, A.; Sampath, V.; Petroni, D.; Londei, M.; Nadeau, K.C. Phase 2a randomized, placebo-controlled study of anti-IL-33 in peanut allergy. *JCI Insight* **2019**, *4*, e131347. [CrossRef] [PubMed]

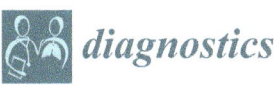

Review

Epidermolysis Bullosa—A Different Genetic Approach in Correlation with Genetic Heterogeneity

Monica-Cristina Pânzaru [1], Lavinia Caba [1,*], Laura Florea [2,3,*], Elena Emanuela Braha [4] and Eusebiu Vlad Gorduza [1]

1. Department of Medical Genetics, Faculty of Medicine, "Grigore T. Popa" University of Medicine and Pharmacy, 16 University Street, 700115 Iasi, Romania; monica.panzaru@yahoo.com (M.-C.P.); vgord@mail.com (E.V.G.)
2. Department of Nephrology-Internal Medicine, Faculty of Medicine, "Grigore T. Popa" University of Medicine and Pharmacy, 16 University Street, 700115 Iasi, Romania
3. Department of Nephrology-Internal Medicine, "Dr. C. I. Parhon" Clinical Hospital, Carol I Street, No 50, 700503 Iasi, Romania
4. "C. I. Parhon" National Institute of Endocrinology, 410087 Bucharest, Romania; elenabraha@yahoo.com
* Correspondence: lavinia_zanet@yahoo.com (L.C.); lflorea68@yahoo.com or laura.florea@umfiasi.ro (L.F.)

Abstract: Epidermolysis bullosa is a heterogeneous group of rare genetic disorders characterized by mucocutaneous fragility and blister formation after minor friction or trauma. There are four major epidermolysis bullosa types based on the ultrastructural level of tissue cleavage: simplex, junctional, dystrophic, and Kindler epidermolysis bullosa. They are caused by mutations in genes that encode the proteins that are part of the hemidesmosomes and focal adhesion complex. Some of these disorders can be associated with extracutaneous manifestations, which are sometimes fatal. They are inherited in an autosomal recessive or autosomal dominant manner. This review is focused on the phenomena of heterogeneity (locus, allelic, mutational, and clinical) in epidermolysis bullosa, and on the correlation genotype–phenotype.

Keywords: epidermolysis bullosa; mutation; heterogeneity

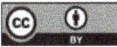

1. Introduction

Epidermolysis bullosa (EB) is a heterogeneous group of rare genetic disorders characterized by mucocutaneous fragility and blister formation after minimal trauma [1]. EB presents a variable expression with a wide phenotypic spectrum ranging from localized, mild, acral blistering, and normal life expectancy, to generalized, severe blistering and extracutaneous involvement, which could lead to infections, electrolyte imbalances, or respiratory distress, as well as poor prognosis. Nail dystrophy, keratoderma, and atrophic scarring are common features. Major extracutaneous complications may develop in some subtypes of EB: laryngeal or esophageal stenosis, ectropion, corneal opacification, pseudosyndactyly, and microstomia. Pyloric atresia, nephropathy, muscular dystrophy, cardiomyopathy, and interstitial lung disease, are encountered in rare forms of EB. Some forms of EB (e.g., severe and intermediate recessive dystrophic EB) are associated with an increased risk of developing cutaneous squamous cell carcinoma [1,2].

Four major EB types are described based on the level of skin cleavage: EB simplex (EBS)—with changes at intraepidermal (epidermolytic) level, junctional EB (JEB)—with changes at the intra-lamina lucida (lamina lucidolytic) level, dystrophic EB (DEB)—with changes at the sub-lamina densa (dermolytic) level, and Kindler EB—with multiple changes at the cutaneous level [1]. Precise diagnosis requires the correlation of clinical data with immunofluorescence antigen mapping (IAM), transmission electron microscopy (TEM), and mutational analysis [2]. In EBS the structure and function of keratin intermediate filaments are altered and the intracellular components of the hemidesmosomes are mutated or missing [2]. In JEB, the transmembrane and extracellular proteins of the hemidesmosomes and the anchoring filaments are modified [2]. In DEB, the anchoring fibrils can be absent, reduced in number, or abnormal. In KS, there are multiple cleavage planes (intraepidermal, junctional, or dense sub-lamina) determined by abnormal fermitin family homolog 1, which is a component in the focal adhesion complexes [2].

Research in recent decades has deciphered some of the pathogenic changes in EB, mainly through histological and genetic studies. These researches proved an important genetic heterogeneity and changed the classification of disorders. Our paper is trying to present synthetically the gene mutations and their implications on the cellular level in connection with their clinical features.

2. Genes and Proteins Involved in Epidermolysis Bullosa

In EB, cell–matrix interactions are mainly altered. Normally cell–matrix interactions are achieved through two elements: hemidesmosomes and focal adhesion.

Hemidesmosomes (HD) are specialized structures that stably anchor the keratinocytes of the epidermis to the basement membranes. This is done by assembly between the intracellular and transmembrane proteins [2]. HD type I (the classic one) is present in the pseudo-stratified epithelium where interactions between intracellular proteins (plectin, dystonin) and transmembrane protein integrin ($\alpha6\beta4$, collagen XVII) and CD151 antigen normally occur. HD type II is found in simple epithelial tissue and consists only of $\alpha6\beta4$ integrin and plectin [3].

The focal adhesion is allowed by different proteins: integrin $\alpha3\beta1$, transmembrane collagen XIII, and fermitin family homolog 1 (FFH1) [2,4].

Table 1 summarizes the main genes involved in the pathogenesis of EB and the encoded proteins.

Table 1. Genes and proteins involved in epidermolysis bullosa [1,5,6].

Gene (Previous/Symbol)	Approved Name (Previous/Alternative Name)	Chromosomal Location	Protein—Recommended Name (Previous/Alternative Name)	Epidermolysis Bullosa Type
KRT5 (EBS2, KRT5A, CK-5)	keratin 5 (epidermolysis bullosa simplex 2 Dowling–Meara/Kobner/Weber–Cockayne types; keratin 5 (epidermolysis bullosa simplex, Dowling–Meara/Kobner/Weber–Cockayne types); keratin 5, type II)	12q13.13	Keratin, type II cytoskeletal 5 (58 kDa cytokeratin; Cytokeratin-5; Keratin-5; Type-II keratin Kb5)	EB simplex, AD EB simplex, AR
KRT14 (EBS3, EBS4)	keratin 14 (keratin 14 (epidermolysis bullosa simplex, Dowling–Meara, Koebner); keratin 14, type I))	17q21.2	Keratin, type I cytoskeletal 14 (Cytokeratin-14; Keratin-14)	EB simplex, AD EB simplex, AR
PLEC (EBS1, PLEC1, PCN, PLTN)	Plectin (plectin 1, intermediate filament binding protein, 500 kD; epidermolysis bullosa simplex 1 (Ogna); plectin 1, intermediate filament binding protein 500 kDa)	8q24.3	Plectin (Hemidesmosomal protein 1—Plectin-1)	EB simplex, AD EB simplex, AR
KLHL24 (DRE1, FLJ20059)	Kelch-like family member 24 (kelch-like 24 (Drosophila))	3q27.1	Kelch-like protein 24 (Kainate receptor-interacting protein for GluR6, Protein DRE1)	EB simplex, AD

Table 1. *Cont.*

Gene (Previous/Symbol)	Approved Name (Previous/Alternative Name)	Chromosomal Location	Protein—Recommended Name (Previous/Alternative Name)	Epidermolysis Bullosa Type
DST (BPAG1, BP240, KIAA0 728, FLJ 21489, FLJ 13425, FLJ 32235, FLJ 30627, CATX-15, BPA, MACF2)	Dystonin (bullous pemphigoid antigen 1, 230/240 kDa)	6p12.1	Dystonin (230 kDa bullous pemphigoid antigen; 230/240 kDa bullous pemphigoid antigen; Bullous pemphigoid antigen 1; Dystonia musculorum protein; Hemidesmosomal plaque protein)	EB simplex, AR
EXPH5 (SLAC2-B)	exophilin 5 (synaptotagmin-like homologue lacking C2 domains)	11q22.3	Exophilin-5 (Synaptotagmin-like protein homolog lacking C2 domains b)	EB simplex, AR
CD151 (SFA-1, PETA-3, TSPAN24, RAPH)	CD151 molecule (Raph blood group) (CD151 antigen; CD151 antigen (Raph blood group))	11p15.5	CD151 antigen (GP27; Membrane glycoprotein SFA-1; Platelet-endothelial tetraspan antigen 3; Tetraspanin-24; *CD_antigen*: CD151)	EB simplex, AR
LAMA3 (LAMNA; nicein-150 kDa; kalinin-165 kDa; BM600–150 kDa epiligrin)	laminin subunit alpha 3 (laminin, alpha 3 (nicein (150 kD), kalinin (165 kD) BM600 (150 kD), epiligrin; laminin, alpha 3)	18q11.2	Laminin subunit alpha-3 (Epiligrin 170 kDa subunit; Epiligrin subunit alpha; Kalinin subunit alpha; Laminin-5 subunit alpha; Laminin-6 subunit alpha; Laminin-7 subunit alpha; Nicein subunit alpha)	Junctional EB, AR
LAMB3 (LAMNB1, nicein-125 kDa, kalinin-140 kDa, BM600–125 kDa)	laminin subunit beta 3 (laminin, beta 3 (nicein (125 kD), kalinin (140 kD), BM600 (125 kD)); laminin, beta 3)	1q32.2	Laminin subunit beta-3 (Epiligrin subunit bata; Kalinin B1 chain; Kalinin subunit beta; Laminin B1k chain; Laminin-5 subunit beta; Nicein subunit beta)	Junctional EB, AR
LAMC2 (EBR2, LAMB2T, LAMNB2, EBR2A, nicein-100 kDa, kalinin-105 kDa, BM600–100 kDa)	laminin subunit gamma 2 laminin, gamma 2 (nicein (100 kD), kalinin (105 kD), BM600 (100 kD), Herlitz junctional epidermolysis bullosa)); laminin, gamma 2	1q25.3	Laminin subunit gamma-2 (Cell-scattering factor 140 kDa subunit; Epiligrin subunit gamma; Kalinin subunit gamma; Kalinin/nicein/epiligrin 100 kDa subunit; Ladsin 140 kDa subunit; Laminin B2t chain; Laminin-5 subunit gamma; Large adhesive scatter factor 140 kDa subunit; Nicein subunit gamma)	Junctional EB, AR
COL17A1 (BPAG2, BP180)	collagen type XVII alpha 1 chain (collagen, type XVII, alpha 1)	10q25.1	Collagen alpha-1 (XVII) chain (180 kDa bullous pemphigoid antigen 2; Bullous pemphigoid antigen 2)	Junctional EB, AR
ITGA6 (CD49f)	integrin subunit alpha 6 (integrin, alpha 6)	2q31.1	Integrin alpha-6 (CD49 antigen-like family member F VLA-6; *CD_antigen*: CD49f)	Junctional EB, AR
ITGB4 (CD104)	integrin subunit beta 4 (integrin, beta 4)	17q25.1	Integrin beta-4 (GP150, *CD_antigen*: CD104)	Junctional EB, AR
ITGA3 (MSK18, CD49c, VLA3a, VCA-2, GAP-B3)	integrin subunit alpha 3 (antigen identified by monoclonal antibody J143; integrin, alpha 3 (antigen CD49C, alpha 3 subunit of VLA-3 receptor))	17q21.33	Integrin alpha-3 (CD49 antigen-like family member C, FRP-2; Galactoprotein B3; VLA-3 subunit alpha; *CD_antigen*: CD49c; CD49 antigen-like family member C)	Junctional EB, AR
COL7A1 (EBDCT, EBD1, EBR1)	Collagen type VII alpha 1 chain (epidermolysis bullosa, dystrophic, dominant and recessive; collagen, type VII, alpha 1; collagen VII, alpha-1 polypeptide; LC collagen)	3p21.31	Collagen alpha-1 (VII) chain (Long-chain collagen)	Dystrophic EB, AD Dystrophic EB, AR

Table 1. Cont.

Gene (Previous/Symbol)	Approved Name (Previous/Alternative Name)	Chromosomal Location	Protein—Recommended Name (Previous/Alternative Name)	Epidermolysis Bullosa Type
FERMT1 (C20orf42, FLJ20116, URP1, KIND1, UNC112A)	FERM domain containing kindlin 1 (chromosome 20 open reading frame 42; fermitin family homolog 1 (Drosophila); fermitin family member 1; kindlin-1; kinderlin)	20p12.3	Fermitin family homolog 1 (Kindlerin; Kindlin syndrome protein, Kindlin-1; Unc-112-related protein 1)	Kindler EB, AR

2.1. Keratins

Keratins are structural proteins. They form obligate heterodimers assembled into intermediate filaments and 3D cytoskeletons. There are two types of keratins: type I and type II. Keratin-5 (type II keratin protein) and keratin 14 (type I) have an α-helical "rod" domain which is flanked by the head and tail domain [7].

2.2. Plectin

Plectin is a cytoskeletal linker protein expressed in skin and skeletal muscle. It links intermediate filaments to hemidesmosomes and in this way functions as a mediator of keratinocyte mechanical stability in the skin [8].

2.3. BTB Domain Containing Kelch-like Protein

Unlike most EBS-associated proteins, the Kelch-like protein 24 (KLHL) is not a structural protein. KLHL proteins are expressed almost ubiquitously at low levels and are involved in cytoskeletal organization, the regulation of cell morphology, cell migration, protein degradation, and gene expression. They contain a BTB domain that binds to cullin 3, a scaffold protein required for the ubiquitination and proteasomal degradation of substrate proteins [7,9].

2.4. Dystonin

Dystonin is one of the largest human proteins and as a member of the plakin family is a structural component of hemidesmosomal inner plaques in basal keratinocytes, a key attachment point for keratin intermediate filaments and the location for other major plaque proteins, such as plectin [10]. The *DST* gene encodes dystonin; alternative splicing produces multiple tissue isoforms expressed in the central nervous system, skin, heart, and skeletal muscle [11,12].

2.5. Exophilin

EXPH5 gene encodes exophilin-5, an effector protein of the Rab27B GTPase. This protein plays a role in intracellular vesicle trafficking and exosome secretion.

2.6. Tetraspanins

Tetraspanins form a protein superfamily widely distributed in the epidermis, renal glomeruli, and proximal and distal tubules. One of its members is the CD151 antigen. In the epidermis, the CD151 antigen participates in the formation of hemidesmosomes and forms very stable laminin-binding complexes with alpha-3beta-11 and alpha-6beta-4 integrins. This allows cell adhesion and the intracellular vesicular transport of integrins. In the kidney, CD151 forms complexes with integrins α3β1 and α6β1 and is essential for the proper assembly of the glomerular and tubular basement membranes [13].

2.7. Laminin Subunits

Laminin 332 is a heterotrimeric molecule that consists of alpha-3, beta-3, and gamma-2 subunits, and is essential for the formation and function of the basement membrane. Laminin 332 interacts with integrin alpha-6beta-4, alpha-3beta-1, and collagen VII, and plays a pivotal role in epidermal adhesion, cell survival, migration, and regeneration. The *LAMA3*, *LAMB3*, and *LAMC2* genes encode the alpha-3, beta-3, and gamma-2 chains of laminin 332 [14,15].

2.8. Collagen XVII

Collagen XVII is expressed in the epithelial hemidesmosomes of the skin, mucous membranes, and eyes [16]. It consists of three identical α1 chains. It has three major domains: a globular intracellular domain, a transmembrane domain, and an extracellular domain. The extracellular domain consists of 15 collagenous domains (cell adhesion domains) and 16 noncollagenous domains (with roles in triple-helix folding) [16]. The collagen XVII binds intracellularly to plectin, dystonin, and β4 integrin, and extracellularly to α6 integrin (that binds to CD151) and laminin 332 [2].

2.9. Collagen VII

Type VII collagen is secreted by keratinocytes as procollagen VII. The procollagen VII is formed by three pro-alpha-1 chains that fold into one molecule. The molecule has an N-terminal noncollagenous 1 (NC1) domain, followed by an extended collagenous domain, and ends with the NC2 domain at the C-terminus. Its role is in anchoring the fibrils that form the cutaneous basement membrane zone adhesion complex [7].

2.10. Integrins

Integrins are transmembrane protein complexes, consisting of alpha and beta chain subunits. The alpha-6 beta-4 integrin is involved in hemidesmosome formation and stability and interacts with laminin, plectin, and dystonin. The activation of integrins mediates extracellular cell–matrix interactions and cytoskeleton organization [17]. *ITGA6* encodes the alpha-6, whereas *ITGB4* encodes the beta-4 subunit of the alpha-6beta-4 integrin. The *ITGA3* gene encodes the integrin alpha-3 subunit that is connected with a beta-1 subunit to form an integrin involved in interactions with extracellular matrix proteins including laminins. The integrin alpha-3 subunit is expressed in basal keratinocytes, podocytes, tubular epithelial cells, alveolar epithelial cells, and many other tissues [7].

2.11. Fermitin Family Homolog 1

The *FFH1* gene is expressed at the dermal–epidermal junction, oral mucosa, and in the gastrointestinal tract [7,18,19]. It is involved in the connection between the actin cytoskeleton and the extracellular matrix by focal adhesion [4]. Also, FFH1 participates in integrins' activation [2].

The main interactions between proteins are shown in Figure 1.

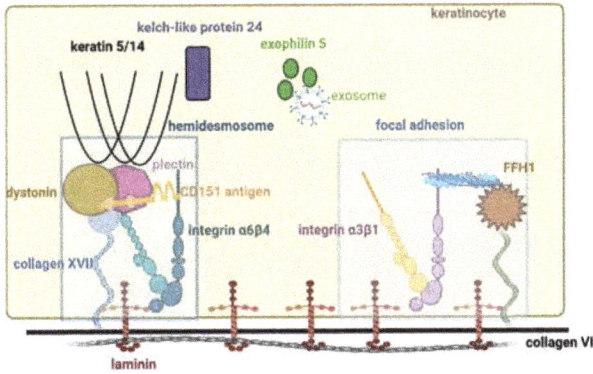

Figure 1. Main proteins involved in epidermolysis bullosa. Created with BioRender.com (accessed on 6 April 2022).

3. Correlations Genotype–Phenotype

3.1. EB Simplex (EBS)

EBS is the most common type of EB accounting for ~70% of all EB [7]. EBS has a prevalence of 6/1,000,000 individuals and an incidence of 7.87 per one million live births [20]. EBS is characterized by skin blistering due to intraepidermal cleavage (within the basal layer of keratinocytes) [7]. In general, blistering is caused by trauma, rarely occurs spontaneously, and tends to heal without scarring. EBS has a variable spectrum of severity ranging from mild blistering of the hands and feet to generalized forms with extracutaneous involvement and is sometimes fatal. Onset varies by subtype and occurs, usually, at birth or during infancy, although patients with localized EBS may not develop their first blisters until adolescence or early adulthood [21,22]. Mutations in the KRT5 and KRT14 genes occur in 75% of cases with EBS [23]. The most recent EB classification includes 14 EBS subtypes based on the distribution and severity of the blisters, specific cutaneous lesions, mode of inheritance, affected gene/protein, and extracutaneous manifestations [1].

3.1.1. EBS, Localized

The most common and mildest subtype of EBS is localized EBS, previously known as Weber–Cockayne disease, with a reported incidence of 3.67 per one million live births [20], but probably a significant percentage of mild cases remain undiagnosed. Localized EBS is characterized by the formation of blisters usually limited to the palms and soles of the feet. The lesions can also appear in other regions of recurrent trauma, such as the knees and shins of a crawling toddler or flexures during hot weather. The age of onset is variable, and the lesions frequently develop in infancy/early childhood and are rarely present at birth or appear in adolescence/adulthood. Nail involvement is uncommon. Common complications are secondary infections, especially foot blisters. Lesions worsen in the warmer months and some patients develop focal palmoplantar keratoderma during adulthood [22,24]. Intraoral blisters or ulcerations are seen during infancy and usually are asymptomatic [22,25]. The disorder has an autosomal dominant inheritance and is produced by missense mutations in the KRT14 and KRT5 genes [26]. The mutations are located outside the highly conserved boundary motifs of the rod domain, usually in the head, tail, or non-helical portions, including the linker area of keratin. They are most frequently found in clusters including in the non-helical L12 linker motif, in the amino-terminal homologous domain (H1) of keratin-5, or in the 2B segment of keratin-14 [27,28]. Hut et al. proposed a genomic mutation detection system for exons 1, 4, and 6 of KRT14 that encode the 1A, L1-2, and 2B domains containing the mutation hotspots [29]. Jiang et al. suggest that in localized EB sequences, coding for the head and the non-helical linker regions of KRT5 should have propriety for the mutation screening [30]. However, mutations were also discovered in the conserved 1A and 2B helix hotspots but with conservative amino acid changes [28]. This is consistent with a report by Cho et al. regarding the influence of polarity on the severity of EBS [31].

3.1.2. EBS, Severe, AD, KRT14/5

Severe EBS, with a reported incidence of 1.16 per one million live births, is characterized by generalized and severe blistering and birth-onset. A suggestive feature is the presence of multiple small blisters in a grouped or arcuate configuration, which explains the previous name "EB herpetiformis". Hemorrhagic blisters are also present. The involvement of the oral mucosa and nail dystrophy are common. Mucosal involvement may interfere with feeding, especially in neonates and infants. Inflammation can occur in hemorrhagic blisters followed by milia and hypo- and hyperpigmentation of the skin. The lesions tend to improve with age or paradoxically, in some cases, during periods of heat or fever. Progressive confluent palmoplantar keratoderma is common, precocious (childhood-onset), and more severe than in other subtypes. This subtype is frequently associated with marked morbidity and in a minority of cases with neonatal/infancy mortality [22,24,32,33]. Dominant-negative mutations in KRT14 and KRT5 have been clustered in regions involved in the highly conserved ends of the rod domains or the helix boundary motifs of keratin. Substitutions are frequently reported and involve highly conserved amino acids within the helix initiation or termination motifs blocking the heterodimerization of keratin polypeptides. Common mutations change the glutamic acid from position 477 of keratin-5 (*KRT5* E477) or the arginine from position 125 of keratin-14 (*KRT14* R125). Both mutations cause the extensive formation of cytoplasmic protein aggregates, a hallmark of severe EBS [22]. Monoallelic in-frame deletion, splice-site, or nonsense mutations were also reported, leading to abnormal proteins with dominant-negative effects. Major changes in polarity or acidity are associated with this subtype [34–36]. Around 70% of cases with severe EBS are generated by one mutation in the *KRT5* gene (c.1429G > A; *p*.Glu477Lys or E477K) and three other in the *KRT14* gene (c.373C > T [*p*.Arg125Cys or R125C]; c.374G > A [*p*.Arg125His or R125H]; c.368A > G [*p*.Asn123Ser or N123S]) [26]. Vahidnezhad et al. reported a case with digenic inheritance, an association of a mutation in the *KRT5* gene and others in the *KRT14* gene [37].

3.1.3. EBS, Intermediate, AD, KRT14/5

This subtype, previously known as Koebner EBS, has an intermediate phenotype, between localized EBS and severe EBS. Blisters appear at birth or in the first few months with generalized distribution, which are milder than those in severe EBS but without a "herpetiform" configuration. The frequency of milia, scarring, nail dystrophy, and oral lesions is intermediate between that of localized EBS and severe EBS. Focal palmoplantar keratoderma can be observed. Lesions worsen in the warmer months. Lesions tend to improve in adolescence when they may become localized to the hands and feet [7,22,24]. Pathogenic variants in the 1A or 2B segments (except the beginning of 1A, 1B, and the end of 1B, which associate severe phenotype) of the rod domain of *KRT5* and *KRT14* are common in intermediate EBS cases. These mutations do not interfere with the elongation process during filament assembly, so filaments essentially appear normal upon ultrastructural examination but are structurally weakened [38,39].

3.1.4. EBS, Intermediate or Severe, AR, KRT14/5

EBS due to *KRT14* or *KRT5* pathogenic variants is frequently inherited in an autosomal dominant mode but autosomal recessive cases were also reported. Most recessive cases are produced by *KRT14* variants and have a phenotype similar to previously described subtypes, but an improvement in blistering with age is not expected. Focal dyskeratotic skin lesions were also reported. Homozygous mutations in *KRT5* lead to severe phenotype, extracutaneous manifestations, and early mortality. Nonsense, missense, splice site, and deletions in *KRT14* have been associated with recessive inheritance. The unaffected parents of each patient were heterozygous for the respective mutations [40]. Rugg et al. consider that these mutations are likely to be associated with a nonsense-mediated messenger RNA decay leading to a functional "knockout" of keratin-14 [41]. Jonkman et al. suggested that increased expression of keratin-5 has a compensatory effect because keratin-14 knockout mice die within the first few weeks after birth [42].

3.1.5. EBS with Mottled Pigmentation

EBS with mottled pigmentation (EBS-MP) with a reported incidence of 0.07 per one million live births, presents generalized blistering from birth but the severity of the lesions is intermediate. The hallmark feature is mottled or reticulate macular pigmentation typically of the neck, upper trunk, and acral skin. Small hyperpigmented macules appear in early childhood, progress over time, and coalesce into a reticulate pattern. Hypopigmented macules are interspersed. The pigmentation does not occur in areas of blistering and often disappears in adult life. Punctate palmar and plantar keratoderma and nail dystrophy may occur. The majority of cases (more than 90%) presented a missense mutation (c.74C > T [*p*.Pro25Leu or P25L]) in the *KRT5* gene [43]. The pigmentary anomalies observed in this EB form could be correlated with the modification of melanosome transport where the non-helical head domain of keratin-5 is involved [44,45]. However, the pathogenic mechanism is incompletely deciphered and some modifiers could interfere with the function of keratin -5. For example, in some cases the pathogenic mutation c.356T > C (*p*.Met119Thr or M119T) in the *KRT14* gene was identified [46].

3.1.6. EBS, Migratory Circinate

EBS, migratory circinate is a rare subtype, previously known as EBS with migratory circinate erythema. It is characterized by generalized blistering from birth with a background of inflammatory migratory circinate erythema that fades and heals with hyperpigmentation (sometimes with a mottled pattern) but without scarring. Nail dystrophy may occur. Some mutations were reported in this form of EB. For example, Gu et al. reported a heterozygous deletion c.1649delG (*p*.Gly550fs) in exon 9 of the *KRT5* gene which leads to a frameshift and delayed termination codon in two unrelated families with EBS, migratory circinate. Lee et al. identified a de novo in-frame 12-bp deletion in exon 7 of the *KRT5* gene, which alters the 2B domain of keratin-5 [47]. Mutations in the keratin-5 tail domain have been related to EBS with unusual features, such as mottled pigmentation and pigmentary disorders, suggesting a possible role of this domain in the regulation of inflammation and pigmentation [48,49].

3.1.7. EBS, AD, with PLEC Mutations

Previously known as Ogna EBS, this subtype presents birth-onset and mild skin blistering, mainly acral and occasionally widespread. The characteristic features are easy skin bruising with the formation of violaceous and hypopigmented macules. Koss-Harnes et al. found the same mutation in exon 31 of the *PLEC* gene (c.6328C > T [*p*.Arg2110Trp or R2110W]) in two unrelated families with Ogna EBS. This mutation changes the plectin polypeptide, which connects the basal keratins to the hemidesmosomal plaque, and generates an aberrant ultrastructure of hemidesmosomes' attachment plates and a frequent fragmentation of hemidesmosomes [50]. Bolling et al. identified mutations in *PLEC* in 6/16 of individuals with biopsy-proven EBS who lack identifiable pathogenic variants in *KRT5* or *KRT14* genes. They suggest that *PLEC* mutations may be more common than previously realized [51].

3.1.8. EBS, AR, with PLEC Mutations

This rare subtype with recessive inheritance has a more severe phenotype than the dominant form. EBS with AR *PLEC* mutations is characterized by generalized skin blistering that heals with scarring and hyperpigmentation. Nail dystrophy is severe. Mucous membranes and the heart and muscles are spared [7]. Gostynska et al. identified homozygosity for a nonsense mutation c.46C > T [*p*.Arg16X] in the first exon of the gene encoding plectin isoform 1a, in two sisters from a consanguineous family. Plectin has eight tissue-specific isoforms in humans, arising from the alternate splicing of the first exon. The isoform 1a is not expressed in striated or cardiac muscle tissue, so muscular dystrophy or cardiomyopathy are not expected to develop in these cases [52].

3.1.9. EBS, Intermediate with Muscular Dystrophy

EBS, intermediate with muscular dystrophy (EBS-MD) is an autosomal recessive disorder characterized by early generalized blistering and variable (usually during childhood) onset of progressive limb-girdle type, muscular dystrophy. Considerable variability in the severity of the muscle weakness, sometimes not noticeable until the fourth decade of the patient's life, is reported. Onychodystrophy, focal plantar keratoderma, and mucosal involvement are common. Abnormal dentition (decay teeth), upper respiratory tract stenosis, urethral strictures, dilated cardiomyopathy, ventricular hypertrophy, and alopecia have been reported [53]. The majority of EBS-MD patients present compound heterozygous or homozygous truncation mutations in exon 31 of the *PLEC* gene, which encodes the rod domain of plectin. Natsuga et al. examined plectin expression in the skin of patients with *PLEC* mutations. In EBS-MD, the expression of the N- and C-terminal domains of plectin remained detectable, although the expression of rod domains was absent or markedly reduced. The alternative splicing of exon 31, resulting in a rodless but still partially functional plectin, was suggested to account for the milder phenotype. Few EBS-MD cases have in-frame mutations in the N-terminal domain of plectin, where the actin-binding domain (ABD) and spectrin repeats are conserved. It is possible that the binding deficits with integrin beta-4 and the collagen alpha-1(XVII) chain, which may explain the phenotype [54–57].

3.1.10. EBS, Severe with Pyloric Atresia

EBS, severe with pyloric atresia (EBS-PA) presents a severe phenotype with widespread generalized blistering or an absence of skin at birth and pyloric atresia. Antenatally, pyloric atresia can manifest with polyhydramnios. Additional features include failure to thrive, aplasia cutis, anemia, sepsis, intraoral blistering, urethral stenosis, and urologic complications. Death usually occurs in infancy [53]. Immunohistochemical studies showed an absent expression of plectin. In contrast to EBS-MD, EBS-PA patients typically have *PLEC* mutations, nonsense or frameshift, outside of exon 31, which leads to loss of both full-length and rodless plectin. Inheritance is autosomal recessive [58].

3.1.11. EBS, Intermediate with Cardiomyopathy

This subtype is characterized by marked erosions in the limbs at birth, healing with dyspigmentation and cribriform atrophic scars, follicular atrophoderma, and late-onset dilated cardiomyopathy. Keratoderma, milia, nail and oral involvement, and progressive diffuse alopecia are reported [7,34,59]. All cases had a heterozygous gain-of-function in *KLHL24* gene start codon mutation, with c.1A-G being the most prevalent. This mutation produces a truncated KLHL24 protein lacking the initial 28 amino acids (KLHL24-ΔN28). The substrate of the KLHL24 protein is keratin-14 and the more stable KLHL24-ΔN28 due to gain-of-function variants inducing the excessive ubiquitination and degradation of keratin-14. Hee et al. consider that *KLHL24* gene mutations disturb the turnover and degradation of intermediate filaments [60]. Schwieger-Briel et al. showed that KHL24 is expressed at similar levels in keratinocytes and cardiomyocytes and may disrupt the degradation of the structural cytoskeletal proteins involved in mechanical resilience [61]. Hedberg-Oldfords et al. reported familial cases with cardiomyopathy due to *KHLH24* gene mutation with polyglucosan accumulation in some cardiomyocytes and with an accumulation of glycogen, desmin, and tubular structures in the cardiomyocytes and in skeletal muscle fibers. They suggest a pivotal role for KLHL24 during cardiogenesis, based on strong *KLHL24* gene expression in early ventricular myocytes and later in the established heart ventricle. As desmin is the cardiac homologue of keratin-14, Vermeer et al. hypothesized that KLHL24-ΔN28 leads to the excessive degradation of desmin, affecting tissue morphology and function. Also, dominant mutations in desmin are associated with a severe form of cardiomyopathy [9,62,63].

3.1.12. EBS, Localized or Intermediate with Dystonin Deficiency

EBS, localized or intermediate with dystonin (BP230) deficiency presents an early-onset with predominantly acral blistering, larger (several centimeters) than in localized EBS. The blisters appear in areas of mechanical trauma but also in non-pressure-prone sites. Blistering could heal without scarring or with post-inflammatory hypo- or hyperpigmentation. Asymptomatic plantar keratoderma was reported [64]. Loss-of-function mutations in the *DST* gene lead to a complete absence of hemidesmosomal plaques, a loss of adhesion, and increased cell spreading and migration. Reduced integrin beta-4 at the cell surface and increased levels of keratin-14 and integrin beta-1 were detected in abnormal cells. Mild phenotype, in contrast to autoimmune bullous pemphigoid who have autoantibodies to dystonin, could be explained by an upregulation of keratin-14 expression. The inheritance is autosomal recessive, but a semi-dominant transmission mode is also plausible because some heterozygous recall some blistering in childhood [34,64,65].

3.1.13. EBS, Localized or Intermediate with Exophilin-5 Deficiency

EBS, localized or intermediate with exophilin-5 deficiency is characterized by localized or generalized intermittent blistering with onset at birth or in early childhood. Skin fragility improves with age, but lesions could heal with hypopigmentation or mottled pigmentation, especially on the trunk and proximal limbs. Skin atrophy and acral blistering with hemorrhagic crusts are cited. Diociaiuti et al. consider that the lack of extracutaneous and adnexal involvement, together with the modest phenotype, differentiates this subtype from the common dominant EBS-MP due to keratin mutations [7,66]. McGrath et al. reported disruption of the keratin filament network, more cortically distributed F-actin, and significantly reduced cell adhesion in keratinocytes from patients with truncating mutations in *EXPH5*. Monteleon et al. demonstrated that exophilin-5 is involved in the delivery of lysosome-related organelles (LROs) to the plasma membrane and is essential for the differentiation of human keratinocytes. LROs are also involved in the packaging and trafficking of melanin, which may explain the pigmentation anomalies. Nonsense and frameshift mutations with autosomal recessive inheritance were reported [1,67–69].

3.1.14. EBS, Localized with Nephropathy

EBS, localized with nephropathy presents early-onset blistering, particularly on pretibial areas associated with nephropathy. Early alopecia, poikiloderma, and nail dystrophy may occur. Involvement of the ocular, oral, gastrointestinal (including esophageal webbing), and urogenital mucosal membranes is reported. Nephropathy manifests with proteinuria and progression to end-stage renal disease [7,34,70]. Homozygous frameshift and splice-site mutations in exon 5 of the *CD151* gene leading to truncated proteins without an integrin-binding domain, were reported [13,53,70,71].

3.2. Junctional EB

Junctional EB (JEB) is a disease with different prevalence in different geographic areas. The USA National EB Registry reported a prevalence of 0.49 per one million population, whereas the Dystrophic Epidermolysis Bullosa Research Association of America showed a prevalence of 3.59 per million per one million population. In Germany, the prevalence of disease was estimated at 6.7 per one million population [20,72,73]. Early lethality of severe forms could explain the differences. The incidence is higher in the Middle East, due to the high inbreeding coefficient. The inheritance is autosomal recessive and germline mosaicism and uniparental isodisomy were reported [74–76]. In JEB skin cleavage occurs within the lamina lucida of the basement membrane zone. The severity of cutaneous and mucosal fragility varies considerably ranging from forms with early lethality to milder phenotypes. A characteristic feature is represented by mature dental enamel anomalies ranging from small pits in the enamel surface to generalized hypoplasia. Impaired adhesion of the odontogenic epithelium from which ameloblasts are derived is involved in abnormal enamel formation [7,22,25]. On a clinical basis, JEB was divided into several categories.

3.2.1. JEB, Severe

In severe JEB, previously known as Herlitz JEB, extensive mucocutaneous blistering with early-onset (at birth or in the neonatal period) may lead to large erosions with extensive loss of proteins, fluids, and iron, which increases susceptibility to infection and electrolyte imbalance. Sometimes, at birth, blisters may be mild and localized to periungual, buttock, or elbow regions [7,22]. The pathognomonic feature is an exuberant granulation tissue located in orofacial (which produces microstomia), periungual, or friction regions, Accumulation of subglottic granulation tissue may lead to a weak, hoarse cry, stridor, and respiratory distress. Alopecia and mature dental enamel defects are common. Involvement of the mucous membranes of the upper respiratory tract, esophagus, bladder, urethra, rectum, and cornea has been reported. Scarring pseudosyndactyly of the hands and feet with severe loss of function has been cited. JEB has the highest risk of infant mortality among the EB subtypes, and the major causes are sepsis, failure to thrive, or tracheolaryngeal obstruction [7,22,24,25,72]. Biallelic mutations in the *LAMA3*, *LAMB3*, and *LAMC2* genes were identified in severe JEB. Varki et al. reported a high proportion of *LAMB3* mutations. The majority lead to premature stop codons, mRNA decay, and synthesis of no protein or to truncated unstable polypeptides. The most frequent mutation in the *LAMB3* gene (45–63%) is c.1903C > T (*p*.Arg635Ter or *p*.R635X) [77]. The distribution of laminin 332 in multiple epithelial basement membranes, including those of the cornea, kidney, lung, thymus, brain, gastrointestinal tract, and lung explains the extracutaneous features [14,15]. However, Abu Sa'd et al. reported a case of severe lethal JEB caused by a homozygous mutation in the *COL17A1* gene [76].

3.2.2. JEB, Intermediate

JEB, intermediate previously called JEB non-Herlitz, presents a less severe clinical phenotype than JEB severe, with a reduced tendency to develop exuberant granulation tissue. Generalized blisters (that predominate in sites exposed to friction, trauma, or heat), heal with atrophy and pigmentation anomalies. Alopecia, enamel defects, and dystrophy or absence of nails are common. Also, a milder involvement of the mucous membranes of the upper respiratory tract (with a lower risk of upper airway occlusion), bladder, and urethra was reported, and adult patients have an increased risk of developing squamous cell carcinoma on their lower extremities in areas of chronic blistering, long-standing erosions, or atrophic scarring [22,24,78]. Specific mutations in the *LAMA3*, *LAMB3*, and *LAMC2* genes (missense or splice-site or compound heterozygosity) that lead to partially functional laminin 332 are reported in this subtype. The intermediate JEB phenotype is also associated with mutations in the *COL17A1* gene. The hallmark of these phenotypes was the total lack of collagen XVII in the skin due to different mutation mechanisms (nonsense/insertions and deletions predicted to result in premature termination/splice site with the production of truncated unstable molecules). The majority of mutations were located in exons 51 and 52. Notably, splice-site mutations occurred preferentially in intron 51 [79]. In this subtype, Jonhman and Pasmooji reported the first cases with revertant mosaicism, both in collagen and laminin deficiency, sustained by the reexpression of the deficient protein on skin specimens. Revertant mosaicism has since been documented in EB forms, implicating the *COL17A1*, *KRT14*, *LAMB3*, *COL7A1*, and *FERMT1* genes [80,81]. Cases with self-improving JEB and milder than expected phenotypes were also reported. The possible underlying molecular mechanisms are an alternative modulation of splicing, a spontaneous readthrough of premature termination codons, or a skipping of exons containing stop codons [1,82–84].

3.2.3. JEB, with Pyloric Atresia

JEB, with pyloric atresia, presents an association between generalized blistering at birth and pyloric atresia. Other gastrointestinal anomalies, such as duodenal and anal atresia, are rarely reported. Aplasia cutis congenita, atrophic scarring, enamel anomalies, oral involvement, and nail dystrophy with patulous nail folds are common. Exuberant granulation tissue in the perioral, neck, and upper back regions may occur. This disorder is associated with a significant risk of genitourinary anomalies (polypoid bladder lesions, urethral stricture, dysplastic kidney, hydronephrosis, ureterocele) and infantile or neonatal death [14,85,86]. JEB with pyloric atresia is associated with mutations in the *ITGA6* or *ITGB4* genes. The majority of the mutations reside in the *ITGB4* gene, being nonsense (with the formation of a premature stop codon) or missense mutations in the amino-terminal extracellular domain that facilitate the association of the alpha-6 or beta-4 subunits. Loss of function mutations in the *ITGA6* gene have been identified in some cases [14,53,87]. The absence of alpha-6 integrins modifies the adhesion of the collecting duct cells to the basal membrane and makes the kidney-collecting system susceptible to degeneration and injury, which explains its renourinary features [88]. DeArcangelis et al. demonstrated by alfa-6 integrin ablation in mice that loss of intestinal epithelial cells/basal membrane interactions initiates the development of inflammatory lesions that progress into high-grade dysplasia and carcinoma [89].

3.2.4. JEB, Localized

Localized JEB is characterized by mild blistering, often acral, variable nail dystrophy, enamel defects, and a tendency to develop cavities. In contrast to the other JEB subtypes, alopecia, extensive atrophic scars, and extracutaneous findings are rarely reported [24,79]. Mutations in the *LAMA3*, *LAMB3*, *LAMC2*, *COL17A1*, *ITGB4*, and *ITGA3* genes were reported. Mutations allowing the expression of a residual protein (usually missense or splicing) lead to this mild phenotype. Condrat and Has stated that as little as 5–10% of residual protein, even if truncated and putatively partially functional, significantly alleviates the phenotype. Some mutations in *COL17A1* that are predicted to lead to a premature stop codon (associated with severe phenotype) escape this outcome because of alternative splicing. Out of the 56 exons of *COL17A1*, 54 are in-frame and can be skipped without shifting the reading frame [57,90,91].

3.2.5. JEB, Inversa

Congenital blistering and erosions confined to flexural areas are suggestive of this rare form of JEB. Blistering is usually severe and may heal with atrophic scarring and milia formation. Nail dystrophy, enamel anomalies and dental caries, oral, esophageal, and vaginal involvement are common. Reduced expression of laminin 332 due to biallelic mutations in the *LAMA3*, *LAMB3*, and *LAMC2* genes was reported [32,92].

3.2.6. JEB, Late-Onset

In contrast to the other subtype of JEB with early-onset, in JEB with late-onset (JEB-lo) the blistering starts in childhood and affects the hands and feet and, to a lesser extent, the elbows, knees, and oral mucosa. Other clinical features are palmoplantar hyperhidrosis, enamel defects, and progressive skin atrophy. The disappearance of dermatoglyphs because of scarring is reported [7]. Yuen et al. reported cases with mutations located in the fourth noncollagenous domain (NC4) of the alpha-1(XVII)-chain gene (c.3908G > A, [*p*.R1303Q or *p*.Arg1303Gln]), which are predicted to affect protein folding and laminin 332 binding. They suggested that missense mutations located in the NC4 domain may be specific for JEB-lo [78].

3.2.7. Laryngo–Onycho–Cutaneous Syndrome

Laryngo–onycho–cutaneous syndrome (LOC), previously called Shabbir syndrome, is characterized by a hoarse cry in the neonatal period, by marked exuberant granulation tissue, in particular affecting the larynx, conjunctiva, and periungual/subungual sites, and by skin blistering and erosions. In contrast to the excessive blistering and erosions described in severe JEB, patients with LOC have minimal blistering but more extensive granulation tissue. Ocular granulation tissue may extend leading to symblepharon and corneal opacification (suggestive features of LOC). Progressive laryngeal granulation can lead to severe respiratory compromise and premature death. Aberrant granulation tissue could also develop on the face, neck, epiglottis, trachea, and main bronchi. Nail dystrophy and enamel anomalies are common [7,32,93,94]. In the affected members of 15 families, McLean et al. identified a homozygous single nucleotide insertion in the *LAMA3* gene (c.151dup; [V51fs]), predicting a stop codon in exon 39 that is specific to laminin alpha-3A, a protein secreted only by the basal keratinocytes of stratified epithelia. They suggested that LOC may be caused by the dysfunction of keratinocyte–mesenchymal communication and hypothesized that the laminin alpha-3A N-terminal domain may be a key regulator of the granulation tissue response. All cases reported are of Punjabi origin, suggesting a possible founder effect. Prodinger et al. reported 3 new mutations in the *LAMA3* gene, outside exon 39 and underscores that molecular diagnostics can be challenging [93,95].

3.2.8. JEB, with Interstitial Lung Disease and Nephrotic Syndrome

The association of congenital nephrotic syndrome, interstitial lung disease, and skin fragility is suggestive of JEB with interstitial lung disease and nephrotic syndrome (ILNEB). The respiratory and renal features predominate and rapid progression usually leads to death in early infancy. The renal anomalies occurring in patients with ILNEB include congenital nephrotic syndrome, focal-segmental glomerulosclerosis, bilateral renal cysts, unilateral kidney hypoplasia, and ectopic conjoint kidney. Patients present variable degrees of cutaneous involvement, nail dystrophy, and sparse hair. Cases with mild phenotypes (without renal anomalies or without lung disease) were reported [34,96,97]. Biallelic mutations (missense, frameshift, or in splice sites) in the *ITGA3* gene were identified. Has et al. reported cases with functionally null mutations and a severe course of disease. Mutations allowing expression of a residual, truncated, or dysfunctional protein may lead to a milder phenotype and improved survival. Lin et al. stated that the phenotype of the *ITGA3* gene mutation may be determined by the residual function of the mutant integrin alpha-3 strain [98,99].

3.3. Dystrophic EB

In dystrophic EB (DEB) the plane of skin cleavage is below the lamina densa in the most superficial portion of the dermis. DEB may be inherited in a dominant (DDEB) or recessive (RDEB) pattern. The prevalence of DDEB and RDEB is quite similar: 1.49 and 1.35 per one million live births respectively [20]. In DEB, blisters, and ulcerations heal with significant scarring and milia formation. Generally, the recessive form is more severe than DDEB; however, there is significant phenotypic overlap between subtypes. All subtypes of DEB are caused by mutations in the *COL7A1* gene, the gene coding collagen VII, the main constituent of the anchoring fibrils at the cutaneous basement membrane zone [1,24,57]. Hovnanian et al. stated that the nature and location of these mutations are important determinants of the phenotype [100]. Mariath et al. suggested that the DEB phenotype is determined by the expression and residual function of collagen VII [24].

3.3.1. DDEB

The majority of DDEB cases result from dominant-negative mutations. Missense substitutions that replace glycine in the collagenous triple-helical domain (frequently in exons 73, 74, and 75) are reported in over 75% of cases. The most common DDEB-causing mutations are c.6100G > A (p.Gly2034Arg or G2034R) and c.6127G > C (p.Gly2043Arg or G2043R) [101,102]. The conservation of glycine residues in every third position of the amino acid sequence is required for the tied packing of the triple helix and these substitutions highly destabilize the triple helix [103]. Other substitutions, insertions, deletions, and splice-site variants have also been described. These mutations involve amino acids essential for the structure of the triple helix and the stability of the anchoring fibrils. However, an inter- and intrafamilial phenotypic variability is reported [86,104,105].

Intermediate DDEB

This subtype presents with generalized blisters from birth or early infancy, milia, albopapuloid lesions, atrophic scarring, and nail dystrophy. Acral sites, elbows, and knees are commonly affected. Mucous membranes may also be involved leading to microstomia, ankyloglossia, and esophageal stenosis, although less commonly than in severe RDEB [1,24].

Localized DDEB

Blistering is confined to the hands, feet, and milia and atrophic scars can also occur. There is no extracutaneous involvement. Rare cases with progressive nail dystrophy and without any other sign of skin fragility are reported [106]. A pretibial form with the development of lesions predominantly in the anterior lower legs is described [107].

3.3.2. RDEB

Severe RDEB

The most severe subtype of DEB, formerly known as Hallopeau-Siemens RDEB, is associated with generalized blistering at birth, progressive extensive scarring, and development of microstomia, ankyloglossia, esophageal stenosis, flexion contractures of limbs, and pseudosyndactyly. Alopecia, milia, and permanent loss of nail plates are common. Eye involvement with corneal erosions, symblepharon, ectropion, and loss of vision is also observed [32,108,109]. The lifetime risk of aggressive squamous cell carcinoma is greater than 90% [110]. Biallelic nonsense or frameshift *COL7A1* gene mutations (insertions/deletions, substitutions, or splice sites) that result in premature termination codons were reported. The consequences for the protein are severe: the absence of or a markedly reduced collagen VII [101,105,110,111].

Intermediate RDEB

Phenotype is similar to intermediate DDEB, but with greater severity of joint contractures and pseudosyndactyly in some cases. Extracutaneous involvement is milder than in severe RDEB. The risk of developing squamous cell carcinomas is also increased (47.5% by age 65) but less common than in severe RDEB and neoplasia occurs later in adulthood [7,108,110]. Many patients are compound heterozygous for a premature stop codon and a glycine substitution within the collagenous domain. The mutations may affect the association of polypeptides and the stability of the triple helix or may cause conformational change [14,86,105].

RDEB, Inversa

This rare subtype is characterized by a peculiar course. Generalized blistering of intermediate severity occurs in the neonatal period, improves with age, and tends to localize to flexure sites in adults. Mucosal involvement (oral, esophageal, anal, genitourinary) is similar but milder than in severe RDEB [32,112,113]. Van den Akker et al. reported specific glycine or arginine substitutions in the carboxyl portion of the triple-helical domain caused by a missense mutation in the *COL7A1* gene. Patients were homozygotes or compound heterozygotes (missense mutation/loss of function mutation). The localization of the amino acid substitutions in specific domains correlates with the synthesis of a thermolabile collagen VII that is specifically less stable in the warm flexural regions [112,113].

RDEB, Localized

The phenotype is similar to localized DDEB. Splice-site mutations and other amino acid (non-glycine) substitutions were reported. In localized RDEB, splice-site mutations result in exon skipping, without altering the remaining protein sequence. This abnormal collagen VII allows the assembly of the anchoring fibrils with small functional defects, which explains the phenotype [61,100,111].

3.3.3. DEB, Pruriginosa

DEB, pruriginosa (*DEB-Pr*) is an unusual subtype that presents blistering in infancy and late-onset (adolescence/adulthood) of intense pruritus and linear cords of lesions (papules, nodules), especially on the extensor surfaces of the limbs (initially on the lower legs). Nail dystrophy, milia, and atrophic scarring are common [7]. Cases with autosomal dominant and autosomal recessive inheritance have been described and glycine substitutions in the collagenous domain, splice-site mutations, and small deletions have been reported. Some of these mutations have been reported in cases with other subtypes of DEB, without pruritus. No specific correlation of the genotype–phenotype has been established. Patients were shown to synthesize a normal or variably reduced amount of type VII collagen, which was correctly deposited at the dermal–epidermal junction [104,114–117]. Studies have excluded other triggering factors, including atopy, elevated IgE levels, matrix metalloproteinase 1 gene polymorphisms, filaggrin gene mutations, and interleukin 31 gene haplotypes [117–120].

3.3.4. DEB, Self-Improving

Previously known as transient bullous dermolysis in a newborn, this rare subtype is characterized by generalized blistering at birth followed by significant improvement within the first 2 years of life [22]. Both dominant and recessive inheritance have been reported in cases of self-improving DEB. The most frequently reported mutations are glycine substitutions and splice-site variants resulting in the skipping of exons (e.g., exon 36). The immunofluorescence shows the accumulation of granular intraepidermal deposits of collagen VII, which regresses with time [121,122]. Christiano et al. suggested that with advancing age, the abnormal polypeptides become degraded at an increasing rate, thus diminishing their dominant-negative effects. The genotype–phenotype relationship remains unclear because of the limited number of cases [123–125].

3.3.5. DEB, Severe, Dominant, and Recessive (Compound Heterozygosity)

The phenotype is indistinguishable from severe RDEB, with severe mucocutaneous involvement from birth. Compound heterozygosity for dominant *COL7A1* glycine substitution mutation and recessive mutation (frameshift leading to a premature termination codon) on the second allele has been reported [14,126–128].

3.4. Kindler EB

In contrast to other types of EB, Kindler EB (KEB) presents a blister formation at different levels of the dermal–epidermal junction: below the lamina densa, within the lamina lucida, or within basal keratinocytes. A single or multiple cleavage planes may be seen within the same sample of skin. KEB manifests with generalized blistering (more prominent on extremities) at birth followed by the development of photosensitivity and progressive poikiloderma. Palmoplantar keratoderma and skin atrophy may occur. Extracutaneous findings include chronic gingivitis, periodontitis, esophageal strictures, ectropion, anal stenosis, and colitis. Pseudosyndactyly has been reported. Patients with KEB have an increased risk of developing cutaneous squamous cell carcinoma (66.7% in those >60 years of age), usually occurring in the fourth to fifth decade of life [22,129]. KEB is caused by a homozygous mutation in the *FERMT1* gene. Zhang et al. suggested that fermitin family homolog 1 is also important for the suppression of UV-induced inflammation and DNA repair [130]. The protein is predominantly expressed in the epithelial cells in the skin, oral mucosa, and the gastrointestinal tract, explaining the distribution of manifestations [131,132]. Deletions, insertions, nonsense, splice-site, and missense mutations (majority loss-of-function) have been reported. Has et al. suggested that mutations compatible with the expression of an abnormal protein (e.g., in-frame) will translate into mild phenotypes, whereas null mutations cause severe forms [133].

4. Current Molecular Approach in Therapeutics

Molecular therapies for EB are conducted in correlation with the mutant genes and specific mutations. They are represented by gene-replacement therapies, gene editing, natural gene therapy, exon skipping, protein therapy, read-through therapies, and small molecules repurposed to relieve symptoms [134]. However, all these treatment methods are still in the phase of therapy trials. Has et al. summarize these gene therapy trials. Mainly recessive dystrophic EB and the type VII collagen and type XVII collagen proteins are targeted. There are ongoing trials in phase I/II in which interventions consist of the ex vivo grafting of gene-corrected epidermal sheets with a gamma-retroviral vector carrying *COL17A1* cDNA or *COL7A1* cDNA [134,135]. The gene-editing strategies are in the preclinical phase and use gene correction in keratinocytes or fibroblasts from patients with RDEB and the skin grafts are transplanted into immunocompromised mice. There are also studies for the JEB and *LAMB3* genes and the EBS and *KRT14* genes [134].

RNA-based therapies use antisense oligonucleotides (ASO) for in-frame exon skipping in the *COL7A1* gene. There are preclinical studies with good results in the skipping exons 13, 70, 73, 80, or 105 in the *COL7A1* gene. A clinical trial testing the ASO-targeting exon 73 in *COL7A1* is currently ongoing [134].

Protein therapy uses recombinant type VII collagen and a phase I/II clinical trial is ongoing in order to evaluate its safety and tolerability in adults with RDEB [134].

The read-through therapies use small molecular-weight compounds, which incorporate an amino acid in a place of a stop codon and in such a way as to suppress the nonsense mutations. Gentamicin was used in clinical studies for RDEB and JEB and also amlexanox to induce the read-through of *COL7A1* [134].

A small molecule used in clinical trials for the reduction of fibrosis (a major complication of RDEB) is losartan [134,136].

5. Conclusions

Epidermolysis bullosa is characterized by high-clinical, allelic, and locus heterogeneity. These features could be explained by the multitude of proteins that are involved in communication and signaling at the basal layers of the skin. In addition, the phenotypes are overlapping and different mutations in the same genes produce the different forms of the disease. The deciphering of pathogenic mechanisms corroborated with the discovery of the genotype–phenotype correlations and will form the basis of personalized management and the prevention of complications.

Author Contributions: All authors contributed equally to this article-type review. All authors have read and agreed to the published version of the manuscript.

Funding: This research received no external funding.

Institutional Review Board Statement: Not applicable.

Informed Consent Statement: Not applicable.

Conflicts of Interest: The authors declare no conflict of interest.

References

1. Has, C.; Bauer, J.W.; Bodemer, C.; Bolling, M.C.; Bruckner-Tuderman, L.; Diem, A.; Fine, J.-D.; Heagerty, A.; Hovnanian, A.; Marinkovich, M.P.; et al. Consensus reclassification of inherited epidermolysis bullosa and other disorders with skin fragility. *Br. J. Dermatol.* **2020**, *183*, 614–627. [CrossRef]
2. Rimoin, D.L.; Pyeritz, R.E.; Korf, B. (Eds.) *Emery and Rimoin's Essential Medical Genetics*; Elsevier: Amsterdam, The Netherlands, 2013.
3. Wang, W.; Zuidema, A.; Te Molder, L.; Nahidiazar, L.; Hoekman, L.; Schmidt, T.; Coppola, S.; Sonnenberg, A. Hemidesmosomes modulate force generation via focal adhesions. *J. Cell Biol.* **2020**, *219*, e201904137. [CrossRef]
4. Sawamura, D.; Nakano, H.; Matsuzaki, Y. Overview of epidermolysis bullosa. *J. Dermatol.* **2010**, *37*, 214–219. [CrossRef]
5. HGNC, HUGO Gene Nomenclature Committee Home Page. Available online: http://www.genenames.org/ (accessed on 28 March 2022).
6. UniProt. Available online: https://www.uniprot.org/ (accessed on 25 March 2022).
7. Bardhan, A.; Bruckner-Tuderman, L.; Chapple, I.L.C.; Fine, J.-D.; Harper, N.; Has, C.; Magin, T.M.; Marinkovich, M.P.; Marshall, J.F.; McGrath, J.A.; et al. Epidermolysis bullosa. *Nat. Rev. Dis. Prim.* **2020**, *6*, 78. [CrossRef]
8. Kiritsi, D.; Tsakiris, L.; Schauer, F. Plectin in Skin Fragility Disorders. *Cells* **2021**, *10*, 2738. [CrossRef]
9. Hedberg-Oldfors, C.; Abramsson, A.; Osborn, D.P.S.; Danielsson, O.; Fazlinezhad, A.; Nilipour, Y.; Hübbert, L.; Nennesmo, I.; Visuttijai, K.; Bharj, J.; et al. Cardiomyopathy with lethal arrhythmias associated with inactivation of KLHL24. *Hum. Mol. Genet.* **2019**, *28*, 1919–1929. [CrossRef]
10. Guo, L.; Degenstein, L.; Dowling, J.; Yu, Q.-C.; Wollmann, R.; Perman, B.; Fuchs, E. Gene targeting of BPAG1: Abnormalities in mechanical strength and cell migration in stratified epithelia and neurologic degeneration. *Cell* **1995**, *81*, 233–243. [CrossRef]
11. Ferrier, A.; Sato, T.; De Repentigny, Y.; Gibeault, S.; Bhanot, K.; O'Meara, R.W.; Lynch-Godrei, A.; Kornfeld, S.F.; Young, K.G.; Kothary, R. Transgenic expression of neuronal dystonin isoform 2 partially rescues the disease phenotype of the dystonia musculorum mouse model of hereditary sensory autonomic neuropathy VI. *Hum. Mol. Genet.* **2014**, *23*, 2694–2710. [CrossRef]

12. Cappuccio, G.; Pinelli, M.; Torella, A.; Alagia, M.; Auricchio, R.; Staiano, A.; Nigro, V.; Brunetti-Pierri, N. Expanding the phenotype of *DST*-related disorder: A case report suggesting a genotype/phenotype correlation. *Am. J. Med. Genet. Part A* **2017**, *173*, 2743–2746. [CrossRef]
13. Crew, V.K.; Burton, N.; Kagan, A.; Green, C.A.; Levene, C.; Flinter, F.; Brady, R.L.; Daniels, G.; Anstee, D.J. CD151, the first member of the tetraspanin (TM4) superfamily detected on erythrocytes, is essential for the correct assembly of human basement membranes in kidney and skin. *Blood* **2004**, *104*, 2217–2223. [CrossRef]
14. Varki, R.; Sadowski, S.; Pfendner, E.; Uitto, J. Epidermolysis bullosa. I. Molecular genetics of the junctional and hemidesmosomal variants. *J. Med. Genet.* **2006**, *43*, 641–652. [CrossRef]
15. Kiritsi, D.; Has, C.; Bruckner-Tuderman, L. Laminin 332 in junctional epidermolysis bullosa. *Cell Adhes. Migr.* **2013**, *7*, 135–141. [CrossRef]
16. Sun, S.; Karsdal, M.A. Type VI collagen. In *Biochemistry of Collagens, Laminins and Elastin*; Academic Press: Cambridge, MA, USA, 2016; pp. 49–55.
17. Larjava, H.; Plow, E.F.; Wu, C. Kindlins: Essential regulators of integrin signalling and cell–matrix adhesion. *EMBO Rep.* **2008**, *9*, 1203–1208. [CrossRef]
18. Lai-Cheong, J.E.; Tanaka, A.; Hawche, G.; Emanuel, P.; Maari, C.; Taskesen, M.; Akdeniz, S.; Liu, L.; McGrath, J.A. Kindler syndrome: A focal adhesion genodermatosis. *Br. J. Dermatol.* **2009**, *160*, 233–242. [CrossRef]
19. Ashton, G.H.; McLean, W.H.I.; South, A.P.; Oyama, N.; Smith, F.J.; Al-Suwaid, R.; Al Ismaily, A.; Atherton, D.J.; Harwood, C.; Leigh, I.M.; et al. Recurrent Mutations in Kindlin-1, a Novel Keratinocyte Focal Contact Protein, in the Autosomal Recessive Skin Fragility and Photosensitivity Disorder, Kindler Syndrome. *J. Investig. Dermatol.* **2004**, *122*, 78–83. [CrossRef]
20. Fine, J.-D. Epidemiology of Inherited Epidermolysis Bullosa Based on Incidence and Prevalence Estimates from the National Epidermolysis Bullosa Registry. *JAMA Dermatol.* **2016**, *152*, 1231–1238. [CrossRef]
21. Sánchez-Jimeno, C.; Escámez, M.; Ayuso, C.; Trujillo-Tiebas, M.; del Río, M. Genetic Diagnosis of Epidermolysis Bullosa: Recommendations from an Expert Spanish Research Group. *Actas Dermo-Sifiliográficas* **2018**, *109*, 104–122. [CrossRef]
22. Fine, J.-D. Inherited epidermolysis bullosa. *Orphanet J. Rare Dis.* **2010**, *5*, 12. [CrossRef]
23. Lane, E.B.; Rugg, E.L.; Navsaria, H.; Leigh, I.M.; Heagerty, A.H.M.; Ishida-Yamamoto, A.; Eady, R.A.J. A mutation in the conserved helix termination peptide of keratin 5 in hereditary skin blistering. *Nature* **1992**, *356*, 244–246. [CrossRef]
24. Mariath, L.M.; Santin, J.T.; Schuler-Faccini, L.; Kiszewski, A.E. Inherited epidermolysis bullosa: Update on the clinical and genetic aspects. *An. Bras. Dermatol.* **2020**, *95*, 551–569. [CrossRef]
25. Wright, J.T. Oral Manifestations in the Epidermolysis Bullosa Spectrum. *Dermatol. Clin.* **2010**, *28*, 159–164. [CrossRef] [PubMed]
26. Pfendner, E.G.; Sadowski, S.G.; Uitto, J. Epidermolysis Bullosa Simplex: Recurrent and De Novo Mutations in the KRT5 and KRT14 Genes, Phenotype/Genotype Correlations, and Implications for Genetic Counseling and Prenatal Diagnosis. *J. Investig. Dermatol.* **2005**, *125*, 239–243. [CrossRef] [PubMed]
27. Szeverenyi, I.; Cassidy, A.J.; Chung, C.W.; Lee, B.T.K.; Common, J.E.A.; Ogg, S.C.; Chen, H.; Sim, S.Y.; Goh, W.L.P.; Ng, K.W.; et al. The Human Intermediate Filament Database: Comprehensive information on a gene family involved in many human diseases. *Hum. Mutat.* **2008**, *29*, 351–360. [CrossRef] [PubMed]
28. Chamcheu, J.C.; Siddiqui, I.A.; Syed, D.N.; Adhami, V.M.; Liovic, M.; Mukhtar, H. Keratin gene mutations in disorders of human skin and its appendages. *Arch. Biochem. Biophys.* **2011**, *508*, 123–137. [CrossRef]
29. Hut, P.H.; Vlies, P.V.; Verlind, E.; Buys, C.H.; Scheffer, H.; Jonkman, M.F.; Shimizu, H. Exempting Homologous Pseudogene Sequences from Polymerase Chain Reaction Amplification Allows Genomic Keratin 14 Hotspot Mutation Analysis. *J. Investig. Dermatol.* **2000**, *114*, 616–619. [CrossRef]
30. Jiang, X.; Zhu, Y.; Sun, H.; Gu, F. A Novel Mutation p.L461P in KRT5 Causing Localized Epidermolysis Bullosa Simplex. *Ann. Dermatol.* **2021**, *33*, 11–17. [CrossRef]
31. Cho, J.-W.; Ryu, H.-W.; Kim, S.-A.; Nakano, H.; Lee, K.-S. Weber-Cockayne Type Epidermolysis Bullosa Simplex Resulting from a Novel Mutation (c. 608T>C) in the Keratin 5 Gene. *Ann. Dermatol.* **2014**, *26*, 739–742. [CrossRef]
32. Fine, J.-D.; Eady, R.A.; Bauer, E.A.; Bauer, J.W.; Bruckner-Tuderman, L.; Heagerty, A.; Hintner, H.; Hovnanian, A.; Jonkman, M.F.; Leigh, I.; et al. The classification of inherited epidermolysis bullosa (EB): Report of the Third International Consensus Meeting on Diagnosis and Classification of EB. *J. Am. Acad. Dermatol.* **2008**, *58*, 931–950. [CrossRef]
33. Pfendner, E.G.; Bruckner, A.L. Epidermolysis Bullosa Simplex. In *GeneReviews®*; Adam, M.P., Ardinger, H.H., Pagon, R.A., Wallace, S.E., Eds.; University of Washington: Seattle, WA, USA, 1998. Available online: https://www.ncbi.nlm.nih.gov/books/NBK1369/ (accessed on 5 March 2022).
34. Has, C.; Fischer, J. Inherited epidermolysis bullosa: New diagnostics and new clinical phenotypes. *Exp. Dermatol.* **2019**, *28*, 1146–1152. [CrossRef]
35. Sathishkumar, D.; Orrin, E.; Terron-Kwiatkowski, A.; Browne, F.; Martinez, A.E.; Mellerio, J.E.; Ogboli, M.; Hoey, S.; Ozoemena, L.; Liu, L.; et al. The p.Glu477Lys Mutation in Keratin 5 Is Strongly Associated with Mortality in Generalized Severe Epidermolysis Bullosa Simplex. *J. Investig. Dermatol.* **2016**, *136*, 719–721. [CrossRef]
36. Coulombe, P.A.; Kerns, M.L.; Fuchs, E. Epidermolysis bullosa simplex: A paradigm for disorders of tissue fragility. *J. Clin. Investig.* **2009**, *119*, 1784–1793. [CrossRef] [PubMed]

37. Vahidnezhad, H.; Youssefian, L.; Saeidian, A.H.; Mozafari, N.; Barzegar, M.; Sotoudeh, S.; Daneshpazhooh, M.; Isaian, A.; Zeinali, S.; Uitto, J. KRT5 and KRT14 Mutations in Epidermolysis Bullosa Simplex with Phenotypic Heterogeneity, and Evidence of Semidominant Inheritance in a Multiplex Family. *J. Investig. Dermatol.* **2016**, *136*, 1897–1901. [CrossRef] [PubMed]
38. Arin, M.J. The molecular basis of human keratin disorders. *Qual. Life Res.* **2009**, *125*, 355–357. [CrossRef] [PubMed]
39. Müller, F.B.; Küster, W.; Wodecki, K.; Almeida, H.; Bruckner-Tuderman, L.; Krieg, T.; Korge, B.P.; Arin, M.J. Novel and recurrent mutations in keratin *KRT5* and *KRT14* genes in epidermolysis bullosa simplex: Implications for disease phenotype and keratin filament assembly. *Hum. Mutat.* **2006**, *27*, 719–720. [CrossRef]
40. Has, C.; Chang, Y.-R.; Volz, A.; Hoeping, D.; Kohlhase, J.; Bruckner-Tuderman, L. Novel Keratin 14 Mutations in Patients with Severe Recessive Epidermolysis Bullosa Simplex. *J. Investig. Dermatol.* **2006**, *126*, 1912–1914. [CrossRef]
41. Rugg, E.L.; McLean, W.H.; Lane, E.B.; Pitera, R.; McMillan, J.R.; Dopping-Hepenstal, P.J.; A Navsaria, H.; Leigh, I.M.; A Eady, R. A functional "knockout" of human keratin 14. *Genes Dev.* **1994**, *8*, 2563–2573. [CrossRef]
42. Jonkman, M.F.; Heeres, K.; Pas, H.H.; van Luyn, M.J.; Elema, J.D.; Corden, L.D.; Smith, F.J.; McLean, W.I.; Ramaekers, F.C.; Burton, M.; et al. Effects of Keratin 14 Ablation on the Clinical and Cellular Phenotype in a Kindred with Recessive Epidermolysis Bullosa Simplex. *J. Investig. Dermatol.* **1996**, *107*, 764–769. [CrossRef]
43. Moog, U.; de Die-Smulders, C.E.; Scheffer, H.; van der Vlies, P.; Henquet, C.J.; Jonkman, M.F. Epidermolysis bullosa sim-plex with mottled pigmentation: Clinical aspects and confirmation of the P24L mutation in the KRT5 gene in further pa-tients. *Am. J. Med. Genet.* **1999**, *86*, 376–379. [CrossRef]
44. Irvine, A.; Rugg, E.; Lane, E.; Hoare, S.; Peret, C.; Hughes, A.; Heagerty, A. Molecular confirmation of the unique phenotype of epidermolysis bullosa simplex with mottled pigmentation. *Br. J. Dermatol.* **2001**, *144*, 40–45. [CrossRef]
45. Uitto, J.; Richard, G.; McGrath, J. Diseases of epidermal keratins and their linker proteins. *Exp. Cell Res.* **2007**, *313*, 1995–2009. [CrossRef]
46. Harel, A.; Bergman, R.; Indelman, M.; Sprecher, E. Epidermolysis Bullosa Simplex with Mottled Pigmentation Resulting from a Recurrent Mutation in KRT14. *J. Investig. Dermatol.* **2006**, *126*, 1654–1657. [CrossRef] [PubMed]
47. Lee, S.E.; Choi, J.Y.; Kim, S.-E.; Kim, S.-C. A novel deletion mutation in the 2B domain of KRT5 in epidermolysis bullosa simplex with childhood-onset migratory circinate erythema. *Eur. J. Dermatol.* **2018**, *28*, 123–125. [CrossRef] [PubMed]
48. Gu, L.-H.; Kim, S.-C.; Ichiki, Y.; Park, J.; Nagai, M.; Kitajima, Y. A usual frameshift and delayed termination codon muta-tion in keratin 5 causes a novel type of epidermolysis bullosa simplex with migratory circinate erythema. *J. Investig. Dermatol.* **2003**, *121*, 482–485. [CrossRef] [PubMed]
49. Kumagai, Y.; Umegaki-Arao, N.; Sasaki, T.; Nakamura, Y.; Takahashi, H.; Ashida, A.; Tsunemi, Y.; Kawashima, M.; Shimizu, A.; Ishiko, A.; et al. Distinct phenotype of epidermolysis bullosa simplex with infantile migratory circinate erythema due to frameshift mutations in the V2 domain of KRT5. *J. Eur. Acad. Dermatol. Venereol.* **2017**, *31*, e241–e243. [CrossRef]
50. Koss-Harnes, D.; Høyheim, B.; Anton-Lamprecht, I.; Gjesti, A.; Jørgensen, R.S.; Jahnsen, F.L.; Olaisen, B.; Wiche, G.; Gedde-Dahl, T. A Site-Specific Plectin Mutation Causes Dominant Epidermolysis Bullosa Simplex Ogna: Two Identical De Novo Mutations. *J. Investig. Dermatol.* **2002**, *118*, 87–93. [CrossRef]
51. Bolling, M.C.; Jongbloed, J.D.; Boven, L.G.; Diercks, G.F.; Smith, F.J.; McLean, W.H.I.; Jonkman, M.F. Plectin Mutations Underlie Epidermolysis Bullosa Simplex in 8% of Patients. *J. Investig. Dermatol.* **2014**, *134*, 273–276. [CrossRef]
52. Gostyńska, K.B.; Nijenhuis, M.; Lemmink, H.; Pas, H.; Pasmooij, A.M.; Lang, K.K.; Castañón, M.J.; Wiche, G.; Jonkman, M.F. Mutation in exon 1a of PLEC, leading to disruption of plectin isoform 1a, causes autosomal-recessive skin-only epidermolysis bullosa simplex. *Hum. Mol. Genet.* **2015**, *24*, 3155–3162. [CrossRef]
53. Vahidnezhad, H.; Youssefian, L.; Saeidian, A.H.; Uitto, J. Phenotypic Spectrum of Epidermolysis Bullosa: The Paradigm of Syndromic versus Non-Syndromic Skin Fragility Disorders. *J. Investig. Dermatol.* **2019**, *139*, 522–527. [CrossRef]
54. Pfendner, E.; Rouan, F.; Uitto, J. Progress in epidermolysis bullosa: The phenotypic spectrum of plectin mutations. *Exp. Dermatol.* **2005**, *14*, 241–249. [CrossRef]
55. Sawamura, D.; Goto, M.; Sakai, K.; Nakamura, H.; McMillan, J.R.; Akiyama, M.; Shirado, O.; Oyama, N.; Satoh, M.; Kaneko, F.; et al. Possible Involvement of Exon 31 Alternative Splicing in Phenotype and Severity of Epidermolysis Bullosa Caused by Mutations in PLEC1. *J. Investig. Dermatol.* **2007**, *127*, 1537–1540. [CrossRef]
56. Natsuga, K.; Nishie, W.; Shinkuma, S.; Arita, K.; Nakamura, H.; Ohyama, M.; Osaka, H.; Kambara, T.; Hirako, Y.; Shimizu, H. Plectin deficiency leads to both muscular dystrophy and pyloric atresia in epidermolysis bullosa simplex. *Hum. Mutat.* **2010**, *31*, E1687–E1698. [CrossRef] [PubMed]
57. Has, C.; Nyström, A.; Saeidian, A.H.; Bruckner-Tuderman, L.; Uitto, J. Epidermolysis bullosa: Molecular pathology of connective tissue components in the cutaneous basement membrane zone. *Matrix Biol.* **2018**, *71–72*, 313–329. [CrossRef] [PubMed]
58. Natsuga, K. Plectin-related skin diseases. *J. Dermatol. Sci.* **2015**, *77*, 139–145. [CrossRef] [PubMed]
59. Has, C. The "Kelch" Surprise: KLHL24, a New Player in the Pathogenesis of Skin Fragility. *J. Investig. Dermatol.* **2017**, *137*, 1211–1212. [CrossRef]
60. He, Y.; Maier, K.; Leppert, J.; Hausser, I.; Schwieger-Briel, A.; Weibel, L.; Theiler, M.; Kiritsi, D.; Busch, H.; Boerries, M.; et al. Monoallelic Mutations in the Translation Initiation Codon of KLHL24 Cause Skin Fragility. *Am. J. Hum. Genet.* **2016**, *99*, 1395–1404. [CrossRef]

61. Schwieger-Briel, A.; Fuentes, I.; Castiglia, D.; Barbato, A.; Greutmann, M.; Leppert, J.; Duchatelet, S.; Hovnanian, A.; Burattini, S.; Yubero, M.J.; et al. Epidermolysis Bullosa Simplex with KLHL24 Mutations Is Associated with Dilated Cardiomyopathy. *J. Investig. Dermatol.* **2019**, *139*, 244–249. [CrossRef]
62. Yenamandra, V.; Akker, P.V.D.; Lemmink, H.; Jan, S.; Diercks, G.; Vermeer, M.; Berg, M.V.D.; van der Meer, P.; Pasmooij, A.; Sinke, R.; et al. Cardiomyopathy in patients with epidermolysis bullosa simplex with mutations in KLHL24. *Br. J. Dermatol.* **2018**, *179*, 1181–1183. [CrossRef]
63. Vermeer, M.C.; Bolling, M.C.; Bliley, J.M.; Gomez, K.F.A.; Pavez-Giani, M.G.; Kramer, D.; Romero-Herrera, P.H.; Westenbrink, B.D.; Diercks, G.F.; van den Berg, M.P.; et al. Gain-of-function mutation in ubiquitin ligase KLHL24 causes desmin degradation and dilatation in hiPSC-derived engineered heart tissues. *J. Clin. Investig.* **2021**, *131*, e140615. [CrossRef]
64. McGrath, J.A. Recently Identified Forms of Epidermolysis Bullosa. *Ann. Dermatol.* **2015**, *27*, 658–666. [CrossRef]
65. Ganani, D.; Malovitski, K.; Sarig, O.; Gat, A.; Sprecher, E.; Samuelov, L. Epidermolysis bullosa simplex due to bi-allelic DST mutations: Case series and review of the literature. *Pediatr. Dermatol.* **2021**, *38*, 436–441. [CrossRef]
66. Diociaiuti, A.; Pisaneschi, E.; Rossi, S.; Condorelli, A.; Carnevale, C.; Zambruno, G.; El Hachem, M. Autosomal recessive epidermolysis bullosa simplex due to EXPH5 mutation: Neonatal diagnosis of the first Italian case and literature review. *J. Eur. Acad. Dermatol. Venereol.* **2020**, *34*, e694–e697. [CrossRef] [PubMed]
67. McGrath, J.A.; Stone, K.L.; Begum, R.; Simpson, M.A.; Dopping-Hepenstal, P.J.; Liu, L.; McMillan, J.R.; South, A.P.; Pourreyron, C.; McLean, W.I.; et al. Germline Mutation in EXPH5 Implicates the Rab27B Effector Protein Slac2-b in Inherited Skin Fragility. *Am. J. Hum. Genet.* **2012**, *91*, 1115–1121. [CrossRef] [PubMed]
68. Turcan, I.; Pasmooij, A.M.G.; Van den Akker, P.C.; Lemmink, H.; Sinke, R.J.; Jonkman, M.F. Association of Epidermolysis Bullosa Simplex with Mottled Pigmentation and EXPH5 Mutations. *JAMA Dermatol.* **2016**, *152*, 1137–1141. [CrossRef]
69. Monteleon, C.L.; Lee, I.Y.; Ridky, T.W. Exophilin-5 Supports Lysosome-Mediated Trafficking Required for Epidermal Differentiation. *J. Investig. Dermatol.* **2019**, *139*, 2219–2222.e6. [CrossRef] [PubMed]
70. Vahidnezhad, H.; Youssefian, L.; Saeidian, A.H.; Mahmoudi, H.; Touati, A.; Abiri, M.; Kajbafzadeh, A.-M.; Aristodemou, S.; Liu, L.; McGrath, J.; et al. Recessive mutation in tetraspanin CD151 causes Kindler syndrome-like epidermolysis bullosa with multi-systemic manifestations including nephropathy. *Matrix Biol.* **2018**, *66*, 22–33. [CrossRef] [PubMed]
71. Naylor, R.W.; Watson, E.; Williamson, S.; Preston, R.; Davenport, J.B.; Thornton, N.; Lowe, M.; Williams, M.; Lennon, R. Basement membrane defects in CD151-associated glomerular disease. *Pediatr. Nephrol.* **2022**, 1–11. [CrossRef]
72. Kelly-Mancuso, G.; Kopelan, B.; Azizkhan, R.G.; Lucky, A.W. Junctional epidermolysis bullosa incidence and survival: 5-year experience of the Dystrophic Epidermolysis Bullosa Research Association of America (DebRA) nurse educator, 2007 to 2011. *Pediatr. Dermatol.* **2014**, *31*, 159–162. [CrossRef]
73. Hammersen, J.; Has, C.; Naumann-Bartsch, N.; Stachel, D.; Kiritsi, D.; Söder, S.; Tardieu, M.; Metzler, M.; Bruckner-Tuderman, L.; Schneider, H. Genotype, Clinical Course, and Therapeutic Decision Making in 76 Infants with Severe Generalized Junctional Epidermolysis Bullosa. *J. Investig. Dermatol.* **2016**, *136*, 2150–2157. [CrossRef]
74. Fassihi, H.; Wessagowit, V.; Ashton, G.H.S.; Moss, C.; Ward, R.; Denyer, J.; Mellerio, J.E.; McGrath, J.A. Complete paternal uniparental isodisomy of chromosome 1 resulting in Herlitz junctional epidermolysis bullosa. *Clin. Exp. Dermatol.* **2005**, *30*, 71–74. [CrossRef]
75. Cserhalmi-Friedman, P.B.; Anyane-Yeboa, K.; Christiano, A.M. Paternal germline mosaicism in Herlitz junctional epidermolysis bullosa. *Exp. Dermatol.* **2002**, *11*, 468–470. [CrossRef]
76. Abu Sa'D, J.; Indelman, M.; Pfendner, E.; Falik-Zaccai, T.C.; Mizrachi-Koren, M.; Shalev, S.; Ben Amitai, D.; Raas-Rothshild, A.; Adir-Shani, A.; Borochowitz, Z.-U.; et al. Molecular Epidemiology of Hereditary Epidermolysis Bullosa in a Middle Eastern Population. *J. Investig. Dermatol.* **2006**, *126*, 777–781. [CrossRef] [PubMed]
77. Rousselle, P.; Beck, K. Laminin 332 processing impacts cellular behavior. *Cell Adhes. Migr.* **2013**, *7*, 122–134. [CrossRef] [PubMed]
78. Yuen, W.Y.; Jonkman, M.F. Risk of squamous cell carcinoma in junctional epidermolysis bullosa, non-Herlitz type: Report of 7 cases and a review of the literature. *J. Am. Acad. Dermatol.* **2011**, *65*, 780–789. [CrossRef]
79. Kiritsi, D.; Kern, J.S.; Schumann, H.; Kohlhase, J.; Has, C.; Bruckner-Tuderman, L. Molecular mechanisms of phenotypic variability in junctional epidermolysis bullosa. *J. Med. Genet.* **2011**, *48*, 450–457. [CrossRef] [PubMed]
80. Jonkman, M.F.; Pasmooij, A.M. Revertant Mosaicism—Patchwork in the Skin. *N. Engl. J. Med.* **2009**, *360*, 1680–1682. [CrossRef] [PubMed]
81. Meyer-Mueller, C.; Osborn, M.J.; Tolar, J.; Boull, C.; Ebens, C.L. Revertant Mosaicism in Epidermolysis Bullosa. *Biomedicines* **2022**, *10*, 114. [CrossRef]
82. Chavanas, S.; Gache, Y.; Vailly, J.; Kanitakis, J.; Pulkkinen, L.; Uitto, J.; Ortonne, J.P.; Meneguzzi, G. Splicing modulation of integrin beta4 pre-mRNA carrying a branch point mutation underlies epidermolysis bullosa with pyloric atresia undergoing spontaneous amelioration with ageing. *Hum. Mol. Genet.* **1999**, *8*, 2097–2105. [CrossRef]
83. McGrath, J.A.; Ashton, G.H.; Mellerio, J.E.; McMillan, J.R.; Eady, R.A.; Salas-Alanis, J.C.; Swensson, O. Moderation of Phenotypic Severity in Dystrophic and Junctional Forms of Epidermolysis Bullosa Through In-Frame Skipping of Exons Containing Non-Sense or Frameshift Mutations. *J. Investig. Dermatol.* **1999**, *113*, 314–321. [CrossRef]
84. Pacho, F.; Zambruno, G.; Calabresi, V.; Kiritsi, D.; Schneider, H. Efficiency of translation termination in humans is highly dependent upon nucleotides in the neighbourhood of a (premature) termination codon. *J. Med. Genet.* **2011**, *48*, 640–644. [CrossRef]

85. Pfendner, E.G.; Lucky, A.W. Epidermolysis Bullosa with Pyloric Atresia. In *GeneReviews®*; Adam, M.P., Ardinger, H.H., Pagon, R.A., Wallace, S.E., Eds.; University of Washington: Seattle, WA, USA, 2008. Available online: https://www.ncbi.nlm.nih.gov/books/NBK1157/ (accessed on 6 March 2022).
86. Chung, H.J.; Uitto, J. Epidermolysis Bullosa with Pyloric Atresia. *Dermatol. Clin.* **2010**, *28*, 43–54. [CrossRef]
87. Lestringant, G.; Allegra, M.; Gagnoux-Palacios, L.; Gache, Y.; Roques, S.; Ortonne, J.-P.; Meneguzzi, G. Rapid Decay of α6 Integrin Caused by a Mis-Sense Mutation in the Propeller Domain Results in Severe Junctional Epidermolysis Bullosa with Pyloric Atresia. *J. Investig. Dermatol.* **2003**, *121*, 1336–1343. [CrossRef] [PubMed]
88. Viquez, O.M.; Yazlovitskaya, E.M.; Tu, T.; Mernaugh, G.; Secades, P.; McKee, K.K.; Georges-Labouesse, E.; De Arcangelis, A.; Quaranta, V.; Yurchenco, P.; et al. Integrin alpha6 maintains the structural integrity of the kidney collecting system. *Matrix Biol.* **2016**, *57–58*, 244–257. [CrossRef] [PubMed]
89. De Arcangelis, A.; Hamade, H.; Alpy, F.; Normand, S.; Bruyère, E.; Lefebvre, O.; Méchine-Neuville, A.; Siebert, S.; Pfister, V.; Lepage, P.; et al. Hemidesmosome integrity protects the colon against colitis and colorectal cancer. *Gut* **2017**, *66*, 1748–1760. [CrossRef] [PubMed]
90. Kowalewski, C.; Bremer, J.; Gostynski, A.; Wertheim-Tysarowska, K.; Wozniak, K.; Bal, J.; Jonkman, M.; Pasmooij, A. Amelioration of junctional epidermolysis bullosa due to exon skipping. *Br. J. Dermatol.* **2016**, *174*, 1375–1379. [CrossRef]
91. Condrat, I.; He, Y.; Cosgarea, R.; Has, C. Junctional Epidermolysis Bullosa: Allelic Heterogeneity and Mutation Stratification for Precision Medicine. *Front. Med.* **2019**, *5*, 363. [CrossRef]
92. Gedde-Dahl, T., Jr.; Dupuy, B.M.; Jonassen, R.; Winberg, J.-O.; Anton-Lamprecht, I.; Olaisen, B.; Olalsen, B. Junctional epidermolysis bullosa inversa (locus EBR2A) assigned to 1q31 by linkage and association to LAMC1. *Hum. Mol. Genet.* **1994**, *3*, 1387–1391. [CrossRef]
93. McLean, W.I.; Irvine, A.D.; Hamill, K.J.; Whittock, N.V.; Coleman-Campbell, C.M.; Mellerio, J.E.; Ashton, G.S.; Dopping-Hepenstal, P.J.; Eady, R.A.; Jamil, T.; et al. An unusual N-terminal deletion of the laminin 3a isoform leads to the chronic granulation tissue disorder laryngo-onycho-cutaneous syndrome. *Hum. Mol. Genet.* **2003**, *12*, 2395–2409. [CrossRef]
94. Siañez-González, C.; Pezoa-Jares, R.; Salas-Alanis, J.C. Congenital epidermolysis bullosa: A review. *Actas Dermo-Sifiliográficas* **2009**, *100*, 842–856. [CrossRef]
95. Prodinger, C.; Chottianchaiwat, S.; Mellerio, J.E.; McGrath, J.A.; Ozoemena, L.; Liu, L.; Moore, W.; Laimer, M.; Petrof, G.; Martinez, A.E. The natural history of laryngo-onycho-cutaneous syndrome: A case series of six pediatric patients and literature review. *Pediatr. Dermatol.* **2021**, *38*, 1094–1101. [CrossRef]
96. Colombo, E.A.; Spaccini, L.; Volpi, L.; Negri, G.; Cittaro, D.; Lazarevic, D.; Zirpoli, S.; Farolfi, A.; Gervasini, C.; Cubellis, M.V.; et al. Viable phenotype of ILNEB syndrome without nephrotic impairment in siblings heterozygous for unreported integrin alpha3 mutations. *Orphanet J. Rare Dis.* **2016**, *11*, 136. [CrossRef]
97. Kinyó, Á.; Kovács, A.L.; Degrell, P.; Kálmán, E.; Nagy, N.; Kárpáti, S.; Gyulai, R.; Saeidian, A.H.; Youssefian, L.; Vahidnezhad, H.; et al. Homozygous ITGA3 Missense Mutation in Adults in a Family with Syndromic Epidermolysis Bullosa (ILNEB) without Pulmonary Involvement. *J. Investig. Dermatol.* **2021**, *141*, 2752–2756. [CrossRef]
98. Has, C.; Spartà, G.; Kiritsi, D.; Weibel, L.; Moeller, M.; Vega-Warner, V.; Waters, A.; He, Y.; Anikster, Y.; Esser, P.; et al. Integrin α3 Mutations with Kidney, Lung, and Skin Disease. *N. Engl. J. Med.* **2012**, *366*, 1508–1514. [CrossRef] [PubMed]
99. Liu, Y.; Yue, Z.; Wang, H.; Li, M.; Wu, X.; Lin, H.; Han, W.; Lan, S.; Sun, L. A novel ITGA3 homozygous splice mutation in an ILNEB syndrome child with slow progression. *Clin. Chim. Acta* **2021**, *523*, 430–436. [CrossRef] [PubMed]
100. Hovnanian, A.; Rochat, A.; Bodemer, C.; Petit, E.; Rivers, C.A.; Prost, C.; Fraitag, S.; Christiano, A.M.; Uitto, J.; Lathrop, M.; et al. Characterization of 18 New Mutations in COL7A1 in Recessive Dystrophic Epidermolysis Bullosa Provides Evidence for Distinct Molecular Mechanisms Underlying Defective Anchoring Fibril Formation. *Am. J. Hum. Genet.* **1997**, *61*, 599–610. [CrossRef] [PubMed]
101. Varki, R.; Sadowski, S.; Uitto, J.; Pfendner, E. Epidermolysis bullosa. II. Type VII collagen mutations and phenotype-genotype correlations in the dystrophic subtypes. *J. Med. Genet.* **2007**, *44*, 181–192. [CrossRef]
102. Hammami-Hauasli, N.; Raghunath, M.; Bruckner-Tuderman, L.; Küster, W. Transient Bullous Dermolysis of the Newborn Associated with Compound Heterozygosity for Recessive and Dominant COL7A1 Mutations. *J. Investig. Dermatol.* **1998**, *111*, 1214–1219. [CrossRef]
103. Persikov, A.V.; Pillitteri, R.J.; Amin, P.; Schwarze, U.; Byers, P.H.; Brodsky, B. Stability related bias in residues replacing glycines within the collagen triple helix (Gly-Xaa-Yaa) in inherited connective tissue disorders. *Hum. Mutat.* **2004**, *24*, 330–337. [CrossRef]
104. Nakamura, H.; Sawamura, D.; Goto, M.; Sato-Matsumura, K.C.; LaDuca, J.; Lee, J.Y.-Y.; Masunaga, T.; Shimizu, H. The G2028R glycine substitution mutation in COL7A1 leads to marked inter-familiar clinical heterogeneity in dominant dystrophic epidermolysis bullosa. *J. Dermatol. Sci.* **2004**, *34*, 195–200. [CrossRef]
105. Dang, N.; Murrell, D.F. Mutation analysis and characterization of COL7A1 mutations in dystrophic epidermolysis bullosa. *Exp. Dermatol.* **2008**, *17*, 553–688. [CrossRef]
106. Yang, R.; Duan, Y.; Kong, Q.; Li, W.; Xu, J.; Xia, X.; Sang, H. What do we learn from dystrophic epidermolysis bullosa, nails only? Idiopathic nail dystrophy may harbor a COL7A1 mutation as the underlying cause. *J. Dermatol.* **2020**, *47*, 782–786. [CrossRef]
107. Christiano, A.M.; Lee, J.Y.-Y.; Chen, W.J.; Laforgia, S.; Uitto, J. Pretibial epidermolysis bullosa: Genetic linkage to COL7A1 and identification of a glycine-to-cysteine substitution in the triple-helical domain of type VII collagen. *Hum. Mol. Genet.* **1995**, *4*, 1579–1583. [CrossRef] [PubMed]

108. Fine, J.-D.; Johnson, L.; Weiner, M.; Stein, A.; Cash, S.; DeLeoz, J.; Devries, D.; Suchindran, C. Pseudosyndactyly and musculoskeletal contractures in inherited epidermolysis bullosa: Experience of the national epidermolysis bullosa registry, 1986–2002. *J. Hand Surg.* **2005**, *30*, 14–22. [CrossRef] [PubMed]
109. Tong, L.; Hodgkins, P.R.; Denyer, J.; Brosnahan, D.; Harper, J.; Russell-Eggitt, I.; Taylor, D.S.; Atherton, D. The eye in epidermolysis bullosa. *Br. J. Ophthalmol.* **1999**, *83*, 323–326. [CrossRef] [PubMed]
110. Fine, J.-D.; Johnson, L.B.; Weiner, M.; Li, K.-P.; Suchindran, C. Epidermolysis bullosa and the risk of life-threatening cancers: The National EB Registry experience, 1986–2006. *J. Am. Acad. Dermatol.* **2009**, *60*, 203–211. [CrossRef] [PubMed]
111. Gardella, R.; Castiglia, D.; Posteraro, P.; Bernardini, S.; Zoppi, N.; Paradisi, M.; Tadini, G.; Barlati, S.; McGrath, J.; Zambruno, G.; et al. Genotype–Phenotype Correlation in Italian Patients with Dystrophic Epidermolysis Bullosa. *J. Investig. Dermatol.* **2002**, *119*, 1456–1462. [CrossRef]
112. Akker, P.C.V.D.; Mellerio, J.E.; Martinez, A.E.; Liu, L.; Meijer, R.; Dopping-Hepenstal, P.J.C.; Van Essen, A.J.; Scheffer, H.; Hofstra, R.; McGrath, J.; et al. The inversa type of recessive dystrophic epidermolysis bullosa is caused by specific arginine and glycine substitutions in type VII collagen. *J. Med. Genet.* **2011**, *48*, 160–167. [CrossRef]
113. Chiaverini, C.; Charlesworth, A.V.; Youssef, M.; Cuny, J.-F.; Rabia, S.H.; Lacour, J.-P.; Meneguzzi, G. Inversa Dystrophic Epidermolysis Bullosa Is Caused by Missense Mutations at Specific Positions of the Collagenic Domain of Collagen Type VII. *J. Investig. Dermatol.* **2010**, *130*, 2508–2511. [CrossRef]
114. McGrath, J.; Schofield, O.; Eady, R. Epidermolysis bullosa pruriginosa: Dystrophic epidermolysis bullosa with distinctive clinicopathological features. *Br. J. Dermatol.* **1994**, *130*, 617–625. [CrossRef]
115. Mellerio, J.E.; Ashton, G.H.; Mohammedi, R.; Eady, R.A.; McGrath, J.A.; Lyon, C.C.; Kirby, B.; Harman, K.E.; Salas-Alanis, J.C.; Atherton, D.J.; et al. Allelic Heterogeneity of Dominant and Recessive COL7A1 Mutations Underlying Epidermolysis Bullosa Pruriginosa. *J. Investig. Dermatol.* **1999**, *112*, 984–987. [CrossRef]
116. Murata, T.; Masunaga, T.; Shimizu, H.; Takizawa, Y.; Ishiko, A.; Hatta, N.; Nishikawa, T. Glycine substitution mutations by different amino acids in the same codon of COL7A1 lead to heterogeneous clinical phenotypes of dominant dystrophic epidermolysis bullosa. *Arch. Dermatol. Res.* **2000**, *292*, 477–481. [CrossRef]
117. Drera, B.; Castiglia, D.; Zoppi, N.; Gardella, R.; Tadini, G.; Floriddia, G.; De Luca, N.; Pedicelli, C.; Barlati, S.; Zambruno, G.; et al. Dystrophic epidermolysis bullosa pruriginosa in Italy: Clinical and molecular characterization. *Clin. Genet.* **2006**, *70*, 339–347. [CrossRef] [PubMed]
118. Almaani, N.; Liu, L.; Harrison, N.; Tanaka, A.; Lai-Cheong, J.E.; Mellerio, J.E.; McGrath, J.A. New Glycine Substitution Mutations in Type VII Collagen Underlying Epidermolysis Bullosa Pruriginosa but the Phenotype is not Explained by a Common Polymorphism in the Matrix Metalloproteinase-1 Gene Promoter. *Acta Dermatol. Venereol.* **2009**, *89*, 6–11. [CrossRef] [PubMed]
119. Schumann, H.; Has, C.; Kohlhase, J.; Bruckner-Tuderman, L. Dystrophic epidermolysis bullosa pruriginosa is not associated with frequentFLGgene mutations. *Br. J. Dermatol.* **2008**, *159*, 464–469. [CrossRef] [PubMed]
120. Nagy, N.; Tanaka, A.; Techanukul, T.; McGrath, J.A. Common IL-31 Gene Haplotype Associated with Non-atopic Eczema is Not Implicated in Epidermolysis Bullosa Pruriginosa. *Acta Dermatol. Venereol.* **2010**, *90*, 631–632. [CrossRef]
121. Fine, J.-D.; Horiguchi, Y.; Stein, D.H.; Esterly, N.B.; Leigh, I.M. Intraepidermal type VII collagen: Evidence for abnormal intracytoplasmic processing of a major basement membrane protein in rare patients with dominant and possibly localized recessive forms of dystrophic epidermolysis bullosa. *J. Am. Acad. Dermatol.* **1990**, *22*, 188–195. [CrossRef]
122. Hatta, N.; Takata, M.; Shimizu, H. Spontaneous disappearance of intraepidermal type VII collagen in a patient with dystrophic epidermolysis bullosa. *Br. J. Dermatol.* **1995**, *133*, 619–624. [CrossRef]
123. Christiano, A.M.; Fine, J.-D.; Uitto, J. Genetic Basis of Dominantly Inherited Transient Bullous Dermolysis of the Newborn: A Splice Site Mutation in the Type VII Collagen Gene. *J. Investig. Dermatol.* **1997**, *109*, 811–814. [CrossRef]
124. Fassihi, H.; Diba, V.C.; Wessagowit, V.; Dopping-Hepenstal, P.J.C.; Jones, C.A.; Burrows, N.P.; McGrath, J.A. Transient bullous dermolysis of the newborn in three generations. *Br. J. Dermatol.* **2005**, *153*, 1058–1063. [CrossRef]
125. Shi, B.-J.; Zhu, X.-J.; Liu, Y.; Hao, J.; Yan, G.-F.; Wang, S.-P.; Wang, X.-Y.; Diao, Q.-C. Transient bullous dermolysis of the newborn: A novel de novo mutation in the *COL7A1* gene. *Int. J. Dermatol.* **2015**, *54*, 438–442. [CrossRef]
126. Christiano, A.M.; Anton-Lamprecht, I.; Amano, S.; Ebschner, U.; Burgeson, R.E.; Uitto, J. Compound heterozygosity for COL7A1 mutations in twins with dystrophic epidermolysis bullosa: A recessive paternal deletion/insertion mutation and a dominant negative maternal glycine substitution result in a severe phenotype. *Am. J. Hum. Genet.* **1996**, *58*, 682–693.
127. Weinel, S.; Lucky, A.W.; Uitto, J.; Pfendner, E.G.; Choo, D. Dystrophic Epidermolysis Bullosa with One Dominant and One Recessive Mutation of the COL7A1 Gene in a Child with Deafness. *Pediatr. Dermatol.* **2008**, *25*, 210–214. [CrossRef] [PubMed]
128. Turczynski, S.; Titeux, M.; Pironon, N.; Cohn, H.; Murrell, D.; Hovnanian, A. Marked intrafamilial phenotypic heterogeneity in dystrophic epidermolysis bullosa caused by inheritance of a mild dominant glycine substitution and a novel deep intronic recessive *COL7A1* mutation. *Br. J. Dermatol.* **2016**, *174*, 1122–1125. [CrossRef] [PubMed]
129. Guerrero-Aspizua, S.; Conti, C.J.; Escamez, M.J.; Castiglia, D.; Zambruno, G.; Youssefian, L.; Vahidnezhad, H.; Requena, L.; Itin, P.; Tadini, G.; et al. Assessment of the risk and characterization of non-melanoma skin cancer in Kindler syndrome: Study of a series of 91 patients. *Orphanet J. Rare Dis.* **2019**, *14*, 183. [CrossRef] [PubMed]
130. Zhang, X.; Luo, S.; Wu, J.; Zhang, L.; Wang, W.-H.; Degan, S.; Erdmann, D.; Hall, R.; Zhang, J.Y. KIND1 Loss Sensitizes Keratinocytes to UV-Induced Inflammatory Response and DNA Damage. *J. Investig. Dermatol.* **2017**, *137*, 475–483. [CrossRef]

131. Jobard, F.; Bouadjar, B.; Caux, F.; Hadj-Rabia, S.; Has, C.; Matsuda, F.; Weissenbach, J.; Lathrop, M.; Prud'Homme, J.-F.; Fischer, J. Identification of mutations in a new gene encoding a FERM family protein with a pleckstrin homology domain in Kindler syndrome. *Hum. Mol. Genet.* **2003**, *12*, 925–935. [CrossRef]
132. Meves, A.; Stremmel, C.; Gottschalk, K.; Fässler, R. The Kindlin protein family: New members to the club of focal adhesion proteins. *Trends Cell Biol.* **2009**, *19*, 504–513. [CrossRef]
133. Has, C.; Castiglia, D.; Del Rio, M.; Diez, M.G.; Piccinni, E.; Kiritsi, D.; Kohlhase, J.; Itin, P.; Martin, L.; Fischer, J.; et al. Kindler syndrome: Extension of FERMT1 mutational spectrum and natural history. *Hum. Mutat.* **2011**, *32*, 1204–1212. [CrossRef]
134. Has, C.; South, A.; Uitto, J. Molecular Therapeutics in Development for Epidermolysis Bullosa: Update 2020. *Mol. Diagn. Ther.* **2020**, *24*, 299–309. [CrossRef]
135. Prodinger, C.; Reichelt, J.; Bauer, J.W.; Laimer, M. Epidermolysis bullosa: Advances in research and treatment. *Exp. Dermatol.* **2019**, *28*, 1176–1189. [CrossRef]
136. Nyström, A.; Thriene, K.; Mittapalli, V.R.; Kern, J.S.; Kiritsi, D.; Dengjel, J.; Bruckner-Tuderman, L. Losartan ameliorates dystrophic epidermolysis bullosa and uncovers new disease mechanisms. *EMBO Mol. Med.* **2015**, *7*, 1211–1228. [CrossRef]

A Positive Dermcidin Expression Is an Unfavorable Prognostic Marker for Extramammary Paget's Disease

Shun Ohmori, Yu Sawada *, Natsuko Saito-Sasaki, Sayaka Sato, Yoko Minokawa, Hitomi Sugino, Hikaru Nanamori, Kayo Yamamoto, Etsuko Okada and Motonobu Nakamura

Department of Dermatology, University of Occupational and Environmental Health, 1-1, Iseigaoka, Yahatanishi-Ku, Kitakyushu, Fukuoka 807-8555, Japan; oh-sh@med.uoeh-u.ac.jp (S.O.); natsuko-saito@med.uoeh-u.ac.jp (N.S.-S.); a0619gacha@gmail.com (S.S.); min.yo5.0628@gmail.com (Y.M.); hsugino@med.uoeh-u.ac.jp (H.S.); hikaru-n@med.uoeh-u.ac.jp (H.N.); kayohama@med.uoeh-u.ac.jp (K.Y.); e-okada@med.uoeh-u.ac.jp (E.O.); motonaka@med.uoeh-u.ac.jp (M.N.)
* Correspondence: long-ago@med.uoeh-u.ac.jp; Tel.: +81-093-691-7445

Abstract: Extramammary Paget's disease is recognized as an apocrine-origin cutaneous tumor and is localized in the intraepithelial skin lesion. However, its advanced form is intractable, and there is currently no therapeutic option with a satisfactory level of clinical outcome. Therefore, it is of great importance to identify a potential biomarker to estimate tumor advancement in extramammary Paget's disease. Dermcidin is an antimicrobial peptide derived from the eccrine gland and is identified as a biomarker in various malignancies. To investigate the potential of dermcidin in extramammary Paget's disease, we investigated dermcidin expression in tumors using the immunostaining technique. Although previous studies have reported that extramammary Paget's disease has no positive staining against dermcidin, 14 out of 60 patients showed positive staining of dermcidin in our study. To clarify the characteristics of positive dermcidin in extramammary Paget's disease, we investigated the clinical characteristics of positive dermcidin extramammary Paget's disease patients. Positive dermcidin patients showed a significantly high frequency of lymph node metastasis. We next investigated the impact of positive dermcidin on overall survival. Univariate analysis identified that positive dermcidin showed a significantly increased hazard ratio in overall survival, suggesting that dermcidin might be a prognostic factor for extramammary Paget's disease.

Keywords: extramammary Paget's disease; dermcidin; prognosis; lymph node metastasis; survival

1. Introduction

The skin is a large surface organ in the human body and is complicatedly organized with various unique cells and glands to adjust to external environmental changes [1–3]. Due to this unique characteristic of skin as a peripheral organ, various types of tumors, including malignancies, have the chance to emerge in it. In the early phase of tumor development, the tumor is localized in the skin, which can be adequately targeted through skin-focused local treatment, such as surgical resection [4]. However, once it progresses to an advanced form and causes distant organ metastasis, it is intractable due to the limited number of therapeutic options against these metastatic skin cancers [5]. Despite recent advancements in immune checkpoint and molecular targeted therapy, this therapeutic approach has still not reached a satisfactory level to obtain positive clinical outcomes [6].

The origin of extramammary Paget's disease is believed to be the apocrine glands. This is because the disease usually arises in the genital, perianal, and axillary regions, where the apocrine glands are located [7]. In agreement with this, previous histological studies have identified that extramammary Paget's disease showed positive immunoreactivity against gross cystic disease fluid protein (GCDFP)-15, carcinoembryonic antigen (CEA), and cytokeratin (CK) 7, all of which receive the same response from the apocrine glands [8]. In general, patients with extramammary Paget's disease have a good prognosis, with a 5-year overall survival of 75% to 95%, because the disease is localized in the epidermis [4,9–12]. In contrast, dermal invasion is closely associated with lymph node metastasis and poor prognosis [8]. However, there is a limited number of biomarkers that can help toward the prognosis of extramammary Paget's disease.

A unique antimicrobial peptide was identified in 2001, i.e., dermcidin., which is constitutively produced by sweat glands. Additionally, an abundance of dermcidin was detected in sweat, showing a beneficial impact on antimicrobial action against microorganisms [13]. In contrast to its beneficial effect on the human body, however, dermcidin can also play an important role in the development of malignant tumors and other diseases. Based on this property of dermcidin, its usefulness as a biomarker for various diseases has been evaluated. Because extramammary Paget's disease is believed to be a malignant tumor derived from the apocrine glands, representing a negative expression of dermcidin in normal tissue, the possible role of dermcidin as a biomarker in patients with extramammary Paget's disease has not been investigated.

In this study, we investigated the potential of dermcidin as a biomarker for the prognosis of extramammary Paget's disease. We identified that there are two groups, dermcidin-positive and -negative extramammary Paget's disease. In addition, dermcidin-positive patients showed an unfavorable clinical behavior and a high frequency of lymph node metastasis. Our results suggest that dermcidin might be an independent prognostic factor in patients with extramammary Paget's disease.

2. Materials and Methods

2.1. Patient Population

In total, 60 patients who underwent surgery as an initial form of treatment for extramammary Paget's disease at the Department of Dermatology, University of Occupational and Environmental Health, were enrolled in this study from December 1979 to August 2017. The diagnosis was based on histopathological analysis carried out by two independent pathologists. Tissue specimens of the tumor were obtained from patients who underwent surgery at our institution. Because of the rarity of this malignant cutaneous tumor [14], it is sometimes difficult for a diagnosis of extramammary Paget's disease to be made, especially as it is hard to distinguish the disease from the pagetoid phenomenon. To exclude a pagetoid phenomenon, perianal extramammary Paget's disease was evaluated via GCDFP15+ and CK20- to determine the correctness of the diagnosis of extramammary Paget's disease. Patients were categorized according to the degree of dermcidin expression, age, sex, and the presence of depigmentation in the skin lesion.

2.2. Immunostaining for Dermcidin

Immunostaining was performed as reported previously [15,16]. In brief, immunochemical staining for dermcidin was conducted using two dermcidin monoclonal antibodies (mAbs) (A-20 and N-20) (Santa Cruz Biotechnology, Santa Cruz, CA, USA) on formalin-fixed, paraffin-embedded specimens. In brief, specimens were cut into 4 μm thick sections and then deparaffinized in xylene and dehydrated through graded alcohol solutions. Antigen retrieval was achieved via boiling in citrate buffer, pH 6.0, using a microwave treatment. All sections were treated with methanol containing 0.3% H_2O_2 for 15 min to block endogenous peroxidase activity. Immunoglobulin G was treated using normal rabbit serum (Nichirei, Tokyo, Japan) to avoid nonspecific antibody binding. After overnight incubation at 4 °C with mouse anti-dermcidin mAb (Lifespan BioSciences, Inc., Seattle, Washington, DC, USA), the sections were incubated with biotinylated rabbit–anti-mouse secondary antibody (Nichirei, Tokyo, Japan) followed by incubation in a streptavidin–peroxidase complex solution for 30 min. Signals were generated via incubation with 3-amino-9-ethyl carbazole to visualize the immunostaining. The expression of dermcidin was classified into 2 groups: dermcidin-positive patients and dermcidin-negative patients. Negative dermcidin indicated absolutely no immunostaining reaction to anti-dermcidin antibody in both specific antibodies.

2.3. Statistical Analyses

Fisher's exact test for unpaired data was used to analyze the association between dermcidin expression and various clinicopathologic factors. Univariate analyses of overall survival were conducted using the log-rank test, and Kaplan–Meier curves were generated. Overall survival was calculated from the date of first diagnosis to the date of death or latest contact with the patient. Univariate analysis was performed using the SPSS software (IBM Corp., Armonk, NY, USA). Kaplan–Meier survival analyses and Fisher's test were performed using GraphPad Prism 4.0. The senser on the survival curve means still alive or discontinuation of follow-up observation during this study period.

2.4. Microarray Data Analysis

For microarray data analysis, dermcidin mRNA expression in healthy subject tissues was obtained from a public data set deposited in the National Center for Biotechnology Information (NCBI) obtained from the Gene Expression Omnibus (GEO) database (GEO accession no. GDS3834) [17]. mRNA was extracted from human tissues, which were purchased from commercial vendors and subjected to microarray analysis.

2.5. Study Approval

Our retrospective study was approved by the Institutional Review Board at the University of Occupational and Environmental Health following the Declaration of Helsinki. Because this study was a retrospective cohort study, the opt-out method of obtaining informed consent was adopted, and informed consent was waived by the Institutional Review Board at the University of Occupational and Environmental Health.

3. Results

3.1. The Finding of Dermcidin-Positive Extramammary Paget's Disease

Dermcidin is produced by the eccrine glands, which are located in the skin. In agreement with this, microarray data set analysis showed that dermcidin expression was highest in the skin from healthy human tissues (Figure 1A). In addition, we confirmed that two antibodies against dermcidin showed a specific positive reaction to the eccrine glands (Figure 1B), suggesting that these antibodies reflect the positivity of dermcidin in the skin.

It has previously been reported that the expression of dermcidin was not identified in epithelial tumors, melanoma, and extramammary Paget's disease [18]. Although there were cases with no staining of dermcidin (Figure 1C), these antibodies showed that several patients diagnosed with extramammary Paget's disease had different expression patterns of dermcidin in the tumor, such as minuscule, average, and strong expression (Figure 1D). These unexpected results prompted us to investigate the characteristics of extramammary Paget's disease with or without dermcidin-positive reaction in further detail.

3.2. The Different Characteristics of Extramammary Paget's Disease Depending on the Expression Degree of Dermcidin

Although extramammary Paget's disease is usually characterized by no expression of dermcidin, as reported previously, we speculated that there were differences in clinical characteristics in extramammary Paget's disease between positive and negative expression of dermcidin.

To clarify this issue, we investigated the differences in age, sex, depigmentation as the manifestation of extramammary Paget's disease, and lymph node metastasis between dermcidin high- and low-expressing groups (Tables 1 and 2). Although there was no significant difference in age, sex, and depigmentation of the tumor, we noticed that the dermcidin-positive group showed a significantly high frequency of nodules and erosion of the tumor upon physical examination. In addition, the dermcidin-positive group also showed a high frequency of dermal invasion and lymph node metastasis. Dermal invasion cases enrolled in this study showed an unfavorable 5-year survival rate of 68.8% ($p < 0.0001$)

(Figure 2). These findings suggest that the positive expression of dermcidin might reflect the extension of tumor development.

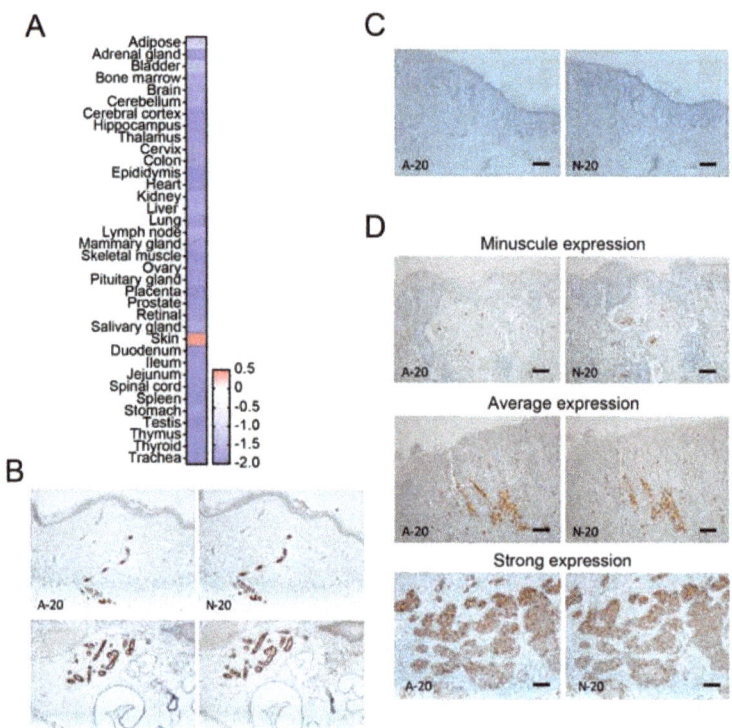

Figure 1. Dermcidin expression in healthy tissue and in the skin and positive staining in extramammary Paget's disease. (**A**) Microarray dataset analysis of dermcidin gene expression; (**B**) representative dermcidin immunostaining for eccrine glands in healthy subjects using two different immunostaining antibodies; (**C,D**) representative negative and (**C,D**) positive staining patterns of dermcidin were observed in extramammary Paget's disease tumor in both intraepithelial and dermal invasive tumors. (**C**) Scale bar: 100 µm; (**D**) scale bar: minuscule expression and average expression were determined at 100 µm, and strong expression was determined at 50 µm.

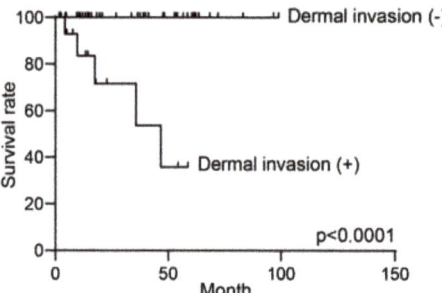

Figure 2. Difference of overall survival curve with or without dermal invasion in extramammary Paget's disease. The overall survival curves were drawn using the Kaplan–Meier method and were compared with the log-rank test.

Table 1. Clinical characteristics of extramammary Paget's disease patients in this study.

Variable		Patients Number
Total		60
Age		
	<60	3
	60–69	13
	70–79	28
	80–89	13
	≥90	3
Sex		
	Male	34
	Female	26
Primary site		
	Genital	54
	Genital and axillary	1
	Genital, axillary, and navel	1
	Perianal	2
	Axillary	1
	Back	1
Clinical manifestations		
	Nodule	9
	Erosion	33
	Depigmentation	21
Dermal invasion		
	Absent	44
	Present	16
Lymph node metastases		
	Absent	52
	Present	8

Table 2. Difference in clinical characteristics in dermcidin expression.

Variable		Total	Dermcidin (+)	Dermcidin (-)	p Value
Total		60	14	46	
Age					0.314
	<70	16	2	14	
	≥70	44	12	32	
Sex					1.000
	Male	34	8	26	
	Female	26	6	20	
Nodule					0.003
	Absent	51	8	43	
	Present	9	6	3	
Erosion					0.013
	Absent	27	2	25	
	Present	33	12	21	
Depigmentation					1.000
	Absent	39	9	30	
	Present	21	5	16	
Dermal invasion					0.006
	Absent	44	6	38	
	Present	16	8	8	
Lymph node metastases					0.013
	Absent	52	9	43	
	Present	8	5	3	

3.3. The Different Prognosis in Extramammary Paget's Disease

We next investigated the prognostic impact of dermcidin in extramammary Paget's disease. The mean survival times were different between positive and negative dermcidin expression in the tumor. Kaplan–Meier curves of overall survival are shown in Figure 3. The overall survival rate in dermcidin-positive patients was significantly lower than that in dermcidin-negative patients. Therefore, a high expression of dermcidin is associated with the poorest prognosis.

Finally, we conducted univariate analyses of dermcidin expression in comparison with clinical variables (Table 3). Univariate analysis showed significantly increased hazard ratios in nodules upon physical examination and dermal invasion and lymph node metastasis in the histological examination, consistent with previous studies [4,19]. In addition, a high expression of dermcidin leads to a significantly increased hazard ratio. Although the impact of dermcidin on prognosis might be limited, dermcidin might become a tool for estimating prognosis in patients with extramammary Paget's disease in some cases.

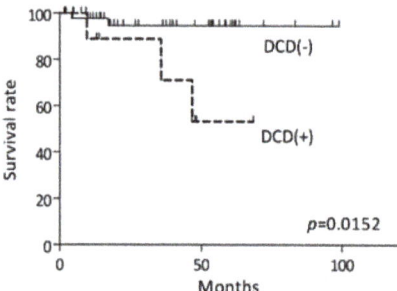

Figure 3. Differences in overall survival curve with or without dermcidin expression in extramammary Paget's disease. The overall survival curves were drawn using the Kaplan–Meier method and were compared with the log-rank test.

Table 3. Univariate analysis of clinical variables.

Variable		HR	95% CI	p Value
Age				0.234
	<70	1		
	≥70	0.3262	0.05144–2.068	
Sex				0.709
	Male	1		
	Female	1.398	0.2406–8.117	
Nodule				<0.0001
	Absent	1		
	Present	7561	338.7–168,800	
Erosion				0.275
	Absent	1		
	Present	2.671	0.4570–15.60	
Depigmentation				0.432
	Absent	1		
	Present	0.4823	0.07834–2.969	
Dermal invasion				<0.0001
	Absent	1		
	Present	240.8	24.80–2338	
Lymph node metastases				<0.0001
	Absent	1		
	Present	442,600	16,480–11,880,000	
dermcidin expression				0.015
	Absent	1		
	Present	16.79	1.721–163.7	

4. Discussion

This study revealed that positive dermcidin expression reflects unfavorable clinical behavior in extramammary Paget's cell tumors. Cancer cell migration into lymph nodes is an important step in the progression toward the advanced stage of malignant tumors. However, the detailed molecular mechanism determining whether dermcidin promotes such tumor cell migration remains unclear.

Our study showed that dermcidin-positive extramammary Page's disease exhibited a high frequency of nodules upon physical examination. One of the reasons behind this might be that dermcidin contributes to the development of the tumor. High dermcidin expression is associated with tumor growth in gastric [20] and breast cancer [21]. Interestingly, dermcidin is also associated with tumor growth and tumor apoptosis in breast cancer. As regards the mechanisms, dermcidin has been found to modulate the HER-2-mediated signal pathway [21], which is one of the major pathways in breast cancer [22]. Because HER-2 signaling is also involved in the pathogenesis of extramammary Paget's disease [23], it is assumed that dermcidin might also activate HER-2 signaling in extramammary Paget's disease and subsequently lead to the development of tumor growth. Because there was no commercially available cell line of extramammary Paget's disease, however, further investigation will be required to clarify the detailed molecular mechanisms.

Several studies have already shown the potential of dermcidin as a biomarker for malignancies. A high expression of dermcidin was identified in approximately 10% of breast cancer patients and has been found to be closely associated with the advanced clinical stage and unfavorable clinical behavior due to regulation of tumor cell growth [24]. Serum dermcidin levels were significantly increased in hepatocellular carcinoma patients and were positively correlated with metastasis [25]. Dermcidin expression in gastric cancer reflects overall survival and is positively correlated with lymph node metastasis [20]. Dermcidin expression is higher in lung cancer patients compared with that in healthy subjects [26]. Among cutaneous malignancies, having high serum levels of dermcidin at the moment of melanoma diagnosis has been associated with the metastatic progression of melanoma among melanoma patients [27,28].

Dermcidin has also been reported as a biomarker in various diseases in addition to malignant tumors. Dermcidin has been identified as a biomarker for Alzheimer's disease (AD) [29], asthma [30], acne vulgaris [31,32], severe obstructive sleep apnea [33], and facioscapulohumeral muscular dystrophy [34]. For example, an abundance of dermcidin was identified in exhaled breath condensate in asthma patients [30]. Therefore, dermcidin may also be a potential biomarker in a variety of skin diseases.

The reason that positive dermcidin expression was observed in clinical patients with unfavorable outcomes who suffered from extramammary Paget's disease remains unclear. A previous study suggested the possibility that one of the characteristics of the eccrine glands might be linked to extramammary Paget's disease. The expressions of histoblood group A type 1, 2, and 3 antigens in normal human skin and extramammary Paget's disease were examined via the immunohistochemical technique [35]. The eccrine glands expressed these antigens, while a negative expression of these antigens was observed in apocrine glands, suggesting that extramammary Paget's disease might be an apocrine-gland-derived tumor stemming from a negative reaction to these antigens. However, 7 out of 16 cases were positive for these antigens, and 6 out of 7 positive cases were associated with dermal invasion. Meanwhile, 5 cases without dermal invasion were negative against these antigens. Although there has been a limited number of studies focusing on this issue to date, the possibility still exists that eccrine gland characteristics include the development of extramammary Paget's disease.

A previous study showed a negative dermcidin expression in patients with extramammary Paget's disease [18]. However, we speculated that the reason behind this result might be that this study did not include any unfavorable clinical cases to show a representative tumor phenotype of extramammary Paget's disease, which is generally located in the epidermis. This previous study may have selected noninvasive extramammary Paget's disease samples to visualize a representative sample of an indolent cutaneous tumor from an extramammary Paget's disease patient.

One possible limitation of our study was that the number of patients involved might not be sufficient to investigate the more detailed characteristics of dermcidin-positive patients with extramammary Paget's disease. Additionally, the detailed molecular role of dermcidin in extramammary Paget's disease for the invasion and metastasis of tumors still needs to be clarified, especially how the degree of dermcidin is associated with the activation of metastatic factors and tumor development, which are involved in the molecular mechanism mediated by HER-2 signaling.

The reason that many of the censored cases are in the dermcidin-negative survival curve may be related to the characteristics of indolent-type cutaneous malignancy. Patients with the nondermal invasion type had their clinical observation follow-up in other hospitals after surgical resection in our department. By contrast, dermal invasion cases are known to have an unfavorable clinical behavior, as shown in Figure 2, and thus, careful follow-up was needed in our hospital or in another hospital where skin oncologists are available.

In conclusion, dermcidin has the potential to help toward the prognosis of extramammary Paget's disease at the moment of surgical resection of the tumor. It is therefore urgently needed to further investigate the actual impact of dermcidin on the molecular mechanism of the development of extramammary Paget's disease.

Author Contributions: S.O. and Y.S. designed, analyzed, and wrote the manuscript. N.S.-S., S.S., Y.M., H.S., H.N., K.Y., and E.O. were extramammary Paget's disease patients treated at our hospital and enrolled in this study who conducted a critical review of this manuscript. M.N. organized this study and wrote the manuscript. All authors have read and agreed to the published version of the manuscript.

Funding: This research received no external funding.

Institutional Review Board Statement: This study was conducted with the approval of and in accordance with the guidelines of the Ethics Committee of the University of Occupational and Environmental Health (approved code H29-211, approved date 20 November 2017), and in accordance with the Declaration of Helsinki. This study was conducted using the opt-out method of obtaining a waiver of informed consent, which was adopted with the Ethics Committee's approval.

Informed Consent Statement: Because this study was a retrospective cohort study, the opt-out method of obtaining informed consent was adopted, and informed consent was waived by the In-stitutional Review Board at the University of Occupational and Environmental Health.

Data Availability Statement: Not applicable.

Conflicts of Interest: This research was conducted in the absence of any commercial or financial relationships that could be construed as a potential conflict of interest.

References

1. Dainichi, T.; Kitoh, A.; Otsuka, A.; Nakajima, S.; Nomura, T.; Kaplan, D.H.; Kabashima, K. The epithelial immune microenvironment (EIME) in atopic dermatitis and psoriasis. *Nat. Immunol.* **2018**, *19*, 1286–1298. [CrossRef] [PubMed]
2. Kabashima, K.; Honda, T.; Ginhoux, F.; Egawa, G. The immunological anatomy of the skin. *Nat. Rev. Immunol.* **2019**, *19*, 19–30. [CrossRef] [PubMed]
3. Sawada, Y.; Gallo, R.L. Role of Epigenetics in the Regulation of Immune Functions of the Skin. *J. Investig. Dermatol.* **2021**, *141*, 1157–1166. [CrossRef] [PubMed]
4. Morris, C.R.; Hurst, E.A. Extramammary Paget's Disease: A Review of the Literature Part II: Treatment and Prognosis. *Dermatol. Surg.* **2020**, *46*, 305–311. [CrossRef]
5. Galloway, T.J.; Ridge, J.A. Management of Squamous Cancer Metastatic to Cervical Nodes With an Unknown Primary Site. *J. Clin. Oncol.* **2015**, *33*, 3328–3337. [CrossRef]
6. Tarhini, A.A. The current state of adjuvant therapy of melanoma. *Lancet Oncol.* **2020**, *21*, 1394–1395. [CrossRef]
7. Sawada, Y.; Bito, T.; Kabashima, R.; Yoshiki, R.; Hino, R.; Nakamura, M.; Shiraishi, M.; Tokura, Y. Ectopic extramammary Paget's disease: Case report and literature review. *Acta Derm. Venereol.* **2010**, *90*, 502–505. [CrossRef]
8. Mazoujian, G.; Pinkus, G.S.; Haagensen, D.E., Jr. Extramammary Paget's disease–evidence for an apocrine origin. An immunoperoxidase study of gross cystic disease fluid protein-15, carcinoembryonic antigen, and keratin proteins. *Am. J. Surg. Pathol.* **1984**, *8*, 43–50. [CrossRef]
9. Hatta, N.; Yamada, M.; Hirano, T.; Fujimoto, A.; Morita, R. Extramammary Paget's disease: Treatment, prognostic factors and outcome in 76 patients. *Br. J. Dermatol.* **2008**, *158*, 313–318. [CrossRef]
10. Ito, Y.; Igawa, S.; Ohishi, Y.; Uehara, J.; Yamamoto, A.I.; Iizuka, H. Prognostic indicators in 35 patients with extramammary Paget's disease. *Dermatol. Surg.* **2012**, *38*, 1938–1944. [CrossRef]
11. van der Zwan, J.M.; Siesling, S.; Blokx, W.A.; Pierie, J.P.; Capocaccia, R. Invasive extramammary Paget's disease and the risk for secondary tumours in Europe. *Eur. J. Surg. Oncol.* **2012**, *38*, 214–221. [CrossRef]

12. Jones, R.E., Jr.; Austin, C.; Ackerman, A.B. Extramammary Paget's disease. A critical reexamination. *Am. J. Dermatopathol.* **1979**, *1*, 101–132. [CrossRef]
13. Schittek, B.; Hipfel, R.; Sauer, B.; Bauer, J.; Kalbacher, H.; Stevanovic, S.; Schirle, M.; Schroeder, K.; Blin, N.; Meier, F.; et al. Dermcidin: A novel human antibiotic peptide secreted by sweat glands. *Nat. Immunol.* **2001**, *2*, 1133–1137. [CrossRef]
14. Dellino, M.; Gargano, G.; Tinelli, R.; Carriero, C.; Minoia, C.; Tetania, S.; Silvestris, E.; Loizzi, V.; Paradiso, A.; Casamassima, P.; et al. A strengthening the reporting of observational studies in epidemiology (STROBE): Are HE4 and CA 125 suitable to detect a Paget disease of the vulva? *Medicine* **2021**, *100*, e24485. [CrossRef]
15. Saito-Sasaki, N.; Sawada, Y.; Okada, E.; Nakamura, M. Cell Adhesion Molecule 1 (CADM1) Is an Independent Prognostic Factor in Patients with Cutaneous Squamous Cell Carcinoma. *Diagnostics* **2021**, *11*, 830. [CrossRef]
16. Mashima, E.; Sawada, Y.; Yamaguchi, T.; Yoshioka, H.; Ohmori, S.; Haruyama, S.; Yoshioka, M.; Okada, E.; Nakamura, M. A high expression of cell adhesion molecule 1 (CADM1) is an unfavorable prognostic factor in mycosis fungoides. *Clin. Immunol.* **2018**, *193*, 121–122. [CrossRef]
17. She, X.; Rohl, C.A.; Castle, J.C.; Kulkarni, A.V.; Johnson, J.M.; Chen, R. Definition, conservation and epigenetics of housekeeping and tissue-enriched genes. *BMC Genom.* **2009**, *10*, 269. [CrossRef]
18. Minami, Y.; Uede, K.; Sagawa, K.; Kimura, A.; Tsuji, T.; Furukawa, F. Immunohistochemical staining of cutaneous tumours with G-81, a monoclonal antibody to dermcidin. *Br. J. Dermatol.* **2004**, *151*, 165–169. [CrossRef]
19. Ito, T.; Kaku, Y.; Nagae, K.; Nakano-Nakamura, M.; Nakahara, T.; Oda, Y.; Hagihara, A.; Furue, M.; Uchi, H. Tumor thickness as a prognostic factor in extramammary Paget's disease. *J. Dermatol.* **2015**, *42*, 269–275. [CrossRef]
20. Zhang, J.; Ding, W.; Kuai, X.; Ji, Y.; Zhu, Z.; Mao, Z.; Wang, Z. Dermcidin as a novel binding protein of lncRNA STCAT3 and its effect on prognosis in gastric cancer. *Oncol. Rep.* **2018**, *40*, 2854–2863. [CrossRef]
21. Bancovik, J.; Moreira, D.F.; Carrasco, D.; Yao, J.; Porter, D.; Moura, R.; Camargo, A.; Fontes-Oliveira, C.C.; Malpartida, M.G.; Carambula, S.; et al. Dermcidin exerts its oncogenic effects in breast cancer via modulation of ERBB signaling. *BMC Cancer* **2015**, *15*, 70. [CrossRef]
22. Slamon, D.J.; Clark, G.M.; Wong, S.G.; Levin, W.J.; Ullrich, A.; McGuire, W.L. Human breast cancer: Correlation of relapse and survival with amplification of the HER-2/neu oncogene. *Science* **1987**, *235*, 177–182. [CrossRef]
23. Tanskanen, M.; Jahkola, T.; Asko-Seljavaara, S.; Jalkanen, J.; Isola, J. HER2 oncogene amplification in extramammary Paget's disease. *Histopathology* **2003**, *42*, 575–579. [CrossRef]
24. Porter, D.; Weremowicz, S.; Chin, K.; Seth, P.; Keshaviah, A.; Lahti-Domenici, J.; Bae, Y.K.; Monitto, C.L.; Merlos-Suarez, A.; Chan, J.; et al. A neural survival factor is a candidate oncogene in breast cancer. *Proc. Natl. Acad. Sci. USA* **2003**, *100*, 10931–10936. [CrossRef]
25. Qiu, F.; Qiu, F.; Liu, L.; Liu, J.; Xu, J.; Huang, X. The Role of Dermcidin in the Diagnosis and Staging of Hepatocellular Carcinoma. *Genet. Test. Mol. Biomark.* **2018**, *22*, 218–223. [CrossRef]
26. Núñez-Naveira, L.; Mariñas-Pardo, L.A.; Montero-Martínez, C. Mass Spectrometry Analysis of the Exhaled Breath Condensate and Proposal of Dermcidin and S100A9 as Possible Markers for Lung Cancer Prognosis. *Lung* **2019**, *197*, 523–531. [CrossRef]
27. Mancuso, F.; Lage, S.; Rasero, J.; Díaz-Ramón, J.L.; Apraiz, A.; Pérez-Yarza, G.; Ezkurra, P.A.; Penas, C.; Sánchez-Diez, A.; García-Vazquez, M.D.; et al. Serum markers improve current prediction of metastasis development in early-stage melanoma patients: A machine learning-based study. *Mol. Oncol.* **2020**, *14*, 1705–1718. [CrossRef]
28. Ortega-Martínez, I.; Gardeazabal, J.; Erramuzpe, A.; Sanchez-Diez, A.; Cortés, J.; García-Vázquez, M.D.; Pérez-Yarza, G.; Izu, R.; Luís Díaz-Ramón, J.; de la Fuente, I.M.; et al. Vitronectin and dermcidin serum levels predict the metastatic progression of AJCC I-II early-stage melanoma. *Int. J. Cancer* **2016**, *139*, 1598–1607. [CrossRef]
29. Kang, S.; Jeong, H.; Baek, J.H.; Lee, S.J.; Han, S.H.; Cho, H.J.; Kim, H.; Hong, H.S.; Kim, Y.H.; Yi, E.C.; et al. PiB-PET Imaging-Based Serum Proteome Profiles Predict Mild Cognitive Impairment and Alzheimer's Disease. *J. Alzheimer's Dis.* **2016**, *53*, 1563–1576. [CrossRef]
30. Bloemen, K.; Van Den Heuvel, R.; Govarts, E.; Hooyberghs, J.; Nelen, V.; Witters, E.; Desager, K.; Schoeters, G. A new approach to study exhaled proteins as potential biomarkers for asthma. *Clin. Exp. Allergy* **2011**, *41*, 346–356. [CrossRef]
31. Alatas, E.T.; Kara Polat, A.; Kalayci, M.; Dogan, G.; Akin Belli, A. Plasma dermcidin levels in acne patients, and the effect of isotretinoin treatment on dermcidin levels. *Dermatol. Ther.* **2019**, *32*, e13044. [CrossRef] [PubMed]
32. El Aziz Ragab, M.A.; Omar, S.S.; Collier, A.; El-Wafa, R.; Gomaa, N. The effect of continuous high versus low dose oral isotretinoin regimens on dermcidin expression in patients with moderate to severe acne vulgaris. *Dermatol. Ther.* **2018**, *31*, e12715. [CrossRef] [PubMed]
33. Kohli, M.; Sharma, S.K.; Upadhyay, V.; Varshney, S.; Sengupta, S.; Basak, T.; Sreenivas, V. Urinary EPCR and dermcidin as potential novel biomarkers for severe adult OSA patients. *Sleep Med.* **2019**, *64*, 92–100. [CrossRef] [PubMed]
34. Corasolla Carregari, V.; Monforte, M.; Di Maio, G.; Pieroni, L.; Urbani, A.; Ricci, E.; Tasca, G. Proteomics of Muscle Microdialysates Identifies Potential Circulating Biomarkers in Facioscapulohumeral Muscular Dystrophy. *Int. J. Mol. Sci.* **2020**, *22*, 290. [CrossRef]
35. Tanaka, A.; Kimura, A.; Yamamoto, Y.; Uede, K.; Furukawa, F. Expression of histo-blood group A type 1, 2 and 3 antigens in normal skin and extramammary Paget's disease. *Acta Histochem. Cytochem.* **2008**, *41*, 165–171. [CrossRef]

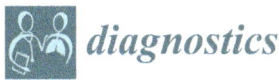

Article

Mechanical Intermittent Compression Affects the Progression Rate of Malignant Melanoma Cells in a Cycle Period-Dependent Manner

Takashi Morikura [1] and Shogo Miyata [2,*]

[1] Graduate School of Science and Technology, Keio University, Yokohama 223-8522, Japan; dnngu-1elife@keio.jp
[2] Department of Mechanical Engineering, Faculty of Science and Technology, Keio University, Yokohama 223-8522, Japan
* Correspondence: miyata@mech.keio.ac.jp

Abstract: Static mechanical compression is a biomechanical factor that affects the progression of melanoma cells. However, little is known about how dynamic mechanical compression affects the progression of melanoma cells. In the present study, we show that mechanical intermittent compression affects the progression rate of malignant melanoma cells in a cycle period-dependent manner. Our results suggest that intermittent compression with a cycle of 2 h on/2 h off could suppress the progression rate of melanoma cells by suppressing the elongation of F-actin filaments and mRNA expression levels related to collagen degradation. In contrast, intermittent compression with a cycle of 4 h on/4 h off could promote the progression rate of melanoma cells by promoting cell proliferation and mRNA expression levels related to collagen degradation. Mechanical intermittent compression could therefore affect the progression rate of malignant melanoma cells in a cycle period-dependent manner. Our results contribute to a deeper understanding of the physiological responses of melanoma cells to dynamic mechanical compression.

Keywords: mechanical intermittent compression; malignant melanoma; in vitro model; cancer progression

1. Introduction

Malignant melanoma is a melanocyte-derived cutaneous skin tumor, which is known as one of the most aggressive cancers and intractable disease with a poor prognosis [1]. The incidence of malignant melanoma is increasing worldwide [2–4], but there are few effective pathological diagnostic techniques to find melanoma [5]. Although a classical "ABCDE" approach is generally considered useful for pathological evaluation of major melanoma subtype such as superficial spreading melanoma (SSM), the pathological evaluation of specific minor subtype is difficult, such as acral lentiginous melanoma (ALM) because the lesions are often heterogeneous and unique [6–8]. The difficulty in diagnosing delays the early detection of lesions, and the associated mortality rate is high because the stage of the disease is often advanced at the time of detection [9,10].

In addition to the lack of effective diagnostics, establishing an effective therapeutic strategy without adverse events remains challenging [11]. Most of the currently available clinical therapies have been developed for major melanoma subtypes, such as SSM, which often occurs in the UV-exposed skin, and there are very few effective treatments for minor subtypes such as ALM, which often occurs on the plantar surface [12,13]. For instance, the molecular targeted drugs and immune checkpoint inhibitors that target mutation, such as BRAF and NRAS gene, are effective for SSM, but ALM has a poor response to these treatments because there are relatively few above-mentioned genetic mutations [14–17]. Therefore, the development of effective treatment and diagnostic strategy for minor melanoma subtypes, such as ALM, is also vitally important.

To establish effective new therapies and diagnostic techniques for cancer, it is important to elucidate the progression mechanisms of the targeted cancer. The development and progression of superficial spreading melanoma, which is common in Caucasoid patients, is correlated with UV exposure, which can cause genetic mutations, such as BRAF and NRAS mutations, which lead to the development and progression of malignant melanoma [18–20]. However, UV exposure of the plantar surface, where ALM commonly occurs, is limited, and some studies have suggested that there is a different mechanism in the progression of melanoma than the genetic mutations caused by UV exposure [12,21]. Recently, the physical environment surrounding malignant melanomas and mechanical stimulus have attracted attention, and the relationship between mechanical stimulation and the progression of malignant melanoma cells has been highlighted.

During tumor growth, cancer cells invade the surrounding interstitial tissue and distantly metastasizes to other tissues by passing through the extracellular matrix (ECM) to infiltrate blood vessels or lymphatics [22–24]. During interstitial tissue invasion, cancer cells are exposed to a variety of mechanical stimuli, such as compression, tension, and shear stimuli. Interestingly, some studies have reported that the behavior of cancer cells changed to adapt to external mechanical stimuli as a biochemical response. Cheng et al. reported that microenvironmental mechanical stimuli regulate tumor size and morphology by inhibiting cell proliferation and promoting apoptosis [25], while Janet et al. showed that mechanical compression contributes to the acquisition of invasive capabilities by cancer cells [26]. Similarly, several previous studies on malignant melanoma have also reported a relationship between the mechanical environment and cancer progression. Importantly, there seems to be a correlation between the area of the plantar surface, where strong mechanical stimuli are applied, and the site of malignant melanoma development, with malignant melanoma size being more expanded in areas under more intense mechanical stimuli [27,28]. We previously reported that static mechanical compression promotes melanoma cell invasion [29]. Those reports suggest that mechanical compression lead a biochemical response associated with progression of melanoma cells. However, little is known about how dynamic mechanical compression affects the progression of melanoma cells. Therefore, in the present study, we investigated the effect of mechanical intermittent compression on the progression of melanoma cells as fundamental research.

The aim of the present study was to elucidate how mechanical intermittent compression affects the progression of malignant melanoma cells in a cell culture model simulating physiological conditions. We established an in vitro cell culture model and cell culture device to apply the mechanical intermittent compression with temporal observation. After the establishment of the cell culture system, the effect of mechanical intermittent compression on the progression of melanoma cells was evaluated.

2. Materials and Methods

2.1. In Vitro Malignant Melanoma Model to Enable Mechanical Intermittent Compression and Temporal Observation of Cell Behavior

A mouse malignant melanoma cell line (B16F10, RIKEN BioResource Center, Tsukuba, Japan) was used to establish an in vitro malignant melanoma model. B16F10 cells were thawed from cryopreserved stock and subcultured twice in Dulbecco's modified Eagle's medium (DMEM)-high glucose, supplemented with 10% fetal bovine serum and 1% antibiotics/antimycotics. The cells were maintained in a 5% CO_2 atmosphere at 37 °C and passaged once in 2–3 days to avoid reaching confluence, which inhibited cell-cell contact.

An in vitro malignant melanoma model was established in our previous study [29]. Briefly, the model was established by seeding B16F10 cells under a type I collagen gel layer, simulating dermal tissue. B16F10 cells were seeded at 1.6×10^5 cells/cm^2 in a 1.5 mm cylindrical area on an f 60 mm cell culture dish (Figure 1a). A type I collagen neutral solution was prepared at a final concentration of 2.4 mg/mL from acid-soluble collagen (I-AC30, KOKEN, Tokyo, Japan). Type I collagen solution (2 mL) was poured into f 60 mm cell culture dishes to cover the B16F10 cells. After polymerization at 37 °C for 20 min, a Cell Culture Insert (pore size; f 8.0 mm, BD Falcon Inc, Franklin Lakes, NJ, USA) was mounted on the gel layer to permit oxygen and nutrient diffusion toward the B16F10 cell-seeded area. The malignant melanoma model was maintained in DMEM-high glucose with 10% FBS and 1% antibiotics/antimycotics at 37 °C in 5% CO_2 for 72 h.

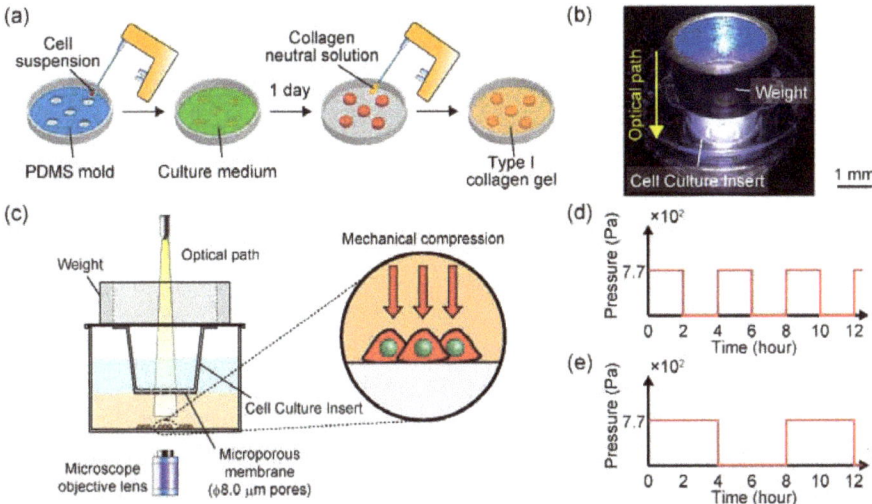

Figure 1. Schematic of the in vitro malignant melanoma model. (**a**) Fabrication of the in vitro malignant melanoma model. B16F10 cells were seeded in a 1.5 mm cylindrical area in the PDMS mold on a cell culture dish. After one day of culture, the mold was removed from the dish and covered with neutralized type I collagen gel. (**b**) Photograph of the experimental set-up. (**c**) Schematic side view of experimental set-up for imposing intermittent mechanical compression and monitoring the cell behavior. (**d**) Mechanical intermittent compression pattern of T = 4 groups. (**e**) Mechanical intermittent compression pattern of T = 8 groups.

A cell culture device was also established to enable intermittent mechanical compression with temporal observation (Figure 1b). To impose mechanical compression onto the gel-covered cells, a cell culture insert with a cylindrical SUS304 weight was mounted on the gel layer (Figure 1c). B16F10 cells were compressed through the collagen gel layer using the Cell Culture Insert with a ring-shaped weight. The melanoma model was subjected to a mechanical intermittent compression of 7.7×10^2 Pa with a cycle of 2 h on/2 h off (T = 4 groups) (Figure 1d) or 4 h on/4 h off (T = 8 groups) (Figure 1e).

Gene expression related to cellular behavior, such as invasion and cell proliferation, fluctuates over time. Gene expression in response to sustained mechanical stimulation is transient, and stabilizes within a few hours. Therefore, we prepared two sample groups that switched mechanical stimuli at the level of several hours. A malignant melanoma model without weights was also prepared similarly for use as the control.

2.2. Creep Phenomenon of Collagen Gel in the Cell Culture Device during Application of Continuous Mechanical Compression

For evaluating the creep in our experimental system, a type I collagen gel containing f 20 mm polystyrene microspheres (Polybead; 18329, Polysciences Inc., Warrington, PA, USA) was prepared. Briefly, a type I collagen neutral solution was prepared at a final concentration of 2.4 mg/mL from I-AC30 acid-soluble collagen. The collagen-neutral solution was mixed with 20 mm polystyrene microspheres to yield a final concentration of 5 v/v% of microspheres. The microspheres were used as markers to evaluate the creep phenomenon of the collagen gel under compression. The type I collagen solution (2 mL) was poured into f 60 mm cell culture dishes, and polymerized at 37 °C for 20 min, and the cell culture insert and ring-shaped weight were mounted on the gel layer, similar to the cell culture experiments.

The prepared creep test specimens were subjected to compressive stimulation for 30 min. Time-lapse images were acquired every minute using a phase contrast microscope (CKX41, Olympus Inc., Tokyo, Japan) equipped with a CCD camera (DP73, Olympus Inc., Tokyo, Japan). Using these images, the temporal strain change in the collagen gel was measured using digital image correlation (DIC), which is a contact-free measurement of material deformation [30,31]. The strain in the collagen gel was measured according to the DIC algorithm at each time point before and after deformation as follows: (1) an interrogation window was set in an arbitrary search area at each time point (Figure 2e). (2) The cross-correlation coefficients of the pixel value pattern in the interrogation window before and after deformation were calculated. (3) The location of the interrogation window where the cross-correlation was maximum was measured as the location after deformation. (4) The displacement of the location between the set interrogation window before and after deformation was calculated as the deformation. (5) Using the measured deformation magnitude, the Green-Lagrange strain was calculated, which contains normal strain and shear strain variables. The normal strain and shear strain in the collagen gel were measured according to the DIC algorithm at each time point before and after deformation, and given as the Green-Lagrange strain. The temporal strain change was measured using the open-source software package Ncorr [32] in the numerical analysis software MATLAB (9.9.0.1570001 (R2020b), MathWorks, Natick, MA, USA).

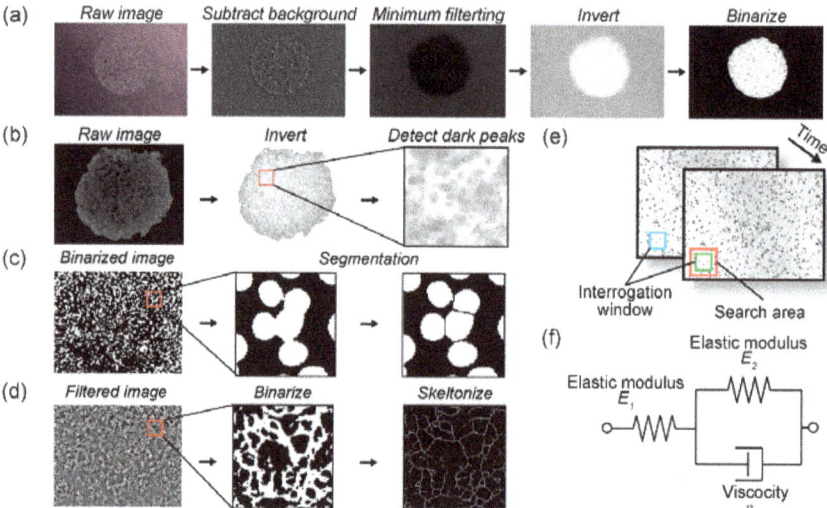

Figure 2. Image analysis and evaluation of creep phenomenon: (**a**) Quantification of cell-occupied area to evaluate cell progression. (**b**) Enumeration of live cells using the ITCN plugin in ImageJ. (**c**) Enumeration of nuclei using binarization and segmentation (**d**) Quantification of total F-actin length using binarization and skeletonization. (**e**) Schematic of digital image correlation method (DIC) (**f**) Three-element generalized Kelvin-Voigt model.

After the representative strain value, defined as the squared norm of the median value of the normal strain in the analyzed area, was calculated, a creep curve was generated. The creep phenomenon of biomaterials, such as biological tissue and collagen gel, is generally described using the generalized Kelvin-Voigt model [33,34]. Nonlinear regression of the creep curve of each sample was performed using a three-element model (Figure 2f). The three-element generalized Kelvin-Voigt model is described as follows:

$$\tau = \frac{\eta}{E_2} \quad (1)$$

$$\gamma = \frac{\sigma_0}{E_1} + \frac{\sigma_0}{E_2}\left(1 - e^{-\frac{t}{\tau}}\right) \qquad (2)$$

where γ is the strain, σ_0 is the applied constant stress, E_i ($i = 1, 2$) is the elastic modulus for each component, and η is the viscosity. The delay time τ of the model, which is defined as Equation (1), was estimated using the Levenberg-Marquardt method in the open-source statistical analysis software R. The fit index between the creep curve and the estimated nonlinear curve using the three-element model was evaluated using Pearson's correlation coefficient.

2.3. Quantification of Cell Progression

The cell behavior was observed for 24 h using a phase-contrast microscope (CKX41, Olympus Inc., Tokyo, Japan) equipped with a CCD camera (DP73, Olympus Inc., Tokyo, Japan). Phase contrast images were continuously acquired at 0 h, 8 h, 16 h, and 24 h under mechanical intermittent compression. Progression was evaluated using the progression distance (l) in the phase-contrast images, which was measured using ImageJ software. To remove the noise within the phase-contrast images, pre-processing was conducted, including filtering and binarization (Figure 2a). The progression distance at each time point (l_t) was calculated as follows:

$$l_t = \sqrt{\frac{a_t}{\pi}} - \sqrt{\frac{a_0}{\pi}} \qquad (3)$$

where a_t is the cell-occupied area at each time and a_0 is the area at 0 h. The radius of the approximate perfect circle, which is equivalent to the cell-occupied area, was calculated, and the difference between the radius of the perfect circle approximating the cell-occupied area at each time and that at the start of culture was defined as the cell progression distance (l_t).

2.4. Cell Viability and Cell Proliferation Assay

To determine the effect of mechanical intermittent compression on cell viability and cell proliferation rate in the malignant melanoma model, a fluorescence live/dead assay was performed after 24 h of culture. The cells were characterized using calcein AM/propidium iodide (PI) double fluorescence staining.

Cell viability was defined as the dead cell rate (DCR), which was calculated as follows:

$$DCR = \frac{N_L}{N_L + N_D} \qquad (4)$$

where N_L is the number of live cells and N_D is the number of dead cells at the end of the culture duration. The number of viable cells (N_L) was measured using the ITCN plugin in ImageJ (Figure 2b). The number of dead cells (N_D) was measured using ImageJ according to the following: (1) grayscale images were binarized using the *Otsu* algorithm, and (2) the nucleus area was segmented using the *watershed* algorithm (Figure 2c).

The cell proliferation rate (CPR) was calculated as follows:

$$CPR = \frac{N_L + N_D}{(N_L + N_D)_{control}} \qquad (5)$$

where N_L and N_D were calculated using the same measurement method as the cell viability assay, and $(N_L + N_D)_{control}$ was defined as the sum of N_L and N_D in the control group.

2.5. Fluorescence Staining of F-Actin and Nuclei

To determine the effect of mechanical intermittent compression on the morphological changes in F-actin filaments in the cell-occupied area, the morphology of F-actin filaments was observed by rhodamine-phalloidin/DAPI fluorescence double staining at 24 h of culture. Briefly, cells in the malignant melanoma model were fixed with 4% paraformaldehyde for 10 min. The cells were then permeabilized with 0.1% Triton X-100 in PBS for 5 min. To stain F-actin filaments, the cells were incubated with 0.7% rhodamine-phalloidin (PHDR1, Cytoskeleton Inc., Denver, CO, USA) for 30 min at 37 °C. After rhodamine-phalloidin staining, 300 nM DAPI solution was added and incubated for 5 min. After removing the DAPI solution, the cells were rinsed with PBS + 1% antimycotic/antibiotic for 5 min three times. F-actin and DAPI were visualized using an inverted fluorescent microscope (CKX41, Olympus Inc., Tokyo, Japan) equipped with a CCD camera (DP73, Olympus Inc., Tokyo, Japan) and fluorescent equipment (U-LH50HG, Olympus Inc., Tokyo, Japan). The length of F-actin filaments was measured to quantitatively evaluate morphological changes in the cytoskeleton. The length of F-actin filaments per single cell (LFC) was calculated as follows:

$$LFC = \frac{L_f}{N_n} \quad (6)$$

where L_f and N_n are the total actin fiber length and number of cell nuclei per acquired image at the end of the culture duration, respectively. The number of cell nuclei per acquired image (N_n) was measured using ImageJ according to the following: (1) grayscale images were binarized using the *mean* algorithm, and (2) the nucleus area was segmented using the *watershed* algorithm (Figure 2c). The total actin fiber length per acquired image (L_f) was measured using ImageJ according to the following: (1) acquired images were pre-processed by a bandpass filter for noise removal and edge-enhancement, (2) grayscale images were binarized using the *Otsu* algorithm, (3) pixels were repeatedly removed from the edges of objects in the binary image until they were reduced to single-pixel-wide shapes, (4) the sum of grayscale in the skeletonized images was equivalent to the total actin fiber length per acquired image (Figure 2d).

2.6. Relative Quantification of mRNA Expression Levels

The relative mRNA expression levels in the cell culture model were quantified by RT-qPCR for matrix metalloproteinase-14 (*Mmp-14*) and glyceraldehyde 3-phosphate dehydrogenase (*Gapdh*), encoding MMP14 and GAPDH, respectively. MMP14 is a key ECM-degrading enzyme, and also a regulator that activates proteins that promote the progression of melanoma cells [35]. GAPDH is a crucial factor in glycolysis and is one of the most commonly used reference genes [36].

Relative mRNA expression levels were measured using total RNA extracted from the cell culture model collected after 24 h of culture. Total RNA was extracted using NucleoSpin RNA kits (740955.50; Takara Bio Inc., Shiga, Japan) and quantified using a Thermal Cycler Dice Real Time System Lite (TP700; Takara Bio Inc., Shiga, Japan). RNA was reverse transcribed into cDNA using the PrimeScript Master Mix (Perfect Real Time) (RR036A; Takara Bio Inc., Shiga, Japan) with an oligo (dT) primer and random hexamer primer for 15 min at 37 °C and 5 s at 85 °C. The concentration of cDNA was quantified using a Biophotometer (6131; Eppendorf, Hamburg, Germany), and then diluted with RNase-free water (9012; Takara Bio Inc., Shiga, Japan) to 10 ng/mL of cDNA. RT-qPCR was conducted in a Thermal Cycler Dice Real Time System Lite using the PCR program 30 s at 95 °C, followed by 60 cycles of 5 s at 95 °C and 30 s at 60 °C. The RT-qPCR reaction mix contained 12.5 µL of TB Green Premix Ex Taq II (Tli RNaseH Plus) (RR820A; Takara Bio Inc., Shiga, Japan), 20 ng of cDNA, 0.4 mM of each forward and reverse primer, and 8.5 µl of RNase-free water. The primer sequences are listed in Table 1. RT-qPCR was performed in technical triplicates for each primer pair and cDNA sample. In addition, the reactions were conducted in biological triplicates under similar conditions. To verify that primer dimers were not responsible for the obtained fluorescence signals, melting curve analysis of the amplicons was performed for each primer pair. Negative control reactions without templates were also included to ensure data quality. Relative mRNA expression was normalized to GAPDH and then calibrated to that of the control group. The fold change was calculated using the $2^{-\Delta\Delta C_t}$ method, where C_t is the threshold cycle.

Table 1. RT-qPCR primer sequences.

Gene Name	Gene Bank Accession Number	Sequence(5'-3')	Tm (°C)	Product Size (bp)
Gapdh	NM_001289726.1	Forward TGTGTCCGTCGTGGATCTGA Reverse TTGCTGTTGAAGTCGCAGGAG	63.9 63.9	3939
Mmp-14	NM_008608.4	Forward CCTCAAGTGGCAGCATAATGAGA Reverse TGGCCTCGAATGTGGCATAC	63.7 64.3	83

2.7. Statistical Analysis

The statistical significance of the differences between experimental groups was evaluated using Dunnett's test. Statistical significance was set at $p < 0.05$ and $p < 0.001$.

3. Results

3.1. Establishment of a Cell Culture Device to Apply Mechanical Intermittent Compression with Temporal Observation

We established a cell culture device to apply mechanical intermittent compression with temporal observation. Prior to observing the progression of melanoma cells in the cell culture device, we evaluated the deformation of collagen gel during applying mechanical compression; the creep phenomenon of the gel.

Representative images of the deformation and strain distribution in the collagen gel are shown in Figure 3a,b. Figure 3c shows the creep curve during mechanical compression and an estimated nonlinear curve fitted by the three-element Kelvin-Voigt model. Regarding the fit index of nonlinear regression, the median of the Pearson correlation coefficients between the creep curves and the estimated nonlinear curves using the generalized Kelvin-Voigt model was 0.968 (Figure 3d). This indicates that the estimation of the creep curve using the models fitted well. As a result of nonlinear regression, the median of the estimated delay time was 7.74 min, which is very small compared to the application time of compression, which was 120 min (Figure 3e). Based on these results, the creep phenomenon horizontal to the surface of the cell culture dish during temporal compression was negligible.

3.2. Progression Rate of Cells in Melanoma Model Was Regulated by Mechanical Intermittent Compression in a Cycle Period-Dependent Manner

Representative microscopic images of B16F10 cells in the control, T = 4, and T = 8 groups are shown in Figure 4a. The white dotted line indicates the cell-occupied area at 0 h of culture, and the yellow dotted line indicates the cell-occupied area at 24 h of culture. The cell-occupied area in the established cell culture model increased during the cultivation period. Figure 4b shows the progression distance at each time, (l_t), during the cultivation period. The slope of the progression distance in the T = 4 group was lower than that in the control group. In contrast, the slope in the T = 8 group was higher than that in the control group. In other words, the progression rate in the T = 4 group decreased, whereas that in the T = 8 group increased. This suggests that intermittent compression with a cycle of 2 h on/2 h off could suppress the progression rate of melanoma cells, while a cycle of 4 h on/4 h off could promote the progression rate.

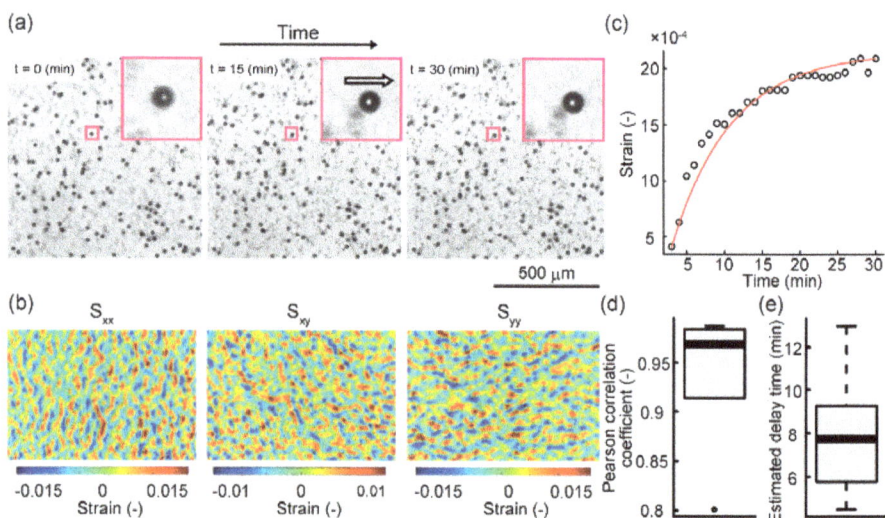

Figure 3. Creep estimation in the collagen gel during mechanical compression: (**a**) Representative time-lapse images acquired by phase contrast microscopy. The black dot object in the image indicates a polystyrene microsphere. The white arrow indicates the direction of displacement. (**b**) Representative images of Green-Lagrange strain. S_{xx} indicates a horizontal normal strain, S_{yy} indicates a vertical normal strain, and S_{xy} indicates a shear strain. (**c**) Representative creep curve and estimated nonlinear curve fitted by the three-element Kelvin-Voigt model. (**d**) Boxplot of Pearson's correlation coefficients. The median of the Pearson's correlation coefficients between the creep curves and the estimated nonlinear curves was 0.968 (n = 6). (**e**) Boxplot of estimated delay time. The median estimated delay time was 7.74 min (n = 6).

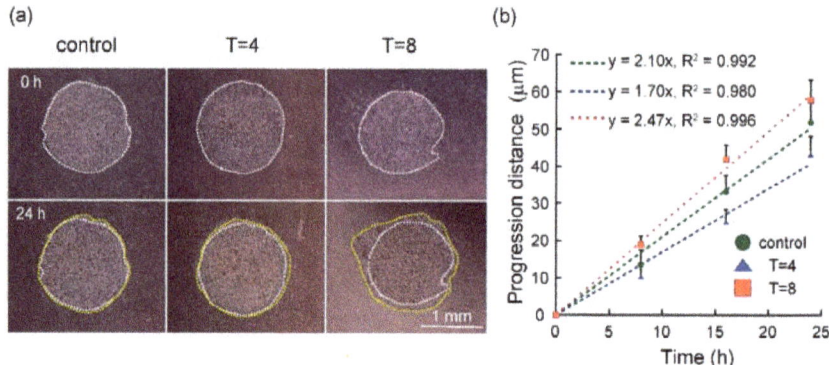

Figure 4. Progression of B16F10 cells in a malignant melanoma model under mechanical intermittent compression. (**a**) Representative phase contrast image. The white dotted lines indicate the cell-adhered area at 0 h of culture, and the yellow dotted lines indicate the cell-adhered area at 24 h of culture. (**b**) Quantification of progression distance. The green circles indicate the progression distance in the control group, the blue triangles indicate the T = 4 group, and red rectangles indicate the T = 8 group. The green, blue, and red dashed lines indicate a regression line to the progression distance in the control, T = 4, and T = 8 groups, respectively (n ≥ 12, data represents the mean ± S.E).

3.3. Cell Viability and Cell Proliferation Rate

Representative fluorescence double staining images using calcein-AM/PI in the control, T = 4, and T = 8 groups are shown in Figure 5a. Most cells in all groups were alive after 24 h of culture. Figure 5b shows the quantitative cell viability, defined as the dead cell rate (DCR). Figure 5c shows the quantitative cell proliferation rate (CPR). There was no significant difference in *DCR* between the control groups and the T = 4 and T = 8 groups. There was no significant difference in *CPR* between the control and T = 4 groups, while the *CPR* in the T = 8 group increased significantly compared to that in the control group. These findings suggest that intermittent compression with a cycle of 2 h on/2 h off did not affect cell viability and proliferation. In contrast, intermittent compression with a cycle of 4 h on/4 h off did not affect cell viability, but promoted cell proliferation.

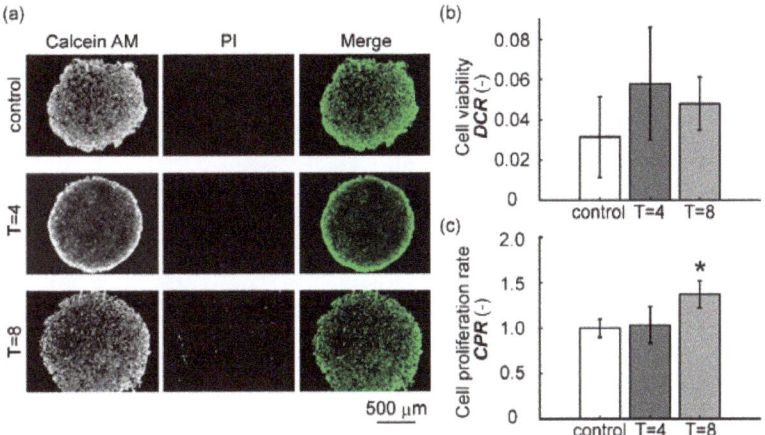

Figure 5. Cell viability and cell proliferation assay. (**a**) Representative fluorescent images stained by calcein AM/PI at 24 h culture duration. The green fluorescence indicates live cells, and the red fluorescence indicates dead cells. (**b**) Quantification of cell viability (*DCR*) (n = 3, mean ± S.D.). (**c**) Quantification of cell proliferation rate (*CPR*) (n = 3, mean ± S.D.). Dunnett's test was used to compare groups. * indicates a significant difference compared to the control group ($p < 0.05$).

3.4. Cell Migration Capacity

Representative rhodamine-phalloidin/DAPI fluorescence staining images in the control, T = 4, and T = 8 groups are shown in Figure 6a. Figure 6b shows the value of the *LFC*, which was defined as the length of F-actin filaments. The *LFC* in the T = 4 group decreased significantly compared to that in the control group, and there was significant decrease between the *LFC* values in the control and T = 8 groups. The LFC in the T = 4 group tended to decrease compared to that in the T = 8 group. In general, elongation of F-actin filaments is correlated with cell motility [37–39]. These results suggest that intermittent compression with a cycle of 2 h on/2 h off could suppress the cell migration capacity rather than a cycle of 4 h on/4 h off.

3.5. Relative mRNA Expression Levels

The relative mRNA expression levels of *Mmp-14* are shown in Figure 6c. The mRNA expression of *Mmp-14* in the T = 4 group was lower than that in the control group, while that in the T = 8 group increased compared to in the control group. Mechanical intermittent compression with a cycle of 2 h on/2 h off might suppress the invasion ability of melanoma cells by regulating the expression of *Mmp-14*. In contrast, compression with a cycle of 4 h on/4 h off might activate the invasive ability of melanoma cells.

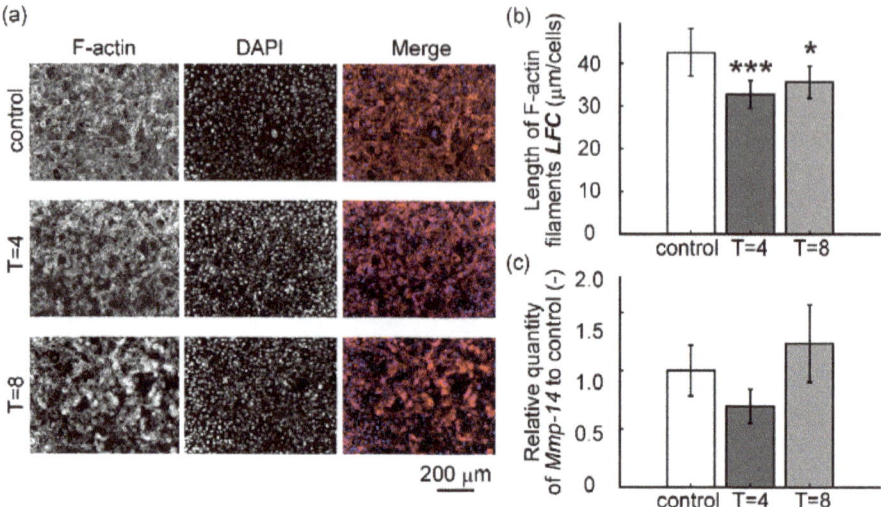

Figure 6. Quantification of cell migration and invasion capacity. (**a**) Representative fluorescence images stained by rhodamine-phalloidin/DAPI at 24 h of culture. The red fluorescence indicates F-actin filaments, and the blue fluorescence indicates nuclei. (**b**) Quantification of the length of F-actin filaments (*LFC*) (n ≥ 3, mean ± S.D.). (**c**) Relative quantity of *Mmp-14* (n = 3, mean ± S.D.). Dunnett's test was used to compare groups. Asterisks indicate a significant difference compared to the control group (*: $p < 0.05$, ***: $p < 0.001$).

4. Discussion

Pathological diagnosis of minor melanoma subtype, which often occurs on the soles of feet, is difficult compared to other melanoma types [6–8]. In addition, the minor subtype responds poorly to current therapy strategies [14–16]. For these reasons, it is important to elucidate the mechanisms by which these minor melanoma progress to establish new pathological diagnostic strategies and therapies. Interestingly, although ultraviolet light is generally thought to be a factor in the development of melanoma, mechanical stimuli may affect the development and progression of melanoma as well as genetic damage caused by UV exposure [12,21]. We previously reported that static mechanical compression promotes the progression of melanoma cells [29]. However, little is known about how dynamic mechanical compression, such as intermittent compression, affects the progression of melanoma cells. The aim of the present study was therefore to elucidate the mechanisms by which mechanical intermittent compression affects the progression of melanoma cells.

We established a cell culture model simulating the physiological conditions of melanomas, and a cell culture device to apply intermittent mechanical compression with temporal observation. In general, it is known that creep occurs when a continuous mechanical force is applied to a viscoelastic material. As a result of the creep phenomenon, the material deforms gradually under continuous force. In the established cell culture device, creep deformation occurred horizontal to the surface of the cell culture dish when a compressive stimulus was applied. The horizontal deformation in response to mechanical compression could apply shear stress to the melanoma cells. If the shear stress is not negligible, it may be a confounding factor in the elucidation of the effects of mechanical intermittent compression on the progression of melanoma cells. Therefore, we evaluated the creep phenomenon of collagen gel in cell culture devices under compression. When the delay time of the creep phenomenon was negligible compared to the observation time, we assumed that the shear stress that the cells were subjected to was also negligible. We measured creep in the collagen gel, and showed that the creep phenomenon in the horizontal direction of the culture dish that was caused by continuous applied compression was negligible. Based on this, we can assume that the effect of intermittent compressive stimulation on melanoma cells can be measured because shear stimulation caused by gel creep can be ignored in the established cell culture device.

We showed that mechanical intermittent compression affects the progression rate of melanoma cells in a cycle period-dependent manner. Interestingly, we found that intermittent compression with a cycle of 2 h on/2 h off suppressed the progression rate of melanoma cells. Under these conditions, the length of F-actin filaments decreased and the mRNA expression level of *Mmp-14*, which is related to collagen degradation, decreased. In general, the cytoskeleton, including F-actin filaments, is reorganized and elongated in the direction of cell migration [40–43]. In other words, the suppression of F-actin filament length correlates with decreased cell motility. In addition, the gene expression level of *Mmp-14*, which promotes collagen degradation, correlates with the invasive ability of melanoma cells in collagen gel [35]. Taken together, these findings suggest that intermittent compression with a cycle of 2 h on/2 h off reduced the progression rate by decreasing the cell migration capacity and invasive ability of melanoma cells through the inhibition of F-actin elongation and collagen degradation, respectively. Here, we should note that the morphological analysis algorithm developed for F-actin has some advantages and limitations compared to conventional analysis approaches. In general, Evaluation of the single-cell level is required to quantify the change of the cytoskeletal morphology. However, in cell culture model simulating biological tissue with high cell density such as our model, it is extremely difficult to segment them even with the advanced mathematical models and machine learning techniques because the cells overlap each other [44]. Hence, to evaluate the morphological changes of the cytoskeleton in the high cell density area, such as our established model, we developed an algorithm to extract the bulk morphological features of the cytoskeleton at the multi-cell level. It has the advantage of being able to measure changes in the cytoskeleton even in regions of high cell density, and the analysis results using our algorithm are sufficient to evaluate the effects between the different stimulus conditions as a fundamental study. On the other hand, the algorithm does not allow for a detailed evaluation of various actin morphologies, such as the filamentous and globular actin. To gain a deeper understanding of cytoskeletal responses under the dynamic mechanical compression, immunofluorescence staining and protein expression analysis are necessary, which is our future work.

In contrast, intermittent compression with a cycle of 4 h on/4 h off could promote the progression rate of melanoma cells. The increasing of the cell-occupied area in the established cell culture model, which indicates the progression of melanoma cells, is caused by the synergistic interaction between cell proliferation, migration, and invasion. The combined effect of those factors causes an increase in the cell-occupied area. As shown in the results from the molecular biological evaluation and image analysis, the cell proliferation and mRNA expression level of *Mmp-14* increased in T = 8 groups. It is also known that the increased mRNA expression level of *Mmp-14* correlates with the promotion of invasion via collagen degradation [45]. Some studies have reported that the collagen degradation by *Mmp-14* is crucial for cancer cells to proliferate and invade in the ECM [46–48]. Shaverdashvili et al. showed that *Mmp-14* is directly contributed to the metastasis of melanoma [49]. In addition, although *Mmp-2* and *Mmp-9* are known to play important roles in the migration and invasion processes of melanoma, *Mmp-14* can activate both [50,51]. Thus, *Mmp-14* is a critical factor in the progression process of melanoma. The result that the expression of *Mmp-14* increased in our melanoma model suggests promoting the progression of melanoma cells. To elucidate the physiological mechanisms of the melanoma progression under the conditions in more detail, the gene expression analysis of other mRNA and protein, such as gene related to cytoskeleton reconstruction, and the metabolic measurements such as glucose consumption are required. In summary, intermittent compression with a cycle of 4 h on/4 h off might promote the progression rate of melanoma cells by accelerating the increase in cell number and invasive ability through the promotion of cell proliferation and collagen degradation, respectively.

We showed for the first time that mechanical intermittent compression affects melanoma cell invasion in a cycle period-dependent manner in this study. However, we should notice that the cell line used in this study is a mouse melanoma cell line, not a human cell line. It is necessary to determine whether the mechanical intermittent compression can affect human melanoma similarly in future work, such as human melanoma cell line and primary melanoma cells collected from the patients. Also, to understand deeply the molecular biological mechanisms more, it is required to conduct comprehensive gene expression analysis and metabolic measurement, and cell culture experiments under cyclic compressive stimulation with different time resolutions in the future.

It may be possible to regulate the invasion of melanoma cells by applying mechanical compressive stimuli with appropriate cycle periods. Mechanical stimuli can be controlled less invasively and more precisely than pharmacokinetic or electromagnetic field control methods. Thus, our results may contribute to establish new therapies that are less invasive and more locally effective than conventional therapies, such as drug therapy, surgery, and radiotherapy. In addition, if a unique relationship between the mechanical stimulation pattern and the progression rate of melanoma is found, new criteria for pathological diagnostic techniques could be established. Our results have the potential to contribute to the establishment of new diagnostic and therapeutic methods.

5. Conclusions

We established an in vitro cell culture model using melanoma cells to simulate the physiological conditions of malignant melanoma, and a cell culture device to apply intermittent mechanical compression with temporal observation.

In the present study, mechanical intermittent compression with a cycle of 2 h on/2 h off could suppress the progression rate of melanoma cells, by suppressing the elongation of F-actin filaments and regulating the levels of mRNA related to collagen degradation. In contrast, mechanical intermittent compression with a cycle of 4 h on/4 h off could promote the progression rate of melanoma cells by promoting cell proliferation and regulating the levels of mRNA related to collagen degradation.

In conclusion, our study revealed that the mechanical intermittent compression affected the progression of melanoma cells in a cycle period-dependent manner. The result will lead to a deeper understanding of melanoma cell behavior under dynamic mechanical compression and could contribute to the establishment of new diagnostics and therapy.

Author Contributions: Conceptualization, T.M. and S.M.; methodology, T.M.; validation, T.M. and S.M.; investigation, T.M.; resources, S.M.; data curation, T.M.; writing—original draft preparation, T.M.; writing—review and editing, S.M.; visualization, T.M.; supervision, S.M.; project administration, S.M.; funding acquisition, T.M. and S.M. Both authors have read and agreed to the published version of the manuscript.

Funding: This research was partially supported by the JSPS KAKENHI (Grant numbers: 17K01369 and 26560222), the Translational Research Network Program from Japan Agency for Medical Research and Development (AMED), and Mori Manufacturing Research and Technology Foundation.

Conflicts of Interest: The authors declare no conflict of interest.

References

1. Kalampokas, E.; Kalampokas, T.; Damaskos, C. Primary Vaginal Melanoma, a Rare and Aggressive Entity. A Case Report and Review of the Literature. *In Vivo* **2017**, *31*, 133–140. [CrossRef] [PubMed]
2. de Vries, E.; Bray, F.I.; Coebergh, J.W.W.; Parkin, D.M. Changing Epidemiology of Malignant Cutaneous Melanoma in Europe 1953–1997: Rising Trends in Incidence and Mortality but Recent Stabilizations in Western Europe and Decreases in Scandinavia. *Int. J. Cancer* **2003**, *107*, 119–126. [CrossRef]
3. Stang, A.; Pukkala, E.; Sankila, R.; Söderman, B.; Hakulinen, T. Time Trend Analysis of the Skin Melanoma Incidence of Finland From 1953 Through 2003 Including 16,414 Cases. *Int. J. Cancer* **2006**, *119*, 380–384. [CrossRef] [PubMed]
4. Koh, D.; Wang, H.; Lee, J.; Chia, K.S.; Lee, H.P.; Goh, C.L. Basal Cell Carcinoma, Squamous Cell Carcinoma and Melanoma of the Skin: Analysis of the Singapore Cancer Registry Data 1968–1997. *Br. J. Dermatol.* **2003**, *148*, 1161–1166. [CrossRef] [PubMed]
5. Domingues, B.; Lopes, J.M.; Soares, P.; Pópulo, H. Melanoma Treatment in Review. *Immuno Targets Ther.* **2018**, *7*, 35–49. [CrossRef]

6. Chang, J.W.C. Acral Melanoma: A Unique Disease in Asia. *JAMA Dermatol.* **2013**, *149*, 1272–1273. [CrossRef]
7. Borkowska, A.M.; Szumera-Ciećkiewicz, A.; Spałek, M.J.; Teterycz, P.; Czarnecka, A.M.; Rutkowski, P.Ł. Clinicopathological Features and Prognostic Factors of Primary Acral Melanomas in Caucasians. *J. Clin. Med.* **2020**, *9*, 2996. [CrossRef]
8. Guo, J.; Si, L.; Kong, Y.; Flaherty, K.T.; Xu, X.; Zhu, Y.; Corless, C.L.; Li, L.; Li, H.; Sheng, X.; et al. Phase II, Open-Label, Single-Arm Trial of Imatinib Mesylate in Patients With Metastatic Melanoma Harboring c-Kit Mutation or Amplification. *J. Clin. Oncol.* **2011**, *29*, 2904–2909. [CrossRef]
9. Bai, X.; Mao, L.L.; Chi, Z.H.; Sheng, X.N.; Cui, C.L.; Kong, Y.; Dai, J.; Wang, X.; Li, S.M.; Tang, B.X.; et al. BRAF Inhibitors: Efficacious and Tolerable in BRAF-Mutant Acral and Mucosal Melanoma. *Neoplasma* **2017**, *64*, 626–632. [CrossRef]
10. Nakamura, Y.; Namikawa, K.; Yoshino, K.; Yoshikawa, S.; Uchi, H.; Goto, K.; Nakamura, Y.; Fukushima, S.; Kiniwa, Y.; Takenouchi, T.; et al. Anti-PD1 Checkpoint Inhibitor Therapy in Acral Melanoma: A Multicenter Study of 193 Japanese Patients. *Ann. Oncol.* **2020**, *31*, 1198–1206. [CrossRef] [PubMed]
11. Hall, K.H.; Rapini, R.P. Acral Lentiginous Melanoma. In *StatPearls*; StatPearls Publishing: Treasure Island, FL, USA, 2021.
12. Bristow, I.R.; Acland, K. Acral Lentiginous Melanoma of the Foot and Ankle: A Case Series and Review of the Literature. *J. Foot Ankle Res.* **2008**, *1*, 11. [CrossRef]
13. Albreski, D.; Sloan, S.B. Melanoma of the Feet: Misdiagnosed and Misunderstood. *Clin. Dermatol.* **2009**, *27*, 556–563. [CrossRef] [PubMed]
14. Bristow, I.R.; de Berker, D.A.; Acland, K.M.; Turner, R.J.; Bowling, J. Clinical Guidelines for the Recognition of Melanoma of the Foot and Nail Unit. *J. Foot Ankle Res.* **2010**, *3*, 25. [CrossRef]
15. Stalkup, J.R.; Orengo, I.F.; Katta, R. Controversies in Acral Lentiginous Melanoma. *Dermatol. Surg.* **2002**, *28*, 1051–1059. [PubMed]
16. Kwon, I.H.; Lee, J.H.; Cho, K.H. Acral Lentiginous Melanoma In Situ: A Study of Nine Cases. *Am. J. Dermatopathol.* **2004**, *26*, 285–289. [CrossRef] [PubMed]
17. Borkowska, A.; Szumera-Ciećkiewicz, A.; Spałek, M.; Teterycz, P.; Czarnecka, A.; Kowalik, A.; Rutkowski, P. Mutation profile of primary subungual melanomas in Caucasians. *Oncotarget* **2020**, *11*, 2404–2413. [CrossRef]
18. Gandini, S.; Sera, F.; Cattaruzza, M.S.; Pasquini, P.; Picconi, O.; Boyle, P.; Melchi, C.F. Meta-Analysis of Risk Factors for Cutaneous Melanoma: II. Sun Exposure. *Eur. J. Cancer* **2005**, *41*, 45–60. [CrossRef] [PubMed]
19. Hodis, E.; Watson, I.R.; Kryukov, G.V.; Arold, S.T.; Imielinski, M.; Theurillat, J.P.; Nickerson, E.; Auclair, D.; Li, L.; Place, C.; et al. A Landscape of Driver Mutations in Melanoma. *Cell* **2012**, *150*, 251–263. [CrossRef]
20. Chang, Y.M.; Barrett, J.H.; Bishop, D.T.; Armstrong, B.K.; Bataille, V.; Bergman, W.; Berwick, M.; Bracci, P.M.; Elwood, J.M.; Ernstoff, M.S.; et al. Sun Exposure and Melanoma Risk at Different Latitudes: A Pooled Analysis of 5700 Cases and 7216 Controls. *Int. J. Epidemiol.* **2009**, *38*, 814–830. [CrossRef]
21. Curtin, J.A.; Fridlyand, J.; Kageshita, T.; Patel, H.N.; Busam, K.J.; Kutzner, H.; Cho, K.H.; Aiba, S.; Bröcker, E.B.; LeBoit, P.E.; et al. Distinct Sets of Genetic Alterations in Melanoma. *N. Engl. J. Med.* **2005**, *353*, 2135–2147. [CrossRef]
22. Wittekind, C.; Neid, M. Cancer Invasion and Metastasis. *Oncology* **2005**, *69* (Suppl. 1), 14–16. [CrossRef]
23. Krakhmal, N.V.; Zavyalova, M.V.; Denisov, E.V.; Vtorushin, S.V.; Perelmuter, V.M. Cancer Invasion: Patterns and Mechanisms. *Acta Nat.* **2015**, *7*, 17–28. [CrossRef]
24. Geiger, T.R.; Peeper, D.S. Metastasis Mechanisms. *Biochim. Biophys. Acta* **2009**, *1796*, 293–308. [CrossRef]
25. Cheng, G.; Tse, J.; Jain, R.K.; Munn, L.L. Micro-Environmental Mechanical Stress Controls Tumor Spheroid Size and Morphology by Suppressing Proliferation and Inducing Apoptosis in Cancer Cells. *PLoS ONE* **2009**, *4*, e4632. [CrossRef]
26. Tse, J.M.; Cheng, G.; Tyrrell, J.A.; Wilcox-Adelman, S.A.; Boucher, Y.; Jain, R.K.; Munn, L.L. Mechanical Compression Drives Cancer Cells Toward Invasive Phenotype. *Proc. Natl. Acad. Sci. USA* **2012**, *109*, 911–916. [CrossRef] [PubMed]
27. Stucke, S.; McFarland, D.; Goss, L.; Fonov, S.; McMillan, G.R.; Tucker, A.; Berme, N.; Cenk Guler, H.; Bigelow, C.; Davis, B.L. Spatial Relationships Between Shearing Stresses and Pressure on the Plantar Skin Surface During Gait. *J. Biomech.* **2012**, *45*, 619–622. [CrossRef] [PubMed]
28. Minagawa, A.; Omodaka, T.; Okuyama, R. Melanomas and Mechanical Stress Points on the Plantar Surface of the Foot. *N. Engl. J. Med.* **2016**, *374*, 2404–2406. [CrossRef]
29. Morikura, T.; Miyata, S. Effect of Mechanical Compression on Invasion Process of Malignant Melanoma Using In Vitro Three-Dimensional Cell Culture Device. *Micromachines* **2019**, *10*, 666. [CrossRef]
30. Chu, T.C.; Ranson, W.F.; Sutton, M.A. Applications of Digital-Image-Correlation Techniques to Experimental Mechanics. *Exp. Mech.* **1985**, *25*, 232–244. [CrossRef]
31. Sutton, M.; Mingqi, C.; Peters, W.; Chao, Y.; McNeill, S. Application of an Optimized Digital Correlation Method to Planar Deformation Analysis. *Image Vis. Comput.* **1986**, *4*, 143–150. [CrossRef]
32. Blaber, J.; Adair, B.; Antoniou, A. Ncorr: Open-Source 2D Digital Image Correlation MATLAB Software. *Exp. Mech.* **2015**, *55*, 1105–1122. [CrossRef]
33. Ortiz, J.S.E.; Lagos, R.E. A Viscoelastic Model to Simulate Soft Tissue Materials. *J. Phys. Conf. Ser.* **2015**, *633*, 012099. [CrossRef]
34. Jayabal, H.; Dingari, N.N.; Rai, B. A Linear Viscoelastic Model to Understand Skin Mechanical Behaviour and for Cosmetic Formulation Design. *Int. J. Cosmet. Sci.* **2019**, *41*, 292–299. [CrossRef] [PubMed]
35. Thakur, V.; Bedogni, B. The Membrane Tethered Matrix Metalloproteinase MT1-MMP at the Forefront of Melanoma Cell Invasion and Metastasis. *Pharmacol. Res.* **2016**, *111*, 17–22. [CrossRef] [PubMed]

36. Barber, R.D.; Harmer, D.W.; Coleman, R.A.; Clark, B.J. GAPDH as a Housekeeping Gene: Analysis of GAPDH mRNA Expression in a Panel of 72 Human Tissues. *Physiol. Genom.* **2005**, *21*, 389–395. [CrossRef] [PubMed]
37. Pollard, T.D.; Borisy, G.G. Cellular Motility Driven by Assembly and Disassembly of Actin Filaments. *Cell* **2003**, *112*, 453–465. [CrossRef]
38. Carlier, M.F.; Pantaloni, D. Control of Actin Assembly Dynamics in Cell Motility. *J. Biol. Chem.* **2007**, *282*, 23005–23009. [CrossRef]
39. Jacquemet, G.; Hamidi, H.; Ivaska, J. Filopodia in Cell Adhesion, 3D Migration and Cancer Cell Invasion. *Curr. Opin. Cell Biol.* **2015**, *36*, 23–31. [CrossRef]
40. Woodrum, D.T.; Rich, S.A.; Pollard, T.D. Evidence for Biased Bidirectional Polymerization of Actin Filaments Using Heavy Meromyosin Prepared by an Improved Method. *J. Cell Biol.* **1975**, *67*, 231–237. [CrossRef]
41. Pollard, T.D.; Cooper, J.A. Actin and Actin-Binding Proteins. A Critical Evaluation of Mechanisms and Functions. *Annu. Rev. Biochem.* **1986**, *55*, 987–1035. [CrossRef]
42. Suetsugu, S. Shaping the Membrane at Submicron Scale by BAR Proteins and the Actin Cytoskeleton. *Seikagaku* **2014**, *86*, 637–649.
43. Gardel, M.L.; Schneider, I.C.; Aratyn-Schaus, Y.; Waterman, C.M. Mechanical Integration of Actin and Adhesion Dynamics in Cell Migration. *Annu. Rev. Cell Dev. Biol.* **2010**, *26*, 315–333. [CrossRef]
44. Peng, H. Bioimage informatics: A new area of engineering biology. *Bioinformatics* **2008**, *24*, 1827–1836. [CrossRef] [PubMed]
45. Altadill, A.; Rodríguez, M.; González, L.O.; Junquera, S.; Corte, M.D.; González-Dieguez, M.L.; Linares, A.; Barbón, E.; Fresno-Forcelledo, M.; Rodrigo, L.; et al. Liver expression of matrix metalloproteases and their inhibitors in hepatocellular carcinoma. *Dig. Liver Dis.* **2009**, *41*, 740–748. [CrossRef]
46. Hotary, K.B.; Allen, E.D.; Brooks, P.C.; Datta, N.S.; Long, M.W.; Weiss, S.J. Membrane type I matrix metalloproteinase usurps tumor growth control imposed by the three-dimensional extracellular matrix. *Cell* **2003**, *114*, 33–45. [CrossRef]
47. Koshikawa, N.; Minegishi, T.; Sharabi, A.; Quaranta, V.; Seiki, M. Membrane-type matrix metalloproteinase-1 (MT1-MMP) is a processing enzyme for human laminin gamma 2 chain. *J. Biol. Chem.* **2005**, *280*, 88–93. [CrossRef] [PubMed]
48. Seiki, M. The cell surface: The stage for matrix metalloproteinase regulation of migration. *Curr. Opin. Cell Biol.* **2002**, *14*, 624–632. [CrossRef]
49. Shaverdashvili, K.; Wong, P.; Ma, J.; Zhang, K.; Osman, I.; Bedogni, B. MT1-MMP modulates melanoma cell dissemination and metastasis through activation of MMP2 and RAC1. *Pigment. Cell Melanoma Res.* **2014**, *27*, 287–296. [CrossRef]
50. Sato, H.; Takino, T.; Okada, Y.; Cao, J.; Shinagawa, A.; Yamamoto, E.; Seiki, M. A matrix metalloproteinase expressed on the surface of invasive tumour cells. *Nature* **1994**, *370*, 61–65. [CrossRef] [PubMed]
51. Ranjan, A.; Kalraiya, R.D. Invasive potential of melanoma cells correlates with the expression of MT1-MMP and regulated by modulating its association with motility receptors via N-glycosylation on the receptors. *Biomed. Res. Int.* **2014**, *2014*, 804680. [CrossRef] [PubMed]

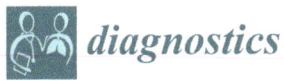

Article

STAT3 Activation in Psoriasis and Cancers

Megumi Kishimoto [1], Mayumi Komine [1,*], Miho Sashikawa-Kimura [1], Tuba Musarrat Ansary [1], Koji Kamiya [1], Junichi Sugai [1], Makiko Mieno [2], Hirotoshi Kawata [3], Ryutaro Sekimoto [4], Noriyoshi Fukushima [3] and Mamitaro Ohtsuki [1]

[1] Department of Dermatology, Jichi Medical University, Shimotsuke-shi 329-0498, Tochigi, Japan; megumihkishimoto@gmail.com (M.K.); sashikawa@jichi.ac.jp (M.S.-K.); tuba2020@jichi.ac.jp (T.M.A.); m01023kk@jichi.ac.jp (K.K.); junsugar1112@gmail.com (J.S.); mamitaro@jichi.ac.jp (M.O.)
[2] Department of Medical Informatics, Center for Information, Jichi Medical University, Shimotsuke-shi 329-0498, Tochigi, Japan; mnaka@jichi.ac.jp
[3] Department of Diagnostic Pathology, Jichi Medical University, Shimotsuke-shi 329-0498, Tochigi, Japan; kawata@jichi.ac.jp (H.K.); nfukushima@jichi.ac.jp (N.F.)
[4] Department of Pathology, Tokyo Metropolitan Cancer and Infectious Diseases Center Komagome Hospital, Bunkyo-ku, Tokyo 113-8677, Japan; rsekimoto@gmail.com
* Correspondence: mkomine12@jichi.ac.jp; Tel.: +81-285-58-7360

Abstract: Activation of signal transducer and activator of transcription (STAT)3 has been reported in many cancers. It is also well known that STAT3 is activated in skin lesions of psoriasis, a chronic skin disease. In this study, to ascertain whether patients with psoriasis have a predisposition to STAT3 activation, we examined phosphorylated STAT3 in cancer cells of psoriasis patients via immunohistochemistry. We selected patients with psoriasis who visited the Department of Dermatology, Jichi Medical University Hospital, from January 2000 to May 2015, and had a history of cancer. We performed immunostaining for phosphorylated STAT3 in tumor cells of five, four, and six cases of gastric, lung, and head and neck cancer, respectively. The results showed that there was no significant difference in STAT3 activation in any of the three cancer types between the psoriasis and control groups. Although this study presents limitations in its sample size and inconsistency in the histology and differentiation of the cancers, results suggest that psoriasis patients do not have a predisposition to STAT3 activation. Instead, STAT3 activation is intricately regulated by each disorder or cellular microenvironment in both cancer and psoriasis.

Keywords: psoriasis; STAT3; cancer; immunohistochemistry

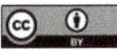

1. Introduction

Psoriasis is a chronic inflammatory skin disease associated with musculoskeletal symptoms in about 25% of patients [1]. Psoriasis is thought to be triggered by environmental factors such as trauma and infection in addition to genetic background, with both innate and acquired immunity involved in its pathogenesis. The pathogenesis of psoriasis has been intensively investigated, but its enigmatic nature has yet to be defined [2]. The relationship between psoriasis and STAT3 was first described by Sano et al. in 2005, when they reported that STAT3 was activated in keratinocytes of psoriasis lesions [3]. Since then, STAT3 hyperactivation has been reported in the cell types involved in psoriasis, including Th17 cells and keratinocytes [4].

STAT3 was first identified in 1993 [5] and known to be an important transcription factor and mediator in a number of different cell biological processes including proliferation, survival, differentiation, and angiogenesis under both physiological and pathological conditions [6,7]. It is one of the members of the seven STAT proteins, STAT 1, 2, 3, 4, 5A, 5B, and 6 [8]. Activation of STAT3 usually occurs through phosphorylation, in response to all IL-6 family members and various other cytokines, growth factors, oncoproteins, and hormones such as leptin [4,5,9]. STAT3 has two phosphorylation sites, namely a tyrosine residue (Tyr705) and a serine residue (Ser727) [10]. The canonical function of STAT3 as a transcription factor is mainly through the phosphorylation of tyrosine [7]. When a ligand binds to its cognate receptor, phosphorylation of Tyr705 occurs, resulting in dimerization of STAT3 and its translocation into the nucleus to exert its function as a transcription factor [5,11]. Non-receptor tyrosine kinases, such as c-Src, MAPK, and Abl are also involved in the activation of STAT3 through Tyr 705 phosphorylation [12]. Phosphorylation of Tyr705 plays a main and important role in the transcriptional function of STAT3, while phosphorylation of Ser727 also has various functions [12]. STAT3 is found in mitochondria, acting as a modulator of mitochondrial respiration and regulator of complex I activity and ROS production. These activities are related to the phosphorylation of Ser727 [13,14].

In recent years, there have been many reports of STAT3 overexpression has been found in cancer cells. Activation of STAT3 in malignant tumors has been implicated in poor prognosis, metastasis, and proliferation of cancers, and several STAT3 inhibitors are currently under development [5].

STAT3 is also involved in inflammation and immunity [15–17]. As mentioned above, Sano et al. reported in 2005 that STAT3 activation was observed in human epidermal keratinocytes in more than 90% ($n = 19$ of 21) of psoriatic lesions and some adjacent uninvolved epidermis by immunohistochemical analyses [3]. They also reported that transgenic mice expressing a constitutively active form of STAT3 in keratinocytes developed skin lesions that closely resembled human psoriasis [3]. STAT3 has recently emerged as a key player in the development and pathogenesis of psoriasis and psoriasis-like inflammatory conditions [4].

The risk of malignancy in patients with psoriasis is thought to be slightly increased compared to that in the normal population; thus, we speculated that STAT3 activation in psoriasis patients is related to malignancy risk.

In this study, we investigated the rate of active STAT3 tumors in patients with psoriasis compared to that in patients with eczema. To the best of our knowledge, very few studies have focused on STAT3 expression in the tumor cells of patients with psoriasis.

2. Materials and Methods

2.1. Patients

We selected Japanese patients with psoriasis and Japanese patients with eczema without psoriasis who presented to the Department of Dermatology in Jichi Medical University Hospital between 1 January 2000 and 31 May 2015. Among these patients, those with a medical history of non-skin cancers were selected for statistical analyses of malignancy risk. For the STAT3 immunohistochemical study, we extracted those who had undergone biopsy or surgery of their tumor at our hospital with a sufficient quantity of paraffin-embedded samples.

All patients with psoriasis and eczema were clinically diagnosed by experienced dermatologists with or without histological examination. All malignant tumors underwent histopathological diagnosis by pathologists. All patients were aged 20 years or above. All protocols were approved by the ethics committee of the Jichi Medical University.

2.2. Immunohistochemical Staining

Formalin-fixed, paraffin-embedded samples were sliced to a thickness of 5 mm. Antigen retrieval was performed by autoclaving sample slides at 120 °C for 10 min in citrate buffer (pH 6.0) and incubated with the primary antibody, rabbit monoclonal anti-phosphorylated STAT3 (Tyr 705) antibody (Cell Signaling Technology, Danvers, MA, USA), at a dilution of 1:100 overnight at 4 °C. Peroxidase staining was then performed with VECTASTAIN®ABC Kit (Vector Laboratories, Inc., Burlingame, CA, USA) following the manufacturer's protocol, with diaminobenzidine (DAB, Dojindo, Kumamoto, Japan) as a chromogenic substrate.

2.3. Immunohistochemical Analysis

The outcomes of the staining were assessed by two factors: the staining intensity and the proportion of positive cells among cancer cells. Since phosphorylated STAT3 usually localizes to the nucleus, the staining of the nucleus was evaluated with anti-phosphorylated STAT3 antibody. The staining intensity was graded with a score of 0 to 3 (0: no staining, 1: mild staining, 2: moderate staining and 3: strong staining), and the proportion of positive cells was graded with a score of 0 to 3 (0: <1%, 1: 1–33%, 2: 34–66% and 3: 67–100%) by three independent experienced researchers under an optical microscope (BX53, Olympus, Tokyo, Japan).

The final score for each specimen was defined as the sum of the intensity score and proportion score.

2.4. Statistical Analysis

Chi-squared test and Student's t-test were used to compare the groups. The Mantel-Haenszel method was used to determine the difference in the frequency of cancer in each organ between the psoriasis and control groups.

The Mann–Whitney U test was used to compare the expression of phosphorylated STAT3 between the groups. Statistical significance was set at $p < 0.05$. Statistical analysis was performed using IBM SPSS software (version 22.0).

3. Results

There was no significant difference in the frequency of malignant tumors in each organ between the psoriasis and eczema groups, but the frequency of patients with multiple malignant tumors was higher in the psoriasis group than in the eczema group.

A total of 103 cancers in 87 psoriasis patients and 135 cancers in 126 control patients were extracted from their medical records. The types of psoriasis patients included 79 cases (91%) of plaque psoriasis, one case (1.1%) of guttata psoriasis, four cases (4.6%) of generalized pustular psoriasis, one case (1.1%) of erythrodermic psoriasis, and two cases (2.3%) of psoriatic arthritis. This proportion is similar to that reported in the epidemiological surveillance of psoriasis patients in Japan from 2009 to 2012 [18]. Table 1 shows the cancer types in the psoriasis and control groups. There was no significant difference in the frequency of occurrence of cancers in any organ between the psoriasis and control groups, but the percentage of multiple cancers was significantly higher in the psoriasis patient group ($p = 0.007$). Among these, we selected cases with paraffin-embedded tumor samples that were able to match the cancer type with the control group.

These included five, four, and six cases in the psoriasis group and 16, six, and six cases in the control group, with gastric, lung, and head and neck cancers, respectively. The backgrounds of patients with psoriasis and control patients are shown in Table 2. All psoriasis patients selected for immunostaining had plaque type psoriasis, and three patients had double cancers: one with gastric cancer and lung cancer, one with lung cancer and lymphoma, and one with head and neck cancer and esophageal cancer. The histological type of each cancer was not completely matched among the groups, but sex ratio and age of onset of cancer were not statistically different.

The frequency of phosphorylated STAT3-positive cancers was not elevated in the psoriasis group compared to eczema group. Immunohistochemical staining images with anti-phosphorylated STAT3 antibodies representing the different scores are shown in Figure 1. There were no statistically significant differences in the staining scores of phosphorylated STAT3 between the psoriasis patient group and the control patient group for gastric, lung, and head and neck cancers.

Table 1. Types of cancer associated with psoriasis and control patients.

Types of Cancer	103 Cancers from 87 Psoriasis Patients			135 Cancers from 126 Control Patients		
		Male (n = 74)	Female (n = 13)		Male (n = 84)	Female (n = 42)
Gastric cancer	15	14	1	22	19	3
Liver cancer	15	13	2	14	12	2
Colon and rectal cancer	11	11	0	16	12	4
Lung cancer	10	10	0	13	9	4
Prostate cancer	8	8	0	13	13	0
Head and neck cancer	8	8	0	11	8	3
Renal cancer	6	4	2	3	2	1
Breast cancer	6	0	6	11	0	11
Esophageal cancer	5	5	0	2	2	0
Urinary tract cancer	5	5	0	7	5	2
Hematologic malignancy	5	5	0	8	4	4
Biliary tract cancer	3	2	1	1	1	0
Uterine cancer	2	0	2	7	0	7
Thyroid cancer	2	1	1	0	0	0
Pancreatic cancer	1	1	0	3	3	0
Mesenchymal tumor	1	1	0	2	2	0
Ovarian cancer	0	0	0	1	0	1
Cecal cancer	0	0	0	1	1	0
percentage of multiple cancers		19.5% *			7.7% *	

* $p = 0.007$.

Table 2. Patients' characteristics.

	Psoriasis Patients					Control Patients			
	Number	Male/Female	Average Age of Onset	Histopathology		Number	Male/Female	Average Age of Onset	Histopathology
gastric cancer	5	4/1	69.8	adenocarcinoma 5		16	14/2	69.7	adenocarcinoma 16
lung cancer	4	3/1	63	squamous cell carcinoma 1 adenocarcinoma 3		6	5/1	66.3	small cell carcinoma 1 squamous cell carcinoma 1 adenocarcinoma 4
head and neck cancer	6	5/1	65.5	squamous cell carcinoma 6		6	4/2	69.0	squamous cell carcinoma 6

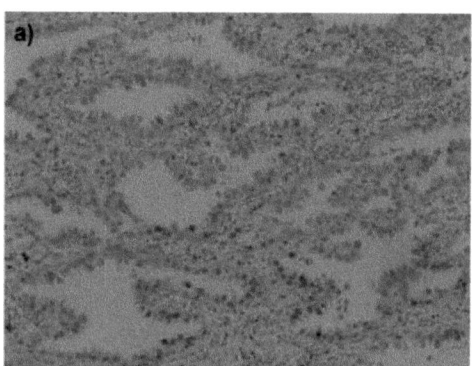
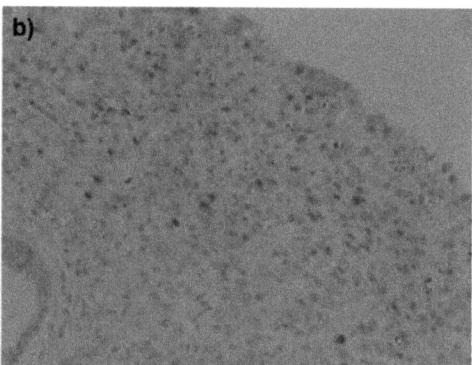

Figure 1. Cont.

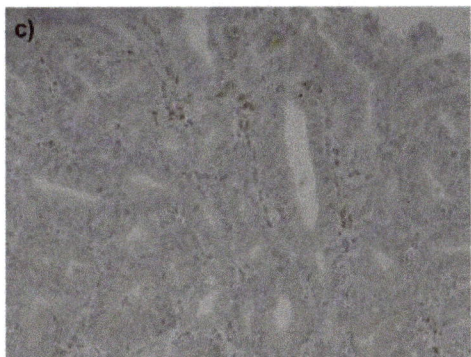
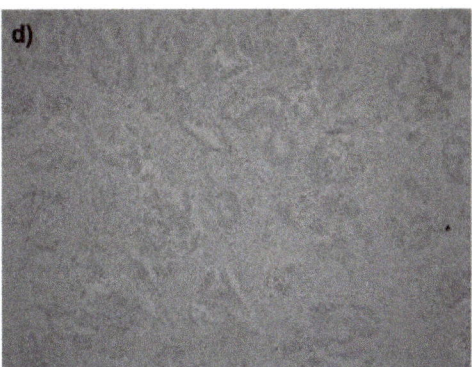

Figure 1. Staining images of phosphorylated STAT3 in cancer cells. (**a**) Expression of phosphorylated STAT3 in lung cancer developed by a control patient (score 5.33), scale bar=50 µm. (**b**) Expression of phosphorylated STAT3 in gastric cancer developed by a psoriasis patient (score 4), scale bar=50 µm. (**c**) Expression of phosphorylated STAT3 in gastric cancer developed by a psoriasis patient (score 3.33), scale bar=50 µm. (**d**) Expression of phosphorylated STAT3 in gastric cancer developed by a control patient (score 0), scale bar=100 µm.

4. Discussion

Many studies have shown that moderate to severe psoriasis are associated with comorbidities, such as cardiovascular disease, hypertension, metabolic syndrome, and psychiatric disorders. Cancer remains a matter of debate. Some cancers present no increased risk, but most studies have demonstrated the association of psoriasis with higher risks for cancer [19,20]. A recent meta-analysis in 2020 concluded that patients with psoriasis appear to have a slightly increased risk of cancer, particularly of keratinocyte cancer, lymphomas, lung cancer, and bladder cancer [21]. A systematic review in 2019 also showed that psoriasis was associated with an increased risk of overall cancer, as well as in site-specific cancers of the colon, colorectal, kidney, laryngeal, liver, lymphoma, keratinocyte, esophageal, oral cavity, and pancreatic cancer [20]. Our study demonstrated that there was no difference in the prevalence of cancer in psoriasis patients compared to eczema patients, but the frequency of patients with multiple cancers was significantly higher in the psoriasis group than in the eczema group, although the limitations of this study include the small sample size at a single institution and the fact that the histological type and grade of cancer were not consistent with those of the control group. Furthermore, the number of patients with sufficient samples at our hospital was limited because some patients underwent surgery at other institutions or did not undergo resection after diagnosis by biopsy. In order to compare psoriasis which is a Th17-balanced inflammatory skin disease, we chose the eczema group as a control, which is usually one of the Th2-balanced inflammatory skin diseases.

Psoriasis causes chronic low inflammation throughout the patient's life, which increases the risk of malignancy. Psoriasis patients also have a higher ratio of smoking and/or alcohol consumption habits and higher body mass index (BMI), which would increase cancer risk. In addition, psoriasis treatment, such as systemic immunosuppressive drugs methotrexate and cyclosporine, and biologics may increase the risk of malignancy. In this study, we were not able to collect all the information on patients' smoking and/or drinking habits, BMI, history of hepatitis B and/or hepatitis C, or their past use of immunosuppressive drugs that could influence the development of cancer. Thus, our data cannot determine whether the accurate risk of malignancies in psoriasis inflammation increased, but results showed that the overall frequency of psoriasis patients who developed cancers did not increase as the frequency of patients with multiple cancers increased, suggesting that the frequency of cancer-prone patients may be increased in the psoriasis population.

In previous reports, activation of STAT3 was detected in a wide variety of human cancer cells, including head and neck, brain, breast, gastric, colorectal, liver, lung, kidney, pancreas, prostate, ovarian, cervical cancer, multiple myeloma, and acute myeloid leukemia [22,23]. STAT3 is thought to be highly involved in cancer invasion, migration, metastasis, and angiogenesis, and plays an important role in cancer immune escape [22]. In relation, phosphorylation of Tyr705 and phosphorylation of Ser727 can then affect cancer metabolism [12]. With regard to gastric, lung, and head and neck cancers, which we examined in this study, previous reports showed that STAT3 activation was associated with negative factors such as poor prognosis of cancers [23–25].

In psoriasis, in addition to the activation of STAT3 in keratinocytes [3], STAT3 is activated by various stimuli in Th17 cells, which play an important role in the pathogenesis of psoriasis [4]. STAT3 is included as one of the genetic risk loci in psoriasis, and was reported as an up-regulated gene in a study of psoriatic patients compared to healthy controls [26,27]. Therefore, we designed this study to determine whether patients with psoriasis are susceptible to STAT3 activation in tumors. In this study, we investigated the activation of STAT3 in cancer cells by immunohistochemistry and found that the frequency of phosphorylated STAT3-positive cancers was not significantly different from that in the eczema group.

In fact, phosphorylated STAT3 in cancer was mostly reported as a cancer promoter, but some studies indicated that it may also act as a suppressor under certain conditions [5]. In lung cancer, STAT3 was shown to play an unexpected tumor-suppressive role in *KRAS*-mutant lung adenocarcinoma [28]. High nuclear STAT3 expression levels are associated with favorable outcomes in head and neck squamous cell carcinomas [29]. Sano et al. reported that transgenic mice with keratinocytes expressing a constitutively active form of STAT3 developed psoriasis spontaneously [3], and that squamous cell carcinoma occurred early after carcinogenic stimuli in these mice [30]. Interestingly, in this transgenic mouse, squamous cell carcinoma avoided skin lesions of psoriasis [31]. These studies indicate that constitutive STAT3 activation in keratinocytes is involved in the pathogenesis of both psoriasis and skin squamous cell carcinoma, but oncogenic activation and inflammatory activation may differ.

Regarding its function in psoriasis, STAT3 activation in psoriatic keratinocytes occurs by IL-17, IL-19, IL-21, IL-22 [4], visfatin [32], and IL-36 [33]. These stimuli phosphorylate Tyr705 in STAT3. For example, activation of STAT3 by IL-22 is involved in the proliferation of keratinocytes [34], and activation of STAT3 by IL22 and IL-17A is involved in the induction of keratin 17, which is overexpressed in psoriasis [35–37]. Recently, it has been reported that oxidative stress caused by reactive oxygen species also promotes psoriasis through activation of STAT3 [38]. Ultraviolet B (UVB) activates STAT3 via phosphorylation of Tyr705 in the skin of mice. STAT3 activation was associated with a decreased UVB-induced apoptotic response and increased leukocyte infiltration and hyperplasia, suggesting a possible link to cancer [39]. In contrast, narrowband UVB irradiation had a suppressive effect on psoriasis by downregulating the expression of keratin 17 through inhibition of STAT3 activation, depending on the irradiation dose [40]. Another study in cultured keratinocytes showed that Jak2-dependent phosphorylation of Tyr705 induced by IL-6 and IL-20 resulted in a strong increase in the transcriptional activity of STAT3, and that ERK1/2- and p38 MAPK-dependent phosphorylation of Ser727 induced by tumor necrosis factor-α and UVB irradiation had a modulatory effect on the transcriptional activity of STAT3 [41]. Patients with psoriasis may have a genetic background that predisposes them to STAT3 activation [42]. The above studies suggest that differences in the mode of stimulation have different effects on STAT3 activation; that is, inflammatory stimuli from cytokines, such as IL-17 and IL-22, may activate STAT3 without influencing cancer risk, but oxidative stress, such as UV, may activate STAT3 with increased cancer risk.

5. Conclusions

The frequency of patients with psoriasis associated with cancer was similar to that of eczema patients, but the frequency of multiple cancers with psoriasis was increased compared to that with eczema patients. STAT3 is activated in psoriasis lesion and many cancers. STAT3 is a multifunctional protein whose function depends on the context of its activation. This means that there is a wide variety of stimuli and pathways that activate STAT3, and there are many different downstream reactions mediated by activated STAT3. STAT3 activation is observed both in psoriasis and cancers, however, STAT3 activation in keratinocytes involved in the pathogenesis of psoriasis; i.e., inflammatory STAT3 activation, may differ from oncogenic stimulation of STAT3 in cancers. The significance of STAT3 activation in inflammatory/oncogenic effects requires further investigation under specific conditions.

Author Contributions: Conceptualization, M.K. (Megumi Kishimoto) and M.K. (Mayumi Komine); Methodology, M.K. (Megumi Kishimoto), M.K. (Mayumi Komine) and M.M.; Formal Analysis, M.K. (Megumi Kishimoto) and M.M.; Investigation, M.K. (Megumi Kishimoto), M.K. (Mayumi Komine), M.S.-K., T.M.A., H.K. and R.S.; Resources, H.K and N.F.; Data Curation, M.K. (Megumi Kishimoto); Writing—Original Draft Preparation, M.K. (Megumi Kishimoto); Writing—Review and Editing, M.K. (Mayumi Komine), K.K., J.S., M.M., H.K. and M.O.; Visualization, M.K. (Megumi Kishimoto); Supervision, N.F. and M.O.; Project Administration, M.K. (Mayumi Komine); Funding Acquisition, M.K. (Mayumi Komine) and M.O. All authors have read and agreed to the published version of the manuscript.

Funding: This research received no external funding.

Institutional Review Board Statement: The study was conducted according to the guidelines of the Declaration of Helsinki and approved by the Ethical Committee of Jichi Medical University (protocol code: A20-003, date of approval: 1 April 2020).

Informed Consent Statement: Informed consent was obtained from all subjects involved in the study.

Data Availability Statement: Data sharing not applicable.

Acknowledgments: This study is supported by The Ministry of Education, Culture, Sports, Science and Technology (MEXT) Grant-in-Aid for Scientific Research (C) 20K08661.

Conflicts of Interest: The authors declare no conflict of interest.

References

1. Alinaghi, F.; Calov, M.; Kristensen, L.E.; Gladman, D.D.; Coates, L.C.; Jullien, D.; Gottlieb, A.B.; Gisondi, P.; Wu, J.J.; Thyssen, J.P.; et al. Prevalence of Psoriatic Arthritis in Patients With Psoriasis: A Systematic Review and Meta-Analysis of Observational and Clinical Studies. *J. Am. Acad. Dermatol.* **2019**, *80*, 251–265.e19. [CrossRef]
2. Hawkes, J.E.; Chan, T.C.; Krueger, J.G. Psoriasis Pathogenesis and the Development of Novel Targeted Immune Therapies. *J. Allergy Clin. Immunol.* **2017**, *140*, 645–653. [CrossRef]
3. Sano, S.; Chan, K.S.; Carbajal, S.; Clifford, J.; Peavey, M.; Kiguchi, K.; Itami, S.; Nickoloff, B.J.; DiGiovanni, J. Stat3 Links Activated Keratinocytes and Immunocytes Required for Development of Psoriasis in a Novel Transgenic Mouse Model. *Nat. Med.* **2005**, *11*, 43–49. [CrossRef]
4. Calautti, E.; Avalle, L.; Poli, V. Psoriasis: A STAT3-Centric View. *Int. J. Mol. Sci.* **2018**, *19*, 171. [CrossRef]
5. Tolomeo, M.; Cascio, A. The Multifaced Role of STAT3 in Cancer and Its Implication for Anticancer Therapy. *Int. J. Mol. Sci.* **2021**, *22*, 603. [CrossRef] [PubMed]
6. Zou, S.; Tong, Q.; Liu, B.; Huang, W.; Tian, Y.; Fu, X. Targeting STAT3 in Cancer Immunotherapy. *Mol. Cancer* **2020**, *19*, 145. [CrossRef] [PubMed]
7. Avalle, L.; Poli, V. Nucleus, Mitochondrion, or Reticulum? STAT3 à La Carte. *Int. J. Mol. Sci.* **2018**, *19*, 2820. [CrossRef]
8. Villarino, A.V.; Kanno, Y.; Ferdinand, J.R.; O'Shea, J.J. Mechanisms of Jak/STAT Signaling in Immunity and Disease. *J. Immunol.* **2015**, *194*, 21–27. [CrossRef] [PubMed]
9. Gao, Y.; Zhao, H.; Wang, P.; Wang, J.; Zou, L. The Roles of SOCS3 and STAT3 in Bacterial Infection and Inflammatory Diseases. *Scand. J. Immunol.* **2018**, *88*, e12727. [CrossRef]
10. Kim, M.; Morales, L.D.; Jang, I.S.; Cho, Y.Y.; Kim, D.J. Protein Tyrosine Phosphatases as Potential Regulators of STAT3 Signaling. *Int. J. Mol. Sci.* **2018**, *19*, 2708. [CrossRef]
11. Banerjee, S.; Biehl, A.; Gadina, M.; Hasni, S.; Schwartz, D.M. JAK-STAT Signaling as a Target for Inflammatory and Autoimmune Diseases: Current and Future Prospects. *Drugs* **2017**, *77*, 521–546. [CrossRef] [PubMed]
12. Chun, K.S.; Jang, J.H.; Kim, D.H. Perspectives Regarding the Intersections between STAT3 and Oxidative Metabolism in Cancer. *Cells* **2020**, *9*, 2202. [CrossRef] [PubMed]
13. Mohammed, F.; Gorla, M.; Bisoyi, V.; Tammineni, P.; Sepuri, N.B.V. Rotenone-Induced Reactive Oxygen Species Signal the Recruitment of STAT3 to Mitochondria. *FEBS Lett.* **2020**, *594*, 1403–1412. [CrossRef] [PubMed]

14. Wegrzyn, J.; Potla, R.; Chwae, Y.J.; Sepuri, N.B.; Zhang, Q.; Koeck, T.; Derecka, M.; Szczepanek, K.; Szelag, M.; Gornicka, A.; et al. Function of Mitochondrial Stat3 in Cellular Respiration. *Science* **2009**, *323*, 793–797. [CrossRef]
15. Hillmer, E.J.; Zhang, H.; Li, H.S.; Watowich, S.S. STAT3 Signaling in Immunity. *Cytokine Growth Factor Rev.* **2016**, *31*, 1–15. [CrossRef]
16. Nguyen, P.M.; Putoczki, T.L.; Ernst, M. STAT3-Activating Cytokines: A Therapeutic Opportunity for Inflammatory Bowel Disease? *J. Interferon Cytokine Res.* **2015**, *35*, 340–350. [CrossRef]
17. Oike, T.; Sato, Y.; Kobayashi, T.; Miyamoto, K.; Nakamura, Y.; Kaneko, Y.; Kobayashi, S.; Harato, K.; Saya, H.; Matsumoto, M.; et al. Stat3 as a Potential Therapeutic Target for Rheumatoid Arthritis. *Sci. Rep.* **2017**, *7*, 10965. [CrossRef]
18. Ito, T.; Takahashi, H.; Kawada, A.; Iizuka, H.; Nakagawa, H. Japanese Society for Psoriasis Research. Epidemiological survey from 2009 to 2012 of psoriatic patients in Japanese Society for Psoriasis Research. *J Dermatol.* **2018**, *45*, 293–301. [CrossRef]
19. Takeshita, J.; Grewal, S.; Langan, S.M.; Mehta, N.N.; Ogdie, A.; Van Voorhees, A.S.; Gelfand, J.M. Psoriasis and Comorbid Diseases: Epidemiology. *J. Am. Acad. Dermatol.* **2017**, *76*, 377–390. [CrossRef]
20. Trafford, A.M.; Parisi, R.; Kontopantelis, E.; Griffiths, C.E.M.; Ashcroft, D.M. Association of Psoriasis With the Risk of Developing or Dying of Cancer: A Systematic Review and Meta-Analysis. *JAMA Dermatol.* **2019**, *155*, 1390–1403. [CrossRef]
21. Vaengebjerg, S.; Skov, L.; Egeberg, A.; Loft, N.D. Prevalence, Incidence, and Risk of Cancer in Patients with Psoriasis and Psoriatic Arthritis: A Systematic Review and Meta-Analysis. *JAMA Dermatol.* **2020**, *156*, 421–429. [CrossRef]
22. Lee, H.; Jeong, A.J.; Ye, S.K. Highlighted STAT3 as a Potential Drug Target for Cancer Therapy. *BMB Rep.* **2019**, *52*, 415–423. [CrossRef]
23. Ji, K.; Zhang, L.; Zhang, M.; Chu, Q.; Li, X.; Wang, W. Prognostic Value and Clinicopathological Significance of p-stat3 Among Gastric Carcinoma Patients: A Systematic Review and Meta-Analysis. *Medicine* **2016**, *95*, e2641. [CrossRef] [PubMed]
24. Mohrherr, J.; Uras, I.Z.; Moll, H.P.; Casanova, E. STAT3: Versatile Functions in Non-Small Cell Lung Cancer. *Cancers* **2020**, *12*, 1107. [CrossRef] [PubMed]
25. Mali, S.B. Review of STAT3 (Signal Transducers and Activators of Transcription) in Head and Neck Cancer. *Oral Oncol.* **2015**, *51*, 565–569. [CrossRef]
26. Tsoi, L.C.; Spain, S.L.; Knight, J.; Ellinghaus, E.; Stuart, P.E.; Capon, F.; Ding, J.; Li, Y.; Tejasvi, T.; Gudjonsson, J.E.; et al. Identification of 15 new psoriasis susceptibility loci highlights the role of innate immunity. *Nat. Genet.* **2012**, *44*, 1341–1348. [CrossRef] [PubMed]
27. Liang, Y.; Sarkar, M.K.; Tsoi, L.C.; Gudjonsson, J.E. Psoriasis: A Mixed Autoimmune and Autoinflammatory Disease. *Curr. Opin. Immunol.* **2017**, *49*, 1–8. [CrossRef]
28. Grabner, B.; Schramek, D.; Mueller, K.M.; Moll, H.P.; Svinka, J.; Hoffmann, T.; Bauer, E.; Blaas, L.; Hruschka, N.; Zboray, K.; et al. Disruption of STAT3 Signalling Promotes KRAS-Induced Lung Tumorigenesis. *Nat. Commun.* **2015**, *6*, 6285. [CrossRef] [PubMed]
29. Pectasides, E.; Egloff, A.M.; Sasaki, C.; Kountourakis, P.; Burtness, B.; Fountzilas, G.; Dafni, U.; Zaramboukas, T.; Rampias, T.; Rimm, D.; et al. Nuclear Localization of Signal Transducer And Activator Of Transcription 3 in Head and Neck Squamous Cell Carcinoma Is Associated With a Better Prognosis. *Clin. Cancer Res.* **2010**, *16*, 2427–2434. [CrossRef] [PubMed]
30. Chan, K.S.; Sano, S.; Kataoka, K.; Abel, E.; Carbajal, S.; Beltran, L.; Clifford, J.; Peavey, M.; Shen, J.; Digiovanni, J. Forced Expression of a Constitutively Active Form of Stat3 in Mouse Epidermis Enhances Malignant Progression of Skin Tumors Induced by Two-Stage Carcinogenesis. *Oncogene* **2008**, *27*, 1087–1094. [CrossRef]
31. Sano, S.; Chan, K.S.; DiGiovanni, J. Impact of Stat3 Activation upon Skin Biology: A Dichotomy of Its Role between Homeostasis and Diseases. *J. Dermatol. Sci.* **2008**, *50*, 1–14. [CrossRef]
32. Hau, C.S.; Kanda, N.; Noda, S.; Tatsuta, A.; Kamata, M.; Shibata, S.; Asano, Y.; Sato, S.; Watanabe, S.; Tada, Y. Visfatin Enhances the Production of Cathelicidin Antimicrobial Peptide, Human β-defensin-2, Human β-defensin-3, and S100A7 in Human Keratinocytes and Their Orthologs in Murine Imiquimod-Induced Psoriatic Skin. *Am. J. Pathol.* **2013**, *182*, 1705–1717. [CrossRef]
33. Müller, A.; Hennig, A.; Lorscheid, S.; Grondona, P.; Schulze-Osthoff, K.; Hailfinger, S.; Kramer, D. IκBζ Is a Key Transcriptional Regulator of IL-36-driven Psoriasis-Related Gene Expression in Keratinocytes. *Proc. Natl. Acad. Sci. USA* **2018**, *115*, 10088–10093. [CrossRef]
34. Wolk, K.; Haugen, H.S.; Xu, W.; Witte, E.; Waggie, K.; Anderson, M.; Vom Baur, E.; Witte, K.; Warszawska, K.; Philipp, S.; et al. IL-22 and IL-20 Are Key Mediators of the Epidermal Alterations in Psoriasis While IL-17 and IFN-Gamma Are Not. *J. Mol. Med.* **2009**, *87*, 523–536. [CrossRef]
35. Komine, M.; Freedberg, I.M.; Blumenberg, M. Regulation of Epidermal Expression of Keratin K17 in Inflammatory Skin Diseases. *J. Investig. Dermatol.* **1996**, *107*, 569–575. [CrossRef] [PubMed]
36. Zhang, W.; Dang, E.; Shi, X.; Jin, L.; Feng, Z.; Hu, L.; Wu, Y.; Wang, G. The Pro-Inflammatory Cytokine IL-22 Up-Regulates Keratin 17 Expression in Keratinocytes via STAT3 and ERK1/2. *PLoS ONE* **2012**, *7*, e40797. [CrossRef] [PubMed]
37. Shi, X.; Jin, L.; Dang, E.; Chang, T.; Feng, Z.; Liu, Y.; Wang, G. IL-17A Upregulates Keratin 17 Expression in Keratinocytes Through STAT1- and STAT3-Dependent Mechanisms. *J. Investig. Dermatol.* **2011**, *131*, 2401–2408. [CrossRef] [PubMed]
38. Lin, X.; Huang, T. Oxidative Stress in Psoriasis and Potential Therapeutic Use of Antioxidants. *Free Radic. Res.* **2016**, *50*, 585–595. [CrossRef] [PubMed]
39. Ahsan, H.; Aziz, M.H.; Ahmad, N. Ultraviolet B Exposure Activates Stat3 Signaling via Phosphorylation at Tyrosine705 in Skin of SKH1 Hairless Mouse: A Target for the Management of Skin Cancer? *Biochem. Biophys. Res. Commun.* **2005**, *333*, 241–246. [CrossRef] [PubMed]

40. Zhuang, Y.; Han, C.; Li, B.; Jin, L.; Dang, E.; Fang, H.; Qiao, H.; Wang, G. NB-UVB Irradiation Downregulates keratin-17 Expression in Keratinocytes by Inhibiting the ERK1/2 and STAT3 Signaling Pathways. *Arch. Dermatol. Res.* **2018**, *310*, 147–156. [CrossRef]
41. Andrés, R.M.; Hald, A.; Johansen, C.; Kragballe, K.; Iversen, L. Studies of Jak/STAT3 Expression and Signalling in Psoriasis Identifies STAT3-Ser727 Phosphorylation as a Modulator of Transcriptional Activity. *Exp. Dermatol.* **2013**, *22*, 323–328. [CrossRef] [PubMed]
42. Chandra, A.; Das, S.; Mazumder, S.; Senapati, S.; Chatterjee, G.; Chatterjee, R. Functional Mapping of Genetic Interactions between Human Leukocyte Antigen (HLA)-Cw6 and Late Cornified Envelope 3A in Psoriasis. *J. Investig. Dermatol.* **2021**. [CrossRef] [PubMed]

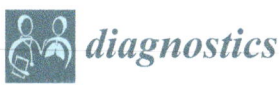

Article

PSORS1 Locus Genotyping Profile in Psoriasis: A Pilot Case-Control Study

Noha Z. Tawfik [1,*], Hoda Y. Abdallah [2,3], Ranya Hassan [4], Alaa Hosny [5], Dina E. Ghanem [5], Aya Adel [5] and Mona A. Atwa [1]

1. Dermatology, Venereology and Andrology Department, Faculty of Medicine, Suez Canal University, Ismailia 41522, Egypt; atwamona@gmail.com
2. Medical Genetics Unit, Histology & Cell Biology Department, Faculty of Medicine, Suez Canal University, Ismailia 41522, Egypt; hoda_ibrahim1@med.suez.edu.eg
3. Center of Excellence in Molecular and Cellular Medicine, Faculty of Medicine, Suez Canal University, Ismailia 41522, Egypt
4. Clinical Pathology Department, Faculty of Medicine, Suez Canal University, Ismailia 41522, Egypt; rania.moustafa@med.suez.edu.eg
5. Ministry of Health, Cairo 11435, Egypt; eng_aliuop@yahoo.com (A.H.); drdinaghanem@gmail.com (D.E.G.); ayadel90@gmail.com (A.A.)
* Correspondence: nohazakaria1@gmail.com; Tel.: +20-127-4504926

Abstract: (1) Background: The psoriasis susceptibility 1 (PSORS1) locus, located within the major histocompatibility complex, is one of the main genetic determinants for psoriasis, the genotyping profile for three single-nucleotide polymorphisms (SNPs) comprising the PSORS1 locus: rs1062470 within *PSORS1C1/CDSN* genes, rs887466 within *PSORS1C3* gene, rs10484554 within *LOC105375015* gene, were investigated and correlated with psoriasis risk and severity. (2) Methods: This pilot case-controlled study involved 100 psoriatic patients and 100 healthy individuals. We investigated three SNPs and assessed the relative gene expression profile for the *PSORS1C1* gene. We then correlated the results with both disease risk and severity. (3) Results: The most significantly associated SNP in PSORS1 locus with psoriasis was rs10484554 with its C/T genotype 5.63 times more likely to develop psoriasis under codominant comparison. Furthermore, C/T and T/T genotypes were 5 times more likely to develop psoriasis. The T allele was 3 times more likely to develop psoriasis under allelic comparison. The relative gene expression of *PSORS1C1* for psoriatic patients showed to be under-expressed compared to normal controls. (4) Conclusions: Our study revealed the association of the three studied SNPs with psoriasis risk and severity in an Egyptian cohort, indicating that rs10484554 could be the major key player in the PSORS1 locus.

Keywords: psoriasis; *PSORS1C3*; *PSORS1C1/CDSN*; *LOC105375015*; rs1062470; rs887466; rs10484554; single-nucleotide polymorphism

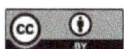

1. Introduction

Psoriasis is a common inflammatory skin disease of multifactorial origin that causes significant stress and morbidity [1]. It most often presents with well-demarcated, scaling and erythematous plaques, often at the extensor surfaces of knees and elbows [2]. Until now, the definite etiopathogenesis of psoriasis is not fully understood, however, it is widely regarded as a multifactorial disorder caused by the interaction between inherited susceptibility alleles and environmental triggers (e.g., stress, mechanical trauma and streptococcal infections) in combination with skin barrier disruption and immune dysfunction [3,4]. Recent advancements for expanding our understanding of psoriasis pathophysiology and targeted therapies are currently a hot topic in research [5,6].

Familial recurrence is also well documented and disease concordance is higher in monozygotic vs. dizygotic twins [7]. The main genetic determinant for psoriasis is the psoriasis susceptibility 1 locus (PSORS1), located within the major histocompatibility complex (MHC) on chromosome 6p21.3 [8] spanning from 180 to 250 kb [9,10]. The PSORS1 locus contains several genes, including protein-coding genes, non-protein-coding genes and pseudogenes. It has been found that some variants of them are associated with psoriasis [10–13].

Single-nucleotide polymorphisms (SNPs) are substitutions of a single nucleotide at a specific position in the genome, which is present in at least 1% of the population [14] and may act as biomarkers for various complex diseases [15]. There are over 500 SNPs related to the PSORS1 locus [16]. Among all those variants, the following three SNPs have been suggested to be associated with psoriasis, namely: rs1062470, rs887466, and rs10484554. These SNPs are located at different points of the PSORS1 locus, as shown in Figure 1.

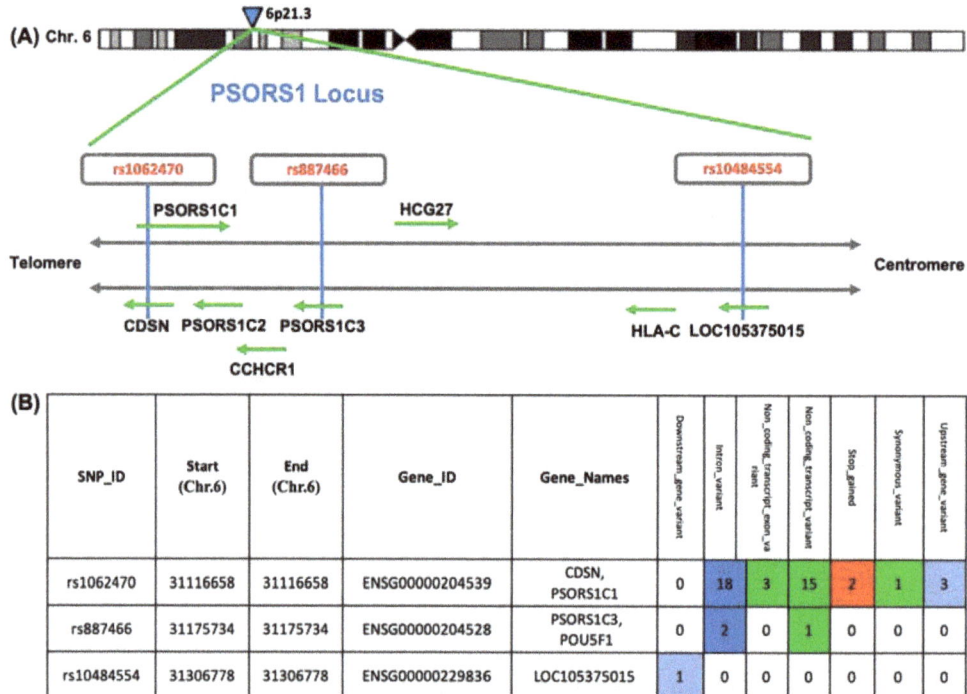

Figure 1. Single nucleotide polymorphisms (SNPs) included in the study. (**A**) Localization of the PSORS1 locus on human chromosome 6. (**B**) List of SNPs in the study to their gene names (official and Ensembl) with chromosomal coordinates and predicted variant effects. The variant effects are described with a color-coded set of variant consequences terms, defined by the sequence ontology and ordered by severity. The SNPs under study have 7 categories which are: downstream gene variant, intron variant, non-coding transcript exon variant, non-coding transcript variant, stop gained, synonymous variant, and upstream gene variant. (This diagram was constructed based on Ensembl https://www.ensembl.org/index.html (accessed on 1 March 2022) [15] and g:profiler tools https://biit.cs.ut.ee/gprofiler/gost (accessed on 1 March 2022) [16].

To date, and to the best of our knowledge, no data has been reported about PSORS1 locus SNPs among any Egyptian cohort, specifically for rs1062470, rs887466 and rs10484554 genetic variants as possible risk factors for psoriasis. Therefore, this study is the first to provide data about the association between these SNPs and psoriasis predisposition in the Egyptian population. This might help in anticipating the disease and early prophylactic measures could be taken.

2. Materials and Methods

A case-control study was conducted on two hundred participants. Written informed consent was taken from each patient before enrollment in the study. The study participants were divided into two groups: 100 Egyptian patients diagnosed with chronic plaque psoriasis of both genders with ages above 16 years old were recruited from the Dermatology Outpatient Clinics, and we excluded patients with psoriatic arthritis (PsA) or autoimmune diseases; and 100 healthy non-related participants of Egyptian descent, matched by age and gender to the patients with no family history of psoriasis or autoimmune diseases. All patients were subjected to full history taking and detailed dermatological examination. The severity of psoriasis was assessed using a PASI score that included an assessment of four body areas: head and neck (H), upper limbs (UL), trunk (T) and lower limbs (LL). Within each area, the severity of three signs, erythema (E), thickness/induration (I) and desquamation/scaling (D), is each assessed on a five-point scale: 0, none; 1, mild; 2, moderate; 3, severe; 4, very severe. According to the European consensus, interpretation of PASI is mild if the PASI score is <10, moderate if the PASI score is 10–20 and severe if PASI is >20 [17]. This study was performed in compliance with the guidelines of the Helsinki Declaration, 2013. Approval was taken from the Research Ethics Committee and the Institutional Review Board.

2.1. SNP Selection

The three studies' SNPs were selected based on the level of evidence demonstrated by the number of publications studied, with each SNP adopted from https://opensnp.org/ (accessed on 1 March 2022) [18]. The rs10484554 exhibited a high level of evidence equivalent to 37 publications, while rs1062470 and rs887466 values were 4 and 7 publications, respectively. Our selection was also based on the latest findings of Wiśniewski et al. [19], who studied the same SNPs with a proven significance in psoriatic Poland patients, supported by the fact that these SNPs were not investigated among Egyptians in any published research.

2.2. Molecular Analysis

Lab work was performed in the Center of Excellence in Molecular and Cellular Medicine & Genetics Unit using three milliliters of venous blood in an EDTA anticoagulant vacutainer. They were kept at $-20\ °C$ till DNA extraction was performed.

2.3. DNA Extraction

Genomic DNA was extracted using the Invitrogen Gene Catcher purification system (Thermofisher, Waltham, MA, USA) from the frozen venous blood according to the manufacturer's instructions. DNA concentration and purity were determined using a NanoDrop 2000 1C spectrophotometer (NanoDrop Tech., Inc. Wilmington, DE, USA).

2.4. Allelic Discrimination Analysis

The chosen genetic variants, rs1062470 (C__2438414_20), rs887466 (C___8941351_1) and rs10484554 (C__29612773_30) were genotyped using the TaqMan SNP Genotyping Assays (Thermofisher, Foster City, CA, USA) according to manufacturer's instructions. The Applied Biosystems StepOnePlus Real-Time PCR detection system was used to conduct reactions and allelic discrimination, respectively.

2.5. PSORS1C1 Relative Gene Expression Analysis

Total RNA was extracted from the plasma of psoriatic patients and controls using the Qiagen miRNeasy mini kit (Qiagen, Hilden, Germany, Cat. no. 217004) following the protocol supplied by the manufacturer. RNA purity and concentration were assessed by a NanoDrop 2000 1C spectrophotometer (NanoDrop Tech., Inc. Wilmington, DE, USA). Complementary DNA (cDNA) was generated from total RNA with the miScript II RT Kit (Qiagen, Cat. no. 218161) in which *PSORS1C1* was polyadenylated by poly (A) polymerase and converted into cDNA by reverse transcriptase with oligo-dT priming. RT was carried out in a Veriti™ 96-Well Thermal Cycler (Applied Biosystems, Bedford, MA, USA) at 37 °C for 1 h, followed by inactivation of the reaction by briefly incubating at 95 °C. *GAPDH* was used as the endogenous control where it exhibited a uniform and stable expression in plasma samples with no significant difference between psoriatic patients and controls. Triplicate PCR reactions were carried out in the StepOne Real-Time PCR system (Applied Biosystems) using the miScript SYBR Green PCR Kit (Qiagen, cat. no 218076) and specific *PSORS1C1* primers: forward primer 5′-CTGACCGACTTTGCCACATGGA-3′, reverse primer 5′-GTGGGAAGAGGGAACCAGGATA-3′ and *GAPDH* primers: forward primer: 5′-GGAGCGAGATCCCTCCAAAAT-3′, reverse primer 5′-GGCTGTTGTCATACTTCTCATGG-3′ with negative controls in each run to exclude amplicon contamination.

The expression levels were done according to the quantitative real-time PCR experiments with minimal information required for publication (MIQE) guidelines. The relative *PSORS1C1* expression levels were calculated using the LIVAK method $2^{(-\Delta\Delta Cq)}$ [20], where Delta–Delta quantitative cycle (C_q) = $(C_q\ PSORS1C1 - C_q\ GAPDH)_{Psoriasis} - (C_q\ PSORS1C1 - C_q\ GAPDH)_{controls}$. The PCR ran initially at 95 °C for 5 min, followed by 40 cycles at 95 °C (15 s), then at 55 °C (1 min), and finally at 72 °C (1 min) for denaturation, annealing and elongation, respectively.

2.6. Statistical Analysis

Data were analyzed using the Statistical Package for the Social Sciences (SPSS), version 20.0 software, and GraphPad Prism version 7.0. Quantitative data were expressed as means ± standard deviation, while qualitative data were expressed as numbers and percentages. Two-sided Chi-square, Student-t, and ANOVA tests were used for parametric data. A *p*-value of <0.05 was considered statistically significant. Analyses of allele frequencies (number of copies of a specific allele divided by the total number of alleles in the group) and carriage rates (number of individuals with at least one copy of the A allele divided by the total number of individuals within the group) was carried out. Genotype frequencies were assessed for deviation from the Hardy–Weinberg equation by the online program (https://www.snpstats.net) (accessed on 1 March 2022) [21]. The relationship between allele frequencies and the presence of psoriasis was determined under different genetic association models using odds ratio with multiple logistic regression analysis after adjustment for psoriasis risk factors was investigated using the same program.

3. Results

3.1. Baseline Characteristics of the Study Population

The age of the patients and controls ranged from 18.0 to 60 years and 20.0 to 62.0 years, respectively, with no statistically significant difference between both groups. Regarding special habits, 77% of patients and 72% of controls were non-smokers. Concerning body mass index (BMI), the mean BMI was 26.80 ± 3.99 kg/m² for patients, while it was 27.70 ± 3.93 kg/m² in controls Table 1.

3.2. Clinical Assessment of Psoriasis Patients

The mean age of disease onset was 35.07 ± 13.43 and the mean duration was 6.75 ± 6.22 years. According to the age of disease onset, the patients were divided into three subgroups: (I) very early-onset psoriasis (vEOP): up to 20 years (21 patients); (II) middle early-onset psoriasis (mEOP): between 21 and 40 years (42 patients); late-onset psoriasis (LOP): above 40 years (37 patients). Forty-five percent of patients showed mild severity, 31% showed moderate severity, and 24% were severe (Table 2). There was a statistically significant difference between the age of onset of psoriasis in subgroups and gender; the vEOP group showed a higher percentage of females, while the median EOP and late EOP groups showed a higher percentage of males. There was no statistically significant difference between the age of onset of psoriasis in groups and the PASI score (Table 3).

Table 1. Baseline characteristics among the study population.

	Cases (n = 100)		Control (n = 100)		p
	No.	%	No.	%	
Age (years)					
• Min.–Max.	18.0–60.0		20.0–62.0		
• Mean ± SD.	41.74 ± 14.08		39.17 ± 11.65		0.134
• Median (IQR)	42.0 (31.50–56.0)		37.0 (30.0–49.0)		
Gender					
• Male	47	47.0	55	55.0	0.258
• Female	53	53.0	45	45.0	
Special habits					
• Non-smoker	77	77.0	72	72.0	0.417
• Smoker	23	23.0	28	28.0	
BMI (kg/m^2)					
• Min.–Max.	19.0–36.21		19.55–35.63		
• Mean ± SD.	26.80 ± 3.99		27.70 ± 3.93		0.112
• Median (IQR)	25.91 (24.13–29.45)		27.43 (25.0–30.8)		

Data are shown as number (percentage) or mean ± SD. p-value < 0.05 was considered as statistically significant.

Table 2. Disease characteristics among psoriatic study population (n = 100).

Disease Characteristic	No.	%
Age of onset		
• vEOP	21	21.0
• mEOP	42	42.0
• LOP	37	37.0
• Min.–Max.	3.0–59.0	
• Mean ± SD.	35.07 ± 13.43	
• Median (IQR)	36.0 (24.13–29.45)	
Severity		
• Mild	45	45.0
• Moderate	31	31.0
• Severe	24	24.0
Duration (years)		
• Min.–Max.	0.50–30.0	
• Mean ± SD.	6.75 ± 6.22	
• Median (IQR)	5.0 (25.0–30.80)	
Family history		
• No	84	84.0
• Yes	16	16.0

Table 2. Cont.

Disease Characteristic	No.	%
Treatment		
• No Treatment	41	41.0
• On Treatment	59	59.0

Data are shown as number (percentage) or mean ± SD; vEOP: very early-onset psoriasis; mEOP: middle early-onset psoriasis; LOP: late-onset psoriasis.

Table 3. Relation between age of onset with gender and PASI in patient group (n = 100).

Age of Onset	vEOP (n = 21)		mEOP (n = 42)		LOP (n = 37)		p
	No.	%	No.	%	No.	%	
Gender							
- Male	3	14.3	22	52.4	22	59.5	0.003 *
- Female	18	85.7	20	47.6	15	40.5	
PASI							
- Min.–Max.	3.50–38.30		2.0–40.50		1.50–35.60		
- Mean ± SD.	12.28 ± 7.84		14.72 ± 9.56		13.29 ± 9.31		0.564
- Median	11.50		12.25		12.50		

Data are shown as number (percentage); p: p-value for comparing between the studied groups; *: statistically significant at $p \leq 0.05$ psoriasis; vEOP: very early-onset psoriasis; mEOP: middle early-onset psoriasis; LOP: late-onset psoriasis.

3.3. Allelic Discrimination Analysis

The three studied polymorphisms were in accordance with Hardy–Weinberg equilibrium (rs887466: p = 0.53, rs1062470: p = 0.31, rs10484554: p = 0.19). On comparing the genotype frequency among the two study groups for rs887466 and rs1062470 genotypes, there was no statistically significant difference between patients and controls. On the contrary, the rs10484554 genotype showed a statistically significant difference between both groups (Figure 2A). Regarding variants comparison between the two study groups, the rs887466 A variant was more frequent among patients (62% in patients versus 52% in the control group), and also for the rs10484554 variant T, which was more frequent among patients (35% in patients versus 15% in the control group). Meanwhile, rs1062470 variants did not show a statistical difference between patients and controls (Figure 2B).

For psoriatic patients, rs887466, rs1062470 and rs10484554 overall minor allele frequencies were 0.62 (A), 0.53 (A), and 0.35 (T), respectively. For controls, rs887466, rs1062470 and rs10484554 overall minor allele frequencies were 0.52 (A), 0.52 (A), and 0.15 (T), respectively. A comparison with other ethnic populations from the 1000Genome Project is shown in Figure 3.

3.4. Association of PSORS1 Locus Gene Variants with Psoriasis Risk

The rs887466 genotype G/G was 0.4 times more likely to protect against psoriasis under a codominant comparison (OR = 0.4, 95% CI = 0.17 to 0.95) and recessive model (OR = 0.5, 95% CI = 0.23 to 1.05). Moreover, allele G, for this polymorphism, was 0.66 times more likely to protect against psoriasis under allelic comparison (OR = 0.66, 95% CI = 0.44 to 0.99).

For the rs1062470 genotype, only A/G was 1.84 times more likely to develop psoriasis under over-dominant comparison (OR = 1.84, 95% CI = 1.09 to 3.13); other genotypes did not show a significant effect on disease risk (Table 4).

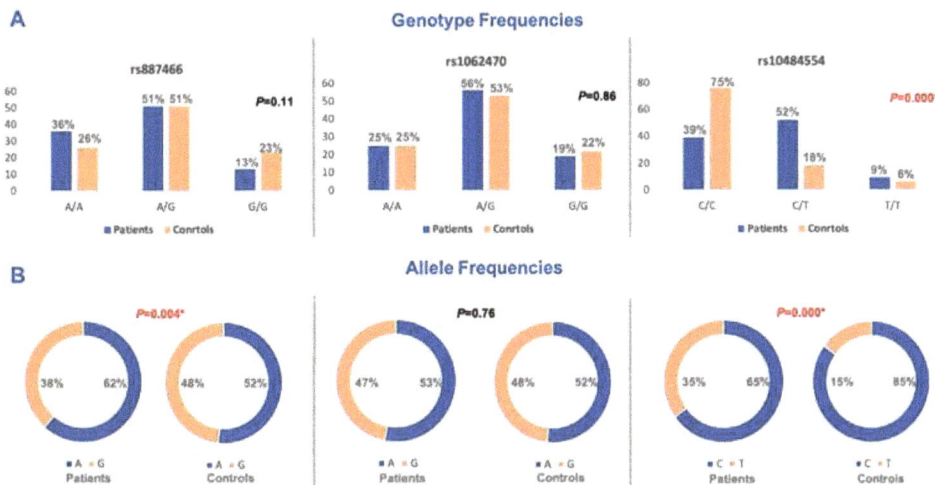

Figure 2. Genotype and allele frequencies of the studied genetic variants for the *PSORS1C3* gene. (**A**) Genotype frequencies of polymorphisms. (**B**) Allele frequencies of polymorphisms. A Chi-square test was applied. Statistical significance was set at $p < 0.05$. Bold red values with * indicate significant value.

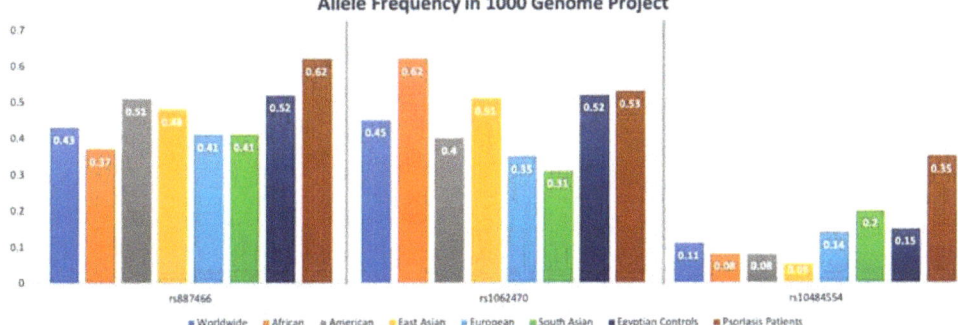

Figure 3. Allele frequencies of *PSORS1C3* gene rs887466, rs1062470 and rs10484554 in 1000Genome Project. This diagram was constructed based on Ensembl https://www.ensembl.org/index.html (accessed on 1 March 2022) [15].

Table 4. Genetic Association Models for *PSORS1C3* Gene Polymorphism with Disease Risk.

SNP	Model	Genotype	Patients	Controls	OR (95% CI)	p-Value
rs887466	Codominant	A/A	36	26	Reference	
		A/G	51	51	0.72 (0.38–1.36)	0.3
		G/G	13	23	0.4 (0.17–0.95)	0.038 *
	Dominant	A/A	36	26	Reference	
		A/G-G/G	64	74	0.62 (0.34–1.14)	0.13
	Recessive	A/A-A/G	87	77	Reference	
		G/G	13	23	0.5 (0.23–1.05)	0.068

Table 4. Cont.

SNP	Model	Genotype	Patients	Controls	OR (95% CI)	p-Value
rs887466	Over-dominant	A/A-G/G	49	49	Reference	
		A/G	51	51	1.0 (0.57–1.74)	1.0
	Allelic Model	A	123	103	Reference	
		G	77	97	0.66 (0.44–0.99)	0.04 *
rs1062470	Codominant	A/A	25	25	Reference	
		A/G	56	53	1.05 (0.54–2.06)	0.87
		G/G	19	22	0.86 (0.37–1.97)	0.72
	Dominant	A/A	25	25	Reference	
		A/G-G/G	75	75	1.04 (0.66–1.62)	0.87
	Recessive	A/A-A/G	81	78	Reference	
		G/G	19	22	0.83 (0.41–1.65)	0.6
	Over-dominant	A/A-G/G	44	77	Reference	
		A/G	56	53	1.84 (1.09–3.13)	0.02 *
	Allelic Model	A	106	103	Reference	
		G	94	97	0.94 (0.63–1.39)	0.76
rs10484554	Codominant	C/C	39	76	Reference	
		C/T	52	18	5.63 (2.9–10.9)	<0.001 *
		T/T	9	6	2.92 (0.97–8.8)	0.05 *
	Dominant	C/C	39	76	Reference	
		C/T-T/T	61	24	5 (2.7–9.1)	<0.001 *
	Recessive	C/C-C/T	91	94	Reference	
		T/T	9	6	1.54 (0.53–4.52)	0.42
	Over-dominant	C/C-T/T	48	82	Reference	
		C/T	52	18	5 (2.59–9.4)	<0.001 *
	Allelic Model	C	130	170	Reference	
		T	70	30	3 (1.88–4.95)	<0.001 *

A: Adenine; C: Cytosine; CI: Confidence Interval; G: Guanine; OR: Odds Ratio; T: Thymine; p: p-value for comparing between the studied groups; *: Statistically significant at $p \leq 0.05$.

The rs10484554 genotype C/T was 5.63 times more likely to develop psoriasis under codominant comparison (OR = 5.63, 95% CI = 2.9 to 10.9). Moreover, the TT genotype was 2.92 times more likely to develop psoriasis under codominant comparison (OR = 2.92, 95% CI = 0.97 to 8.8). Considering the dominant comparison model, C/T and T/T genotypes were 5 times more likely to develop psoriasis (OR = 5, 95% CI = 2.7 to 9.1). For the C/T genotype, it was 5 times more likely to develop psoriasis under over-dominant comparison (OR = 5, 95% CI = 2.59 to 9.4). Finally, allele T for this polymorphism was 3 times more likely to develop psoriasis under allelic comparison (OR = 3, 95% CI = 1.88 to 4.95) See Table 4.

3.5. Association of PSORS1 Locus Haplotypes with Psoriasis Severity

Gene–gene interaction analysis revealed that carriers for GGC genotype combinations had −0.73 times lower disease severity. On the contrary, carriers for GGT genotype combinations had −0.92 times more severe disease form (Table 5). These findings were based on SNPStats [19] web-based platform results, where descriptive statistics were used to estimate the relative frequency for each haplotype. Cumulative frequencies were also calculated to help in the selection of the threshold cut point to group rare haplotypes. The association analysis of haplotypes was either presented using logistic regression results with OR and 95% CI or linear regression results with differences in means and 95% CI. The most frequent haplotype was automatically selected as the reference category and rare haplotypes were pooled together in a group.

Table 5. Haplotype association with Disease Severity.

	rs887466	rs1062470	rs10484554	Frequency	OR (95% CI)	p-Value
1	G	A	C	0.199	Reference	-
2	A	G	C	0.1954	NA (NA–NA)	NA
3	A	A	C	0.1672	0.4 (−0.06–0.85)	0.089
4	A	G	T	0.1508	0.3 (−0.12–0.72)	0.16
5	A	A	T	0.1015	−0.36 (−0.77–0.04)	0.082
6	G	G	C	0.0884	−0.73 (−1.21–−0.24)	0.0038 *
7	G	A	T	0.0623	−0.32 (−0.8–0.17)	0.2
8	G	G	T	0.0354	0.92 (0.18–1.66)	0.015 *

A: Adenine; C: Cytosine; CI: Confidence Interval; G: Guanine; NA: Not Applicable; OR: Odds Ratio; T: Thymine; p: p-value for comparing between the studied groups; *: Statistically significant at $p \leq 0.05$.

3.6. Relative Expression Analysis of Plasma PSORS1C1 in Psoriasis

The relative gene expression of plasma *PSORS1C1* for psoriatic patients showed to be under-expressed compared to normal controls with log-transformed values for median and quartile levels equivalent to −7.24 (−10.35–−2.07) (Figure 4A). There were also significant differential expression levels among *PSORS1C1* SNP rs1062470 genotypes ($p < 0.001$) (Figure 4B).

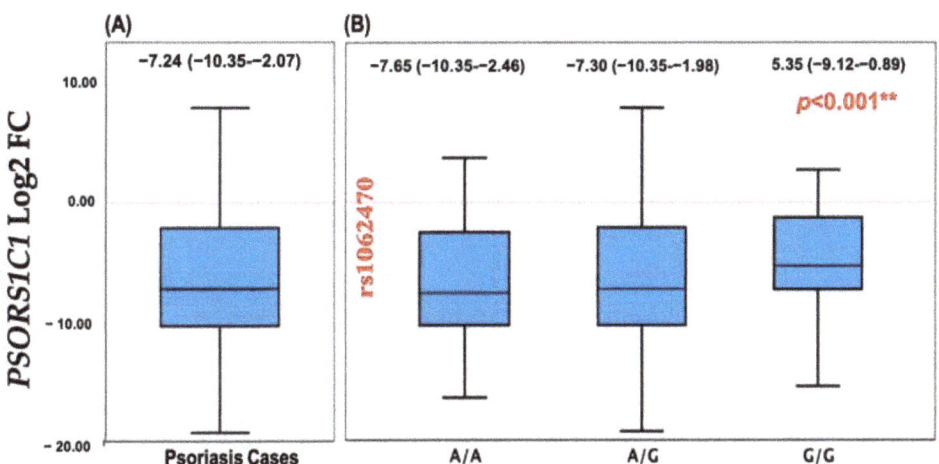

Figure 4. The relative expression profile of the *PSORS1C1* gene in psoriasis plasma samples. Data are shown as medians and quartiles. Box plot values were log-transformed, as data was non-parametric. The red dotted line represents the control level. Mann–Whitney U and Kruskal–Wallis tests were applied. (**A**) Overall psoriatic samples. (**B**) Stratified by rs1062470 genotype. ** Indicate highly significant value.

3.7. Association of the Studied SNPs, PSORS1C1 Gene Expression, and Clinicopathological Features

A heatmap of the inter-relationship between the studied SNPs, *PSORS1C1* gene expression, and clinicopathological features is presented in Figure 5, and the correlation matrix in Table 6. Age was directly and significantly correlated with age of onset (r = 0.896; $p < 0.001$ ***), BMI (0.416; $p < 0.001$ ***), and duration (r = 0.367; $p < 0.001$***). BMI was directly and significantly correlated with age (0.416; $p < 0.001$ ***), age of onset (0.375; $p < 0.001$ ***), and duration (0.279; $p < 0.005$ **). PASI showed a highly significant, direct and very strong correlation with severity and vice versa (0.993; $p < 0.001$ ***).

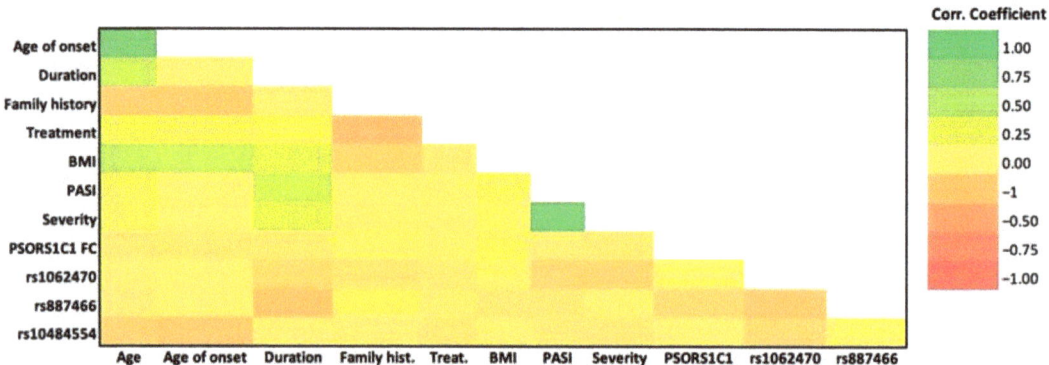

Figure 5. Heatmap presents the inter-relationship among the studied SNPs, *PSORS1C1* gene expression, and clinicopathological features. (BMI, Body Mass Index; PASI, Psoriasis Area and Severity Index).

Table 6. Correlation matrix showing the inter-relationships among the studied SNPs, *PSORS1C1* gene expression, and clinicopathological features.

		Age	Age of Onset	Duration	Family History	Treatment	BMI	PASI	Severity	PSORS1C1 FC	rs1062470	rs887466	rs10484554
Age	R	1	0.896 **	0.367 **	−0.237 *	0.175	0.416 **	0.163	0.164	−0.056	−0.021	−0.039	−0.184
	P	.	<0.001	<0.001	0.018	0.083	<0.001	0.106	0.103	0.583	0.832	0.698	0.067
Age of onset	R	0.896 **	1	−0.023	−0.225 *	0.158	0.375 **	0.022	0.054	−0.05	0.022	0.046	−0.227 *
	P	<0.001	.	0.824	0.024	0.118	<0.001	0.831	0.596	0.624	0.83	0.653	0.023
Duration	R	0.367 **	−0.023	1	−0.017	0.125	0.279 **	0.354 **	0.275 **	−0.034	−0.111	−0.251 *	0.033
	P	<0.001	0.824	.	0.866	0.218	0.005	<0.001	0.006	0.736	0.27	0.012	0.745
Family history	R	−0.237 *	−0.225 *	−0.017	1	−0.310 **	−0.15	0.005	−0.005	0.075	−0.071	0.084	−0.018
	P	0.018	0.024	0.866	.	0.002	0.147	0.963	0.96	0.46	0.483	0.407	0.855
Treatment	R	0.175	0.158	0.125	−0.310 **	1	−0.06	0.062	0.056	0.027	−0.038	−0.013	−0.046
	P	0.083	0.118	0.218	0.002	.	0.578	0.542	0.581	0.788	0.706	0.9	0.649
BMI	R	0.416 **	0.375 **	0.279 **	−0.146	−0.057	1	0.147	0.082	0.118	0.076	−0.051	−0.001
	P	<0.001	<0.001	0.005	0.147	0.578	.	0.145	0.417	0.242	0.454	0.612	0.994
PASI	R	0.163	0.022	0.354 **	0.005	0.062	0.147	1	0.930 **	−0.037	−0.134	−0.049	−0.038
	P	0.106	0.831	<0.001	0.963	0.542	0.145	.	<0.001	0.716	0.183	0.63	0.705
Severity	R	0.164	0.054	0.275 **	−0.005	0.056	0.082	0.930 **	1	−0.051	−0.156	0.015	−0.062
	P	0.103	0.596	0.006	0.96	0.581	0.417	<0.001	.	0.611	0.12	0.881	0.539
PSORS1C1 FC	R	−0.056	−0.05	−0.034	0.075	0.027	0.118	−0.037	−0.051	1	0.074	−0.126	0.008
	P	0.583	0.624	0.736	0.46	0.788	0.242	0.716	0.611	.	0.465	0.212	0.938
rs1062470	R	−0.021	0.022	−0.111	−0.071	−0.038	0.076	−0.134	−0.156	0.074	1	−0.231 *	−0.127
	P	0.832	0.83	0.27	0.483	0.706	0.454	0.183	0.12	0.465	.	0.021	0.209
rs887466	R	−0.039	0.046	−0.251 *	0.084	−0.013	−0.05	−0.049	0.015	−0.126	−0.231 *	1	0.081
	P	0.698	0.653	0.012	0.407	0.9	0.612	0.63	0.881	0.212	0.021	.	0.425
rs10484554	R	−0.184	−0.227 *	0.033	−0.018	−0.046	−0	−0.038	−0.062	0.008	−0.127	0.081	1
	P	0.067	0.023	0.745	0.855	0.649	0.994	0.705	0.539	0.938	0.209	0.425	.

Correlation coefficient (R) represents the value for Spearman's correlation analysis and its *p*-values (P). Shaded boxes enclose values which are statistically significant at either $p < 0.05$ (*) or $p < 0.01$ (**). Abbreviations: BMI, Body Mass Index; FC, Fold Change; PASI, Psoriasis Area and Severity Index.

4. Discussion

To date, there was only one comprehensive genome-wide association study (GWAS) done on the Egyptian population [22], identifying an association between MHC SNPs and psoriasis in a large Egyptian cohort, however, no data was reported from this study on the PSORS1 locus SNPs. The summary of the estimated genotype and allele frequency for each studied SNP based on worldwide previous publications was presented in Table 7.

Table 7. Summary of the estimated genotype and allele frequency for each studied SNP based on worldwide previous publications (Data adopted from https://opensnp.org/ (accessed on 1 March 2022) [18]).

SNP	Genotype Frequency	Allele Frequency	Level of Evidence
rs1062470	GG 43%, AG 13%, AA 44% (TT, CT, --)	A 65%, T 35% (G, C, -)	4 publications
rs887466	GG 47%, AG 15%, AA 38% (CT)	A 61%, T 39% (G, C)	7 publications
rs10484554	CC 22%, TT 76% (CT, --, 00)	A 87%, G 13% (T, C, -, 0)	39 publications

In this study, we found significant associations for the three selected SNPs located within the PSORS1 locus with psoriasis risk and severity, both in single SNP and gene-gene interactions haplotype approaches. Table 5 describes the average genotype and allele frequency for each studied SNP based on the level of evidence demonstrated by a number of publications that included each SNP.

The rs10484554 genetic variant within *LOC105375015* was the most significantly associated with the disease, similar to that reported by Liu et al. [23], Képíró et al. [24], Kisiel et al. [25], Villarreal-Martínez et al. [26], and Strange et al. [27]. Our study odds ratio for the rs10484554 (T) minor allele (OR = 3, 95% CI = 1.88–4.95) was nearly the same as previously reported by Wiśniewski et al. [19] (OR = 2.68) and Villarreal-Martínez et al. [26] (OR=3). In comparing the minor allele frequency (MAF) for genetic variant (T) with other populations, the psoriatic patients in our study reported a MAF = 0.35, which is significantly higher than that reported worldwide (0.11); among Africans (0.08), Americans (0.08), East Asians (0.05), Europeans (0.14), and South Asians (0.2) [15]. In a comparison of different genotypes for this polymorphism with previous studies, the C/T genotype in our study was 5.63 times more likely to develop psoriasis under codominant comparison (OR = 1.84, 95% CI = 2.9–10.9); this is a much higher risk in comparison to Wiśniewski et al. [19] (OR = 3.38, 95% CI = 2.53–4.52). In contrast, the T/T genotype was 2.92 times more likely to develop psoriasis under codominant comparison (OR = 2.92, 95% CI = 0.97–8.8), and this is much lower than that reported by Wiśniewski et al. [19] (OR = 6.82, 95% CI = 4.11–11.30). In line with earlier publications [23,24,28–31], rs10484554 SNP in our study showed a significant correlation with early disease onset. This repetitive finding suggests that rs10484554 could play a role in early-onset psoriasis. However, Hébert et al. revealed that HLA-Cw*06 is associated with late-onset psoriasis using dense genotyping [32]. From a gene perspective, there are no published data about the possible role of *LOC105375015* in the pathogenesis of psoriasis. As rs10484554 belongs to a gene encoding lncRNA—*LOC105375015*—we assume that it might predispose to psoriasis via interacting with mRNA, DNA, protein and miRNA and consequently regulate gene expression at the epigenetic, transcriptional, post-transcriptional, translational, and post-translational levels in a variety of ways [33]. The function of this SNP is also unknown, but being in close proximity to the exon/intron junction, this may suggest a role in the splicing process. However, an explanation of this point requires further studies.

The genetic variant rs887466 from *PSORS1C3* was the only SNP associated with a protective effect in our study. We observed a protective effect only for the G/G genotype, which was 0.4 times more likely to protect against psoriasis under codominant comparison (OR = 0.4, 95% CI = 0.17 to 0.95) and recessive comparison (OR = 0.5, 95% CI = 0.23 to 1.05). In contrast, Wiśniewski et al. [19] reported that the A/A genotype was the protective one. Moreover, allele (G) for this polymorphism was 0.66 times more likely to protect against psoriasis under allelic comparison (OR = 0.66, 95% CI = 0.44 to 0.99), while Wiśniewski et al. [19] reported that the minor allele (A) was 0.77 times more protective against psoriasis, and De Bakker et al. [34] reported that the (G) allele was 5 times more likely to predispose to psoriasis and is considered a risk allele. Thus, the question is whether the (A) or (G) allele is the true marker of protection involving the *PSORS1C3* gene and is still to be investigated in future studies. In comparing the MAF for this genetic variant (A) with other populations, the psoriatic patients in our study reported a MAF = 0.62. This is higher than that reported worldwide (0.43); among Africans (0.37), Americans (0.51), East Asians (0.48), Europeans (0.41), and South Asians (0.41) [15]. The function of the relatively novel *PSORS1C3* gene is still under investigation. Specifically, nothing is known about the role of intronic rs887466. Previously, several SNPs in this gene have been tested in psoriasis in Swedish and Chinese populations [35,36], but rs887466 was just examined once in psoriasis. In our study, we found no significant association between rs887466 SNP and gender of patients or family history, contrasting Wiśniewski et al. [19]. In addition, when we stratified rs887466 SNP genotypes by both the age and gender of patients, we did not find any significant association between them, except with females aged from 41 to 50 years old. In consistence with Wiśniewski et al. [19], we found no statistically significant association between genotype frequencies of the rs887466 polymorphism and PASI score in both genders.

For the rs1062470 genetic variant, only the A/G genotype was 1.84 times more likely to develop psoriasis under over-dominant comparison (OR = 1.84, 95% CI = 1.09 to 3.13); other genotypes did not show a significant effect on disease risk. These results are contradicting those reported by Lesueur et al. [37] and Wiśniewski et al. [19] who stated that the AA genotype increased the risk of psoriasis over fivefold and was significantly associated with higher PASI score in males and explained it by the double effect of the (A) allele in the AA genotype, that may potentially elevate the expression of corneodesmosin in the skin and may result in increased severity of psoriasis. However, they were not able to explain why this effect was observed in males only. In comparing the MAF for this genetic variant (A) with other populations, the psoriatic patients in our study reported a MAF = 0.53, which is considered close to the reported range worldwide (0.45); among Africans (0.62), Americans (0.4), East Asians (0.51) and higher than that of the Europeans (0.35), and South Asians (0.31) [15].

We further assessed the association between the rs1062470 genetic variant and disease severity, and we observed a statistically significant association between rs1062470, and gender stratified by PASI. Interestingly, Wiśniewski et al. [19], Sakai et al. [38], and Hägg et al. [39] also observed that male patients, independently of rs1062470 genotype, had significantly higher PASI scores than female patients except for the earliest onset of disease.

Our study is among few available studies describing a possible gender-dependent association of the rs1062470 genotype with psoriasis severity worldwide and the first to report this finding in Egypt; therefore, further larger-scale studies are needed, including also other polymorphisms in the *CDSN* gene, to confirm our findings. In addition, corneodesmosin expression levels in the psoriatic skin in both genders should be compared and its correlation with the rs1062470 genotype is mandatory to evaluate the gender-dependent effect of this SNP on disease severity.

In haplotype analysis, we observed that carriers for GGC genotype combinations had lower disease severity and carriers for GGT genotype combinations had a more severe disease form. Unfortunately, we were unable to determine whether these haplotypes correspond to other *HLA-C* alleles.

Although the PSORS1C1 gene is located within the PSORS1 locus and is considered one of the potential psoriasis susceptibility genes, the function of its gene product remains unclear in this disease. The relative gene expression level of the *PSORS1C1* gene in our cohort was significantly under-expressed, as shown in Figure 4A, opposing the expected assumption to be over-expressed. This can be justified by our cohort exclusion criteria, where we excluded psoriatic arthritis patients so as to decrease the study confounders. Our justification was based on Sun et al.'s findings which reported over-expression of the *PSORS1C1* gene in blood and synovial tissues [40], supporting the hypothesis that *PSORS1C1* plays a role in rheumatoid arthritis (RA) and is not in close association with the known HLA alleles.

In conclusion, our results demonstrated that rs10484554, rs887466 and rs1062470 genetic variants within the PSORS1 locus encompassing the multiple genes *LOC105375015*, *PSORS1C3* and *PSORS1C1/CDSN*, respectively, are significantly associated with psoriasis. This association is strongly dependent on genotype and less frequently the patient's gender. Because of the complicated and extended LD pattern present in the MHC region, it is not clear whether the markers tested in this study confer the risk of psoriasis dependently or independently of other variants in this region. Our allelic discrimination analysis and association with disease or with the PASI score indicated the possibility that rs10484554 has a higher effect than rs887466 and rs1062470 on the risk and severity of psoriasis, and it is the major key player genetic variant in the PSORS1 locus. Finally, our results suggest that *PSORS1C1* gene under-expression might be in psoriatic patients free from arthritis. However, confirmation of this requires additional studies among Egyptians and other populations. Moreover, the functional consequence of the polymorphism needs to be investigated. Correlation analysis between the single peptide variant and expression levels in patients will add value to future studies outcomes.

Author Contributions: Conceptualization, N.Z.T., R.H. and H.Y.A.; methodology, H.Y.A., N.Z.T. and D.E.G.; software, A.H. and A.A.; validation, M.A.A. and R.H.; formal analysis, N.Z.T., H.Y.A. and R.H.; investigation, H.Y.A. and D.E.G.; resources, A.A. and A.H.; data curation, H.Y.A. and N.Z.T.; writing—original draft preparation, R.H. and N.Z.T.; writing—review and editing, H.Y.A. and N.Z.T.; visualization, M.A.A.; supervision, M.A.A.; project administration, H.Y.A., N.Z.T. and R.H.; funding acquisition, M.A.A., N.Z.T., R.H. and H.Y.A. All authors have read and agreed to the published version of the manuscript.

Funding: This research received no external funding. There are no sponsors or funds for the research.

Institutional Review Board Statement: The study was conducted in accordance with the Declaration of Helsinki, and approved by the Institutional Review Board and the Research Ethics Committee (protocol code #3974) (20 October 2020).

Informed Consent Statement: A written informed consent was taken from each patient before enrollment in the study. Written informed consent has been obtained from the patients to publish this paper.

Data Availability Statement: The data that supports the findings of this study are available from the corresponding author upon reasonable request.

Acknowledgments: We are thankful to all the participants who were very cooperative and welcomed to be part of this study. The patients in this manuscript have given written informed consent to the publication of their case details. There are no sponsors or funds for the research.

Conflicts of Interest: The authors declare no conflict of interest. The funders had no role in the design of the study; in the collection, analyses, or interpretation of data; in the writing of the manuscript, or in the decision to publish the results.

References

1. Springate, D.A.; Parisi, R.; Kontopantelis, E.; Reeves, D.; Griffiths, C.E.M.; Ashcroft, D.M. Incidence, Prevalence and Mortality of Patients with Psoriasis: A U.K. Population-Based Cohort Study. *Br. J. Dermatol.* **2017**, *176*, 650–658. [CrossRef] [PubMed]
2. Pasch, M.C. Nail Psoriasis: A Review of Treatment Options. *Drugs* **2016**, *76*, 675–705. [CrossRef] [PubMed]
3. Boehncke, W.-H.; Schön, M.P. Psoriasis. *Lancet* **2015**, *386*, 983–994. [CrossRef]
4. Strickland, F.M.; Richardson, B.C. Epigenetics in Human Autoimmunity. *Autoimmunity* **2008**, *41*, 278–286. [CrossRef] [PubMed]
5. Ruggiero, A.; Fabbrocini, G.; Cinelli, E.; Megna, M. Efficacy and safety of guselkumab in psoriasis patients who failed ustekinumab and/or anti-interleukin-17 treatment: A real-life 52-week retrospective study. *Dermatol. Ther.* **2021**, *34*, e14673. [CrossRef]
6. Ruggiero, A.; Fabbrocini, G.; Cinelli, E.; Megna, M. Guselkumab and risankizumab for psoriasis: A 44-week indirect real-life comparison. *J. Am. Acad. Dermatol.* **2021**, *85*, 1028–1030. [CrossRef]
7. Generali, E.; Ceribelli, A.; Stazi, M.A.; Selmi, C. Lessons Learned from Twins in Autoimmune and Chronic Inflammatory Diseases. *J. Autoimmun.* **2017**, *83*, 51–61. [CrossRef]
8. Feng, B.-J.; Sun, L.-D.; Soltani-Arabshahi, R.; Bowcock, A.M.; Nair, R.P.; Stuart, P.; Elder, J.T.; Schrodi, S.J.; Begovich, A.B.; Abecasis, G.R.; et al. Multiple Loci within the Major Histocompatibility Complex Confer Risk of Psoriasis. *PLoS Genet.* **2009**, *5*, e1000606. [CrossRef]
9. Nair, R.P.; Stuart, P.; Henseler, T.; Jenisch, S.; Chia, N.V.; Westphal, E.; Schork, N.J.; Kim, J.; Lim, H.W.; Christophers, E.; et al. Localization of Psoriasis-Susceptibility Locus PSORS1 to a 60-Kb Interval Telomeric to HLA-C. *Am. J. Hum. Genet.* **2000**, *66*, 1833–1844. [CrossRef]
10. Clop, A.; Bertoni, A.; Spain, S.L.; Simpson, M.A.; Pullabhatla, V.; Tonda, R.; Hundhausen, C.; Di Meglio, P.; De Jong, P.; Hayday, A.C.; et al. An In-Depth Characterization of the Major Psoriasis Susceptibility Locus Identifies Candidate Susceptibility Alleles within an HLA-C Enhancer Element. *PLoS ONE* **2013**, *8*, e71690. [CrossRef]
11. Capon, F. The Genetic Basis of Psoriasis. *Int. J. Mol. Sci.* **2017**, *18*, 2526. [CrossRef]
12. Capon, F.; Toal, I.K.; Evans, J.C.; Allen, M.H.; Patel, S.; Tillman, D.; Burden, D.; Barker, J.N.W.N.; Trembath, R.C. Haplotype Analysis of Distantly Related Populations Implicates Corneodesmosin in Psoriasis Susceptibility. *J. Med. Genet.* **2003**, *40*, 447–452. [CrossRef] [PubMed]
13. Sherry, S.T.; Ward, M.; Sirotkin, K. DbSNP—Database for Single Nucleotide Polymorphisms and Other Classes of Minor Genetic Variation. *Genome Res.* **1999**, *9*, 677–679. [CrossRef] [PubMed]
14. Ahmad, T.; Valentovic, M.A.; Rankin, G.O. Effects of Cytochrome P450 Single Nucleotide Polymorphisms on Methadone Metabolism and Pharmacodynamics. *Biochem. Pharmacol.* **2018**, *153*, 196–204. [CrossRef] [PubMed]
15. Howe, K.L.; Achuthan, P.; Allen, J.; Allen, J.; Alvarez-Jarreta, J.; Amode, M.R.; Armean, I.M.; Azov, A.G.; Bennett, R.; Bhai, J.; et al. Ensembl 2021. *Nucleic Acids Res.* **2021**, *49*, D884–D891. [CrossRef] [PubMed]
16. Raudvere, U.; Kolberg, L.; Kuzmin, I.; Arak, T.; Adler, P.; Peterson, H.; Vilo, J. G:Profiler: A Web Server for Functional Enrichment Analysis and Conversions of Gene Lists (2019 Update). *Nucleic Acids Res.* **2019**, *47*, W191–W198. [CrossRef]
17. Simpson, M.J.; Chow, C.; Morgenstem, H.; Luger, T.A.; Ellis, C.N. Comparison of 3 Methods for Measuring Psoriasis Severity in Clinical Studies (Part 2 of 2): Use of Quality of Life to Assess Construct Validity of LS-PGA, PASI and Static Physician's Global Assessment. *Eur. Acad. Dermatol. Venereol.* **2015**, *29*, 1415–1420. [CrossRef]
18. Greshake, B.; Bayer, P.E.; Rausch, H.; Reda, J. OpenSNP-a Crowdsourced Web Resource for Personal Genomics. *PLoS ONE* **2014**, *9*, e89204. [CrossRef]
19. Wiśniewski, A.; Matusiak, Ł.; Szczerkowska-Dobosz, A.; Nowak, I.; Kuśnierczyk, P. HLA-C*06:02-Independent, Gender-Related Association of PSORS1C3 and PSORS1C1/CDSN Single-Nucleotide Polymorphisms with Risk and Severity of Psoriasis. *Mol. Genet. Genomics* **2018**, *293*, 957–966. [CrossRef]
20. Livak, K.J.; Schmittgen, T.D. Analysis of Relative Gene Expression Data Using Real-Time Quantitative PCR and the $2^{-\Delta\Delta CT}$ Method. *Methods* **2001**, *25*, 402–408. [CrossRef]
21. Solé, X.; Guinó, E.; Valls, J.; Iniesta, R.; Moreno, V. SNPStats: A Web Tool for the Analysis of Association Studies. *Bioinformatics* **2006**, *22*, 1928–1929. [CrossRef] [PubMed]
22. Bejaoui, Y.; Witte, M.; Abdelhady, M.; Eldarouti, M.; Abdallah, N.M.A.; Elghzaly, A.A.; Tawhid, Z.; Gaballah, M.A.; Busch, H.; Munz, M.; et al. Genome-Wide Association Study of Psoriasis in an Egyptian Population. *Exp. Dermatol.* **2019**, *28*, 623–627. [CrossRef] [PubMed]
23. Liu, Y.; Helms, C.; Liao, W.; Zaba, L.C.; Duan, S.; Gardner, J.; Wise, C.; Miner, A.; Malloy, M.J.; Pullinger, C.R.; et al. A Genome-Wide Association Study of Psoriasis and Psoriatic Arthritis Identifies New Disease Loci. *PLoS Genet.* **2008**, *4*, e1000041. [CrossRef] [PubMed]

24. Képíró, L.; Széll, M.; Kovács, L.; Keszthelyi, P.; Kemény, L.; Gyulai, R. The Association of HLA-C and ERAP1 Polymorphisms in Early and Late Onset Psoriasis and Psoriatic Arthritis Patients of Hungary. *Postepy Dermatol. Alergol.* **2021**, *38*, 43–51. [CrossRef]
25. Kisiel, B.; Kisiel, K.; Szymański, K.; Mackiewicz, W.; Biało-Wójcicka, E.; Uczniak, S.; Fogtman, A.; Iwanicka-Nowicka, R.; Koblowska, M.; Kossowska, H.; et al. The Association between 38 Previously Reported Polymorphisms and Psoriasis in a Polish Population: High Predicative Accuracy of a Genetic Risk Score Combining 16 Loci. *PLoS ONE* **2017**, *12*, e0179348. [CrossRef]
26. Villarreal-Martínez, A.; Gallardo-Blanco, H.; Cerda-Flores, R.; Torres-Muñoz, I.; Gómez-Flores, M.; Salas-Alanís, J.; Ocampo-Candiani, J.; Martínez-Garza, L. Candidate Gene Polymorphisms and Risk of Psoriasis: A Pilot Study. *Exp. Ther. Med.* **2016**, *11*, 1217–1222. [CrossRef]
27. Strange, A.; Capon, F.; Spencer, C.C.; Knight, J.; Weale, M.E.; Allen, M.H.; Barton, A.; Band, G.; Bellenguez, C.; Bergboer, J.G.; et al. Genome-Wide Association Study Identifies New Psoriasis Susceptibility Loci and an Interaction between HLA-C and ERAP1. *Nat. Genet.* **2010**, *42*, 985. [CrossRef]
28. Wiśniewski, A.; Matusiak, Ł.; Szczerkowska-Dobosz, A.; Nowak, I.; Łuszczek, W.; Kuśnierczyk, P. The Association of ERAP1 and ERAP2 Single Nucleotide Polymorphisms and Their Haplotypes with Psoriasis Vulgaris Is Dependent on the Presence or Absence of the HLA-C* 06: 02 Allele and Age at Disease Onset. *Hum. Immunol.* **2018**, *79*, 109–116. [CrossRef]
29. Evans, D.M.; Spencer, C.C.A.; Pointon, J.J.; Su, Z.; Harvey, D.; Kochan, G.; Oppermann, U.; Dilthey, A.; Pirinen, M.; Stone, M.A.; et al. Interaction between ERAP1 and HLA-B27 in Ankylosing Spondylitis Implicates Peptide Handling in the Mechanism for HLA-B27 in Disease Susceptibility. *Nat. Genet.* **2011**, *43*, 761–767. [CrossRef]
30. Das, A.; Chandra, A.; Chakraborty, J.; Chattopadhyay, A.; Senapati, S.; Chatterjee, G.; Chatterjee, R. Associations of ERAP1 Coding Variants and Domain Specific Interaction with HLA-C∗06 in the Early Onset Psoriasis Patients of India. *Hum. Immunol.* **2017**, *78*, 724–730. [CrossRef]
31. Ho, P.Y.P.C.; Barton, A.; Worthington, J.; Thomson, W.; Silman, A.J.; Bruce, I.N. HLA-Cw6 and HLA-DRB1*07 Together Are Associated with Less Severe Joint Disease in Psoriatic Arthritis. *Ann. Rheum. Dis.* **2007**, *66*, 807–811. [CrossRef] [PubMed]
32. Hébert, H.L.; Bowes, J.; Smith, R.L.; Flynn, E.; Parslew, R.; Alsharqi, A.; McHugh, N.J.; Barker, J.N.W.N.; Griffiths, C.E.M.; Barton, A.; et al. Identification of Loci Associated with Late-Onset Psoriasis Using Dense Genotyping of Immune-Related Regions. *Br. J. Dermatol.* **2015**, *172*, 933–939. [CrossRef] [PubMed]
33. Zhang, X.; Wang, W.; Zhu, W.; Dong, J.; Cheng, Y.; Yin, Z.; Shen, F. Mechanisms and Functions of Long Non-Coding RNAs at Multiple Regulatory Levels. *Int. J. Mol. Sci.* **2019**, *20*, 5573. [CrossRef] [PubMed]
34. De Bakker, P.I.W.; McVean, G.; Sabeti, P.C.; Miretti, M.M.; Green, T.; Marchini, J.; Ke, X.; Monsuur, A.J.; Whittaker, P.; Delgado, M.; et al. A High-Resolution HLA and SNP Haplotype Map for Disease Association Studies in the Extended Human MHC. *Nat. Genet.* **2006**, *38*, 1166–1172. [CrossRef] [PubMed]
35. Chang, Y.T.; Chou, C.T.; Shiao, Y.M.; Lin, M.W.; Yu, C.W.; Chen, C.C.; Huang, C.H.; Lee, D.D.; Liu, H.N.; Wang, W.J.; et al. Psoriasis Vulgaris in Chinese Individuals Is Associated with PSORS1C3 and CDSN Genes: Genetics of Psoriasis in Chinese Individuals. *Br. J. Dermatol.* **2006**, *155*, 663–669. [CrossRef] [PubMed]
36. Holm, S.J.; Sánchez, F.; Carlén, L.M.; Mallbris, L.; Ståhle, M.; O'Brien, K.P. HLA-Cw*0602 Associates More Strongly to Psoriasis in the Swedish Population than Variants of the Novel 6p21.3 Gene PSORS1C3. *Acta Derm. Venereol.* **2005**, *85*, 2–8. [CrossRef] [PubMed]
37. Lesueur, F.; Oudot, T.; Heath, S.; Foglio, M.; Lathrop, M.; Prud'homme, J.-F.; Fischer, J. ADAM33, a New Candidate for Psoriasis Susceptibility. *PLoS ONE* **2007**, *2*, e906. [CrossRef]
38. Sakai, R.; Matsui, S.; Fukushima, M.; Yasuda, H.; Miyauchi, H.; Miyachi, Y. Prognostic Factor Analysis for Plaque Psoriasis. *Dermatology* **2005**, *211*, 103–106. [CrossRef]
39. Hägg, D.; Sundström, A.; Eriksson, M.; Schmitt-Egenolf, M. Severity of Psoriasis Differs between Men and Women: A Study of the Clinical Outcome Measure Psoriasis Area and Severity Index (PASI) in 5438 Swedish Register Patients. *Am. J. Clin. Dermatol.* **2017**, *18*, 583–590. [CrossRef]
40. Sun, H.; Xia, Y.; Wang, L.; Wang, Y.; Chang, X. PSORS1C1 May Be Involved in Rheumatoid Arthritis. *Immunol. Lett.* **2013**, *153*, 9–14. [CrossRef]

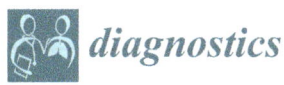

Interesting Images

Secondary Malignant Tumors Arising in Nevus Sebaceus: Two Case Reports

Sohshi Morimura [1], Yasuhiko Tomita [2], Shinichi Ansai [3] and Makoto Sugaya [1,*]

[1] Department of Dermatology, International University of Health and Welfare, Narita 286-8520, Chiba, Japan; morimuras-der@iuhw.ac.jp
[2] Department of Pathology, International University of Health and Welfare, Narita 286-8520, Chiba, Japan; yasuhiko-tomita@iuhw.ac.jp
[3] Division of Dermatology and Dermatopathology, Nippon Medical School Musashi Kosugi Hospital, Kawasaki 211-8533, Kanagawa, Japan; shin8113@nms.ac.jp
* Correspondence: sugayamder@iuhw.ac.jp; Tel.: +81-476-35-5600

Abstract: Nevus sebaceus is a benign tumor that is present at birth and is often seen on the scalp or face. Secondary malignant tumors sometimes occur in nevus sebaceus in adulthood. Herein, we present two malignant tumors arose from nevus sebaceus. One is basal cell carcinoma on the face and the other is sebaceus carcinoma on the lower back, where nevus sebaceus rarely occurs. Basal cell carcinoma sometimes develops in sebaceus nevus after a few decades, seen usually on the scalp or face. Sebaceus carcinoma is a rare malignant tumor that arises in nevus sebaceus.

Keywords: nevus sebaceus; malignant tumor; basal cell carcinoma; sebaceus carcinoma

Nevus sebaceus is a benign hamartoma that is frequently seen on the scalp of infants at birth. Although nevus sebaceus is considered to be a benign tumor, secondary tumors including malignant tumors occur in it after a few decades. Nevus sebaceus usually manifests as a yellowish plaque or a nodule with verrucous appearance, which tends to appear along the Blaschko lines. Pathological features depend on stages. In the early stage, premature pilosebaceus cells are increased while epidermis shows almost no changes. In the following stage, mature pilosebaceus cells with abnormal apocrine glands develop and proliferation of epidermis starts. In the late stage, secondary tumors sometimes develop. Epithelial tumors such as trichoblastoma, syringocystadenoma papilliferum, and basal cell carcinoma sometimes occur secondarily.

In this paper, we show two cases of patients with malignant tumors including basal cell carcinoma and sebaceus carcinoma arising in the nevus sebaceus in adulthood.

A 48-year-old Japanese female was admitted to our department with a skin-colored plaque on the lower jaw (Figure 1A). Multiple black dots were seen on the upper part. Dermatoscopy demonstrated multiple maple-leaf structures. Her laboratory data were not remarkable. The whole plaque was removed by surgery. Histological examination revealed a peripheral palisade of basaloid cells with round nuclei with cleft formation between tumor cells and stroma (Figure 1B,C), which is one of the histopathological features to distinguish basal cell carcinoma from trichoblastoma. Proliferation of mature pilosebaceus tissues and ectopic eccrine glands in the dermis were detected with basaloid cell tumors (Figure 1B). Thus, we diagnosed the skin lesion as basal cell carcinoma generated in nevus sebaceus.

An 82-year-old Japanese female was admitted to our department complaining of bleeding from a red tumor covered with yellow granular papules, which was adjacent to a brown plaque on the right back (Figure 2A). A brown plaque had been present from birth, while it was not clear when the red tumor developed. The red tumor was removed surgically. Histology of the red tumor revealed that atypical basaloid cells form irregular lobular nodules with infiltrative growth pattern in the dermis (Figure 2B). Sebaceus differentiation with a foamy cytoplasm was present in the center of nodules (Figure 2C). The

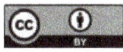

biopsy of brown plaque showed increased multiocular pilosebaceus glands and epidermal papilliform hyperplasia (Figure 2D). Therefore, we diagnosed this tumor as sebaceus carcinoma arising in nevus sebaceus. No extracutaneous metastatic lesions were detected by computed tomography.

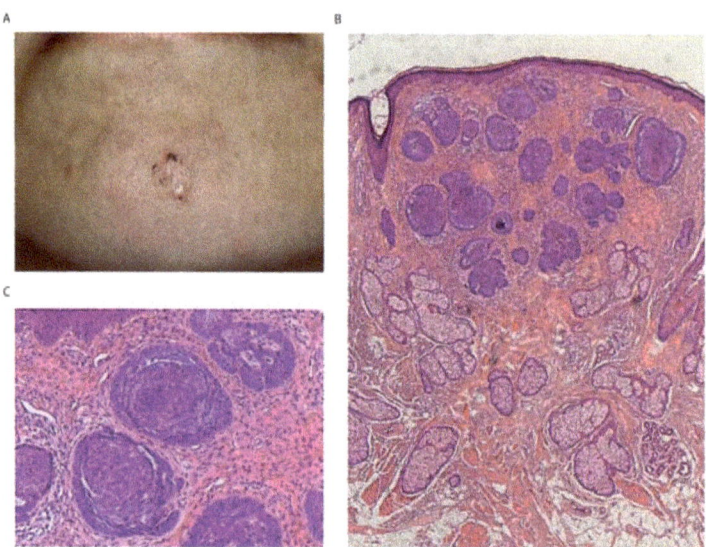

Figure 1. (**A**) A 10 mm skin-colored plaque slightly elevated with several black dots. (**B**) Multiple basaloid cell tumors in the dermis. Proliferation of mature pilosebaceus tissues and ectopic eccrine glands in the dermis. (**C**) Basaloid cell tumors show palisading pattern at the periphery with spaces between the tumor and the surrounding stroma. High magnification of (**B**).

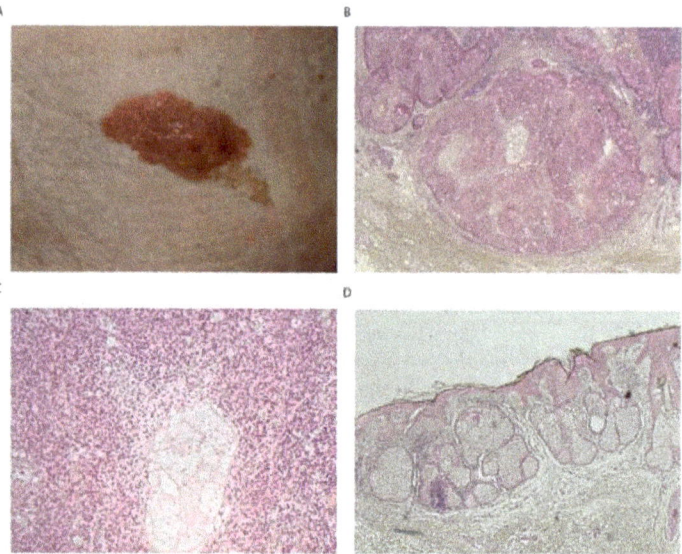

Figure 2. (**A**) A red tumor covered with granular papules adjacent to a brown plaque. (**B**) Atypical basaloid cells form irregular lobular nodules with infiltrative growth pattern in dermis. (**C**) Sebaceus differentiation with a foamy cytoplasm in the center of nodules. High magnification of (**B**). (**D**) Increased multiocular pilosebaceus glands in the dermis.

Nevus sebaceus is a congenital hamartoma, which is clinically a yellowish plaque. Nevus sebaceus frequently occurs on the scalp and face. However, some cases with nevus sebaceus on the chest have been reported [1]. In total, 417 cases (92.6%) out of 450 cases were on the scalp and face, while 4 cases (0.8%) were on the trunk [2]. In one of our cases, nevus sebaceus was detected on the back, which is quite rare. We found only one case with basal cell carcinoma arising in the nevus sebaceus on the upper right back [3].

It has been reported that trichoblastoma is the most common secondary neoplasm that arises within nevus sebaceus [4]. Out of 243 cases with nevus sebaceus, only one case (0.4%) developed sebaceus carcinoma [4]. Another report demonstrated that 38 (8.5%) of 450 cases with nevus sebaceus developed secondary neoplasms, including syringocystadenoma papilliferum (2.7%), the most common tumor [2]. Basal cell carcinoma developed in 4 cases (0.9%) and was the most frequent malignant tumors in nevus sebaceus [2]. Nodular type of basal cell carcinoma arising from nevus sebaceus has been recently reported [5]. Sebaceus carcinoma occurred in only one case (0.2%) out of 450 cases of nevus sebaceus [2].

According to several articles, multiple tumors rarely happen in the nevus sebaceus simultaneously. Sebaceus carcinoma, trichoblastoma, and poroma were detected in one case with nevus sebaceus [6]. Coexistence of adenosquamous carcinoma, trichoblastoma, trichilemmoma, sebaceus adenoma, tumor of follicular infundibulum, and syringocystadenoma papilliferum was also reported [7]. The mechanism of multiple neoplasms happening in nevus sebaceus is still unclear, although diversity and different differentiation status of cells composing nevus sebaceus may be partially responsible for it.

In conclusion, we presented two cases of malignant tumors arising from nevus sebaceus. Nevus sebaceus should be removed in order to avoid malignant transformation. Skin biopsy is essential to avoid overlooking the disease.

Author Contributions: Conceptualization, S.M. and M.S.; data curation, S.M., Y.T., S.A. and M.S.; writing—original draft preparation, S.M. and M.S.; writing—review and editing, S.M. and M.S. All authors have read and agreed to the published version of the manuscript.

Funding: This research received no external funding.

Conflicts of Interest: The authors declare no conflict of interest.

References

1. Gu, A.; Zhang, X.; Zhang, L.; Ma, F. Nevus Sebaceous at an Unusual Location: A Rare Presentation. *Chin. Med. J.* **2017**, *130*, 2897–2898. [CrossRef] [PubMed]
2. Hsu, M.C.; Liau, J.Y.; Hong, J.L.; Cheng, Y.; Liao, Y.H.; Chen, J.S.; Sheen, Y.S.; Hong, J.B. Secondary neoplasms arising from nevus sebaceous: A retrospective study of 450 cases in Taiwan. *J. Dermatol.* **2016**, *43*, 175–180. [CrossRef] [PubMed]
3. Watson, I.T.; DeCrescenzo, A.; Paek, A.Y. Basal cell carcinoma within nevus sebaceous of the trunk. *Proc. Bayl. Univ. Med. Cent.* **2019**, *32*, 392–393. [CrossRef] [PubMed]
4. Ansai, S.; Fukumoto, T.; Kimura, T. A clinicopathological study of nevus sebaceus secondary neoplasms. *Jpn. J. Dermatol.* **2007**, *117*, 2479–2487.
5. Mikoshiba, Y.; Minagawa, A.; Sano, T.; Okuyama, R. Pink nodule accompanied with clustered yellow globules at the periphery. *JAAD Case Rep.* **2017**, *3*, 351–353. [CrossRef] [PubMed]
6. Wang, E.; Lee, J.S.; Kazakov, D.V. A rare combination of sebaceoma with carcinomatous change (sebaceous carcinoma), trichoblastoma, and poroma arising from a nevus sebaceous. *J. Cutan. Pathol.* **2013**, *40*, 676–682. [CrossRef] [PubMed]
7. Manonukul, J.; Omeapinyan, P.; Vongjirad, A. Mucoepidermoid (adenosquamous) carcinoma, trichoblastoma, trichilemmoma, sebaceous adenoma, tumor of follicular infundibulum and syringocystadenoma papilliferum arising within 2 persistent lesions of nevus sebaceous: Report of a case. *Am. J. Dermatopathol.* **2009**, *31*, 658–663. [CrossRef] [PubMed]

MDPI
St. Alban-Anlage 66
4052 Basel
Switzerland
Tel. +41 61 683 77 34
Fax +41 61 302 89 18
www.mdpi.com

Diagnostics Editorial Office
E-mail: diagnostics@mdpi.com
www.mdpi.com/journal/diagnostics

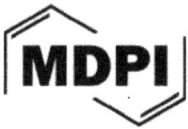

www.ingramcontent.com/pod-product-compliance
Lightning Source LLC
LaVergne TN
LVHW070604100526
838202LV00012B/556